Broken Bones

Second Edition

Broken Bones contains 434 individual cases and 1,101 radiologic images illustrating the typical and less typical appearances of fractures and dislocations throughout the body. The first chapter describes fractures and dislocations of the fingers, starting with fractures of the phalangeal tufts and progressing through the distal, middle, and proximal phalanges and the DIP and PIP joints. Subsequent chapters cover the metacarpals, the carpal bones, the radius and ulna, the elbow and upper arm, and the shoulder and thoracic cage. The cervical spine and the thoracic and lumbosacral spine are covered in separate chapters, followed by the pelvis, the femur, the knee and lower leg, the ankle, the tarsal bones, and the metatarsals and toes. The final three chapters cover the face, fractures and dislocations in children, and fractures and dislocations caused by bullets and nonmilitary blasts.

Felix S. Chew, MD, received his undergraduate degree from Princeton University and his medical degree from the University of Florida. He completed his postgraduate training at SUNY Upstate in Syracuse, NY. He is currently Professor of Radiology at the University of Washington and also serves as section head of musculoskeletal radiology, program director of the musculoskeletal radiology fellowship, and vice chair for academic innovation for the radiology department. He has previously held faculty positions at SUNY Upstate, Massachusetts General Hospital and Harvard Medical School, and Wake Forest University School of Medicine. Dr. Chew has over 200 contributions to the radiology literature, including the textbook *Skeletal Radiology: The Bare Bones*, first published in 1989 and now in its third edition. He is a chief editor of *eMedicine: Radiology* and editor-in-chief of *Radiology Case Reports*. He is a past president of the Association of University Radiologists and his memberships include the International Skeletal Society, the Society for Skeletal Radiology, and the American Academy of Orthopaedic Surgeons.

Email address: fchew@uw.edu

Catherine Maldjian, MD, received her undergraduate degree from Columbia University and her medical degree from UMDNJ-New Jersey Medical School. She completed her diagnostic radiology residency at Icahn School of Medicine at Mount Sinai in New York City. She received fellowship training in Philadelphia, at Temple University and the University of Pennsylvania. She is currently Clinical Professor of Radiology at NYU Langone Medical Center, and has previously held faculty appointments at Temple University, Albert Einstein College of Medicine, and New York Medical College. She has made numerous contributions to the radiology literature, including coauthorships of the first editions of *Musculoskeletal Imaging: A Teaching File* and *Broken Bones: The X-Ray Atlas of Fractures*. Dr. Maldjian is a frequent presenter at national skeletal radiology meetings and has been extensively involved in the training and education of radiology residents and musculoskeletal radiology fellows. She is a member of the International Skeletal Society and the Society for Skeletal Radiology.

Email address: cmaldjian@gmail.com

Hyojeong Mulcahy, MD, received her medical degree from Chonnam National University, College of Medicine, in Kwangju, Korea. She began postgraduate training at the University of Ulsan, Asan Medical Center, in Seoul, Korea, continued at St. Vincent's Medical Center, in Bridgeport, CT, and completed her fellowship in musculoskeletal radiology at the University of Washington in Seattle. She is currently Associate Professor of Radiology at UW. She has many contributions to the radiology literature, including a multi-year series of CME articles explaining current concepts of orthopedic implants that was published in the *American Journal of Roentgenology* and coauthorship of the third edition of *Musculoskeletal Imaging: A Teaching File*. Many of Dr. Mulcahy's educational exhibits have received awards at national and international meetings. She is the director of resident education in musculoskeletal radiology at UW. She is a member of the American Roentgen Ray Society, the Radiologic Society of North America, the International Skeletal Society, the Society for Skeletal Radiology, and the Korean Congress of Radiology.

Email address: hyomul@uw.edu

To our families, without whom nothing would be possible or worthwhile.

Broken Bones

The Radiologic Atlas of Fractures and Dislocations
Second Edition

Felix S. Chew
University of Washington
Catherine Maldjian
New York University
Hyojeong Mulcahy
University of Washington

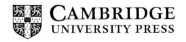

CAMBRIDGE
UNIVERSITY PRESS

University Printing House, Cambridge CB2 8BS, United Kingdom

Cambridge University Press is part of the University of Cambridge.

It furthers the University's mission by disseminating knowledge
in the pursuit of education, learning, and research at the highest
international levels of excellence.

www.cambridge.org
Information on this title: www.cambridge.org/9781107499232

First published 2016

Printed in the United States of America

A catalog record for this publication is available from the British Library.

Library of Congress Cataloging in Publication Data
Names: Chew, Felix S. | Maldjian, Catherine. | Mulcahy, Hyojeong.
Title: Broken bones : the radiologic atlas of fractures and dislocations /
Felix S. Chew, University of Washington, Catherine Maldjian,
New York University, Hyojeong Mulcahy, University
of Washington.
Other titles: Broken bones
Description: Cambridge : Cambridge University Press, 2016. |
Includes bibliographical references and index.
Identifiers: LCCN 2015039551 | ISBN 9781107499232 (pbk.)
Subjects: LCSH: Fractures. | Dislocations. | Human anatomy –
Atlases. | Human keleton – Radiography.
Classification: LCC RD101.C522 2016 | DDC 617.1/5–dc23
LC record available at http://lccn.loc.gov/2015039551

ISBN 978-1-107-49923-2 Paperback

Contents

Contributors

Felix S. Chew, M.D.
Professor and Section Head of Musculoskeletal Radiology
Department of Radiology
University of Washington
Seattle, WA
fchew@uw.edu

Catherine Maldjian, M.D.
Clinical Professor
Department of Radiology
New York University
New York, NY
cmaldjian@gmail.com

Refky Nicola, D.O.
Assistant Professor
Department of Radiology
University of Rochester Medical Center
Rochester, NY
refky_nicola@urmc.rochester.edu

Hyojeong Mulcahy, M.D.
Associate Professor
Department of Radiology
University of Washington
Seattle, WA
hyomul@uw.edu

Christin M.B. Foster, M.D.
CDR MC (FS) USN
Department of Radiology
Naval Medical Center, Portsmouth
Portsmouth, VA
Assistant Professor of Radiology and Radiological Sciences
Uniformed Services University of the Health Sciences
Bethesda, MD
christin.foster@med.navy.mil

Eira Roth, M.D.
Irving Radiological Associates, LLP
Irving, TX
eira.roth@gmail.com

Preface

This book is an atlas of fractures and dislocations, as depicted by radiologic imaging. It was my intention to illustrate all the common and uncommon fractures that may be encountered in clinical practice, and also include as many of the rare injuries as possible. This book is intended for the use of anyone with an interest in the diagnosis, treatment, and management of patients with fractures or dislocations.

When the first edition of *Broken Bones: The X-Ray Atlas of Fractures* was published in 2009, it was the first full-sized radiology textbook written specifically as an e-book for the Amazon Kindle 2 and Apple iPhone 3GS platforms. With the subsequent introduction and proliferation of the Apple iPad and its competitors and of high-resolution large-screen smart phones, many handheld computing devices now rival or exceed clinical radiology workstations in display quality. All of the radiographic images in the new edition were originally acquired with state-of-the-art digital x-ray equipment and faithfully reproduced to provide the reader with images that take advantage of the excellent display technology now available. While retaining its anatomic organization and case-based format, the book has been expanded from 369 to 434 individual cases, 234 of which are new to the second edition. There are now 1,101 radiologic images, increased from the original 939. The new and revised text for each case is self-contained for the reader who is only able to read the book in snippets, yet the organization of cases within each chapter and the organization of the chapters within the book as a whole provide a logical progression and story arc for the reader with longer blocks of time.

The book is organized by anatomic region. The first chapter describes fractures and dislocations of the fingers, starting with fractures of the phalangeal tufts and progressing through the distal, middle, and proximal phalanges and the DIP and PIP joints. Subsequent chapters cover the metacarpals, the carpal bones, the radius and ulna, the elbow and upper arm, and the shoulder and thoracic cage. The cervical spine and the thoracic and lumbosacral spine are covered in separate chapters, followed by the pelvis, the femur, the knee and lower leg, the ankle, the tarsal bones, and the metatarsals and toes. The final three chapters cover the face, fractures and dislocations in children, and fractures and dislocations caused by bullets and nonmilitary blasts.

The radiologic images have been carefully chosen to illustrate the typical and less typical appearances of fractures and dislocations. It would have been ideal but impractical to include all of the images that were obtained for clinical diagnosis in these cases. To meet the limitations of the textbook format, the images have been cropped, resized, reoriented, and re-leveled. Radiographs are presented in standard fashion, generally looking at the hands, wrists, and feet as if they were the viewer's own, and the other body parts as if the patient were facing the viewer. For clarity and ease of correlation, cross-sectional images are presented in the same orientation as the radiographs they accompany. Many fracture classifications are described in the text, but the coverage of classifications is not meant to be exhaustive or even complete. Radiologists are usually not called on to classify fractures, but it is important to know which characteristics of various injuries determine how they would be classified, so that the imaging examination and report can be more useful.

In my work as a diagnostic radiologist at the University of Washington in Seattle, I see the images from thousands of injured patients every year, including many from Harborview Medical Center (Seattle, WA), the Level 1 Trauma Center that serves the states of Washington, Wyoming, Alaska, Montana, and Idaho, and the University of Washington Medical Center, the region's leading academic medical center. Additional cases used in this book were drawn from the teaching collections of the authors. A few images have been previously published and are used with permission.

Fractures and dislocations of the fingers

Felix S. Chew, M.D., and Catherine Maldjian, M.D.

Case 1–1
Phalangeal tuft avulsion fracture

(A)

(B)

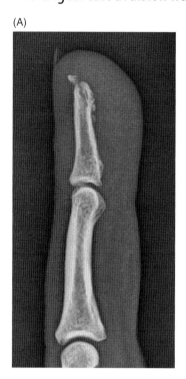

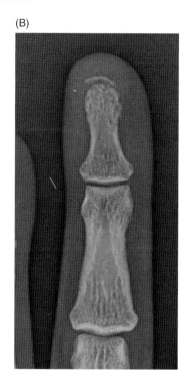

31-year-old woman injured in a ground-level fall. Lateral (A) and PA (B) radiographs of the left middle finger. There is an avulsion fracture of the very tip of the tuft distal phalanx. The fingernail appears to be intact. The connective tissue septae that support the pulp of the fingertip attach to the tuft of the distal phalanx.

Case 1–2
Phalangeal tuft fracture

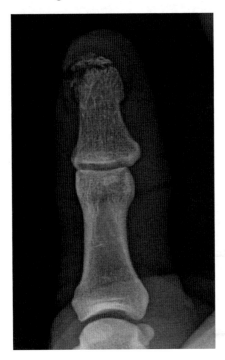

42-year-old man whose thumb was crushed by a tie-down chain while unloading a truck. PA radiograph of the right thumb. There is transverse fracture through the tip of the phalangeal tuft of the thumb with a small amount of comminution. A soft tissue laceration extends from the thumbnail through the fracture site. More than 50% of all phalangeal fractures involve the distal phalanx, most often involving the ungual tuft [1–2]. These may be comminuted or not. The fibrous septae extending from periosteum to the skin resist displacement of fragments.

Case 1–3
Phalangeal tuft fracture

(A)

(B)

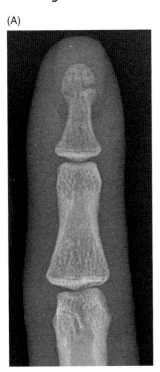 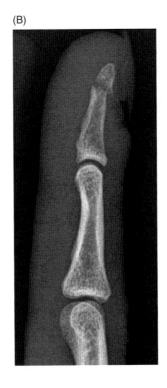

43-year-old woman who was bitten in the hand by an aggressive dog. PA (A) and lateral (B) radiographs of the right index finger. There is a transverse fracture of the distal phalanx through the phalangeal tuft. There is a soft tissue defect in the nailbed on the lateral view.

Case 1–4   Finger amputation

(A)

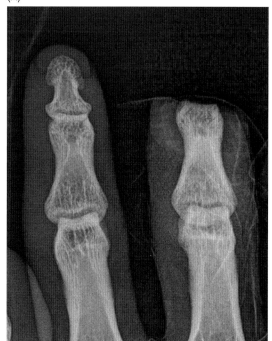

(B)

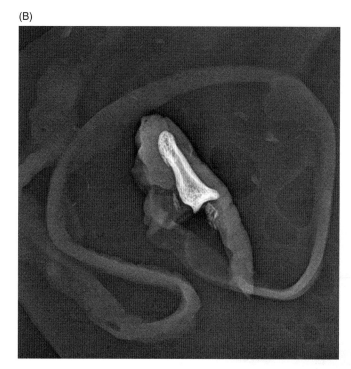

31-year-old man whose hand was trapped in a mechanical laundry press for several seconds. PA radiograph of the right index and middle fingers (A) and of the amputated part of middle finger (B). There has been amputation through the DIP joint of the middle finger with soft tissue degloving injury. The radiograph of the amputated fingertip shows an intact distal phalanx, with fragments of the middle phalanx, and an extensive portion of soft tissues that were degloved from the dorsal aspect of the middle phalanx. The long soft tissue structure coiled around the amputated fingertip is the flexor digitorum profundus tendon to the middle finger with some attached muscle tissue.

Case 1–5   Mallet finger

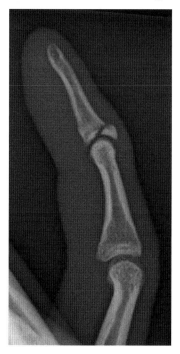

17-year-old man who jammed his small finger. Lateral radiograph of the right small finger. There is a fracture at the dorsal aspect of the base of distal phalanx with slight flexion of the DIP joint. This injury is an avulsion fracture of the common extensor tendon insertion at dorsal base of the distal phalanx. A direct blow to the fingertip with forced flexion at the DIP joint, as from a baseball in flight against an outstretched finger, gives rise to this fracture pattern, also known as mallet finger or baseball finger [1–3].

Case 1–6
Mallet finger

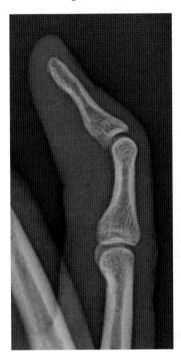

27-year-old man who injured his small finger several months ago. Lateral radiograph of the right small finger. There is an isolated flexion deformity at the DIP joint, without fracture. This lesion is a soft tissue mallet finger. Rupture of the common extensor tendon results in unopposed flexion at the DIP joint, with the flexed distal phalanx likened to a mallet. Most cases of mallet finger are soft tissue avulsion injuries of the tendon; only 25% of cases of mallet finger will demonstrate an avulsion fracture [1–4].

Case 1–7
Mallet finger

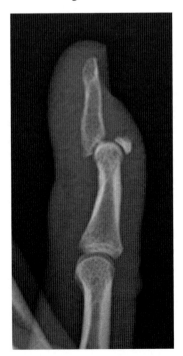

28-year-old woman who injured her small finger in a bicycle crash. Lateral radiograph of the right small finger. There is an intra-articular fracture of the distal phalanx of the small finger. The small dorsal fragment includes the majority of the articular surface and remains located. The large volar fragment has a minority of the articular surface and is subluxated volarly by unopposed tension from the flexor tendon, resulting in displacement of the fragments.

Case 1–8
Complete articular fracture of the distal phalanx

(A)

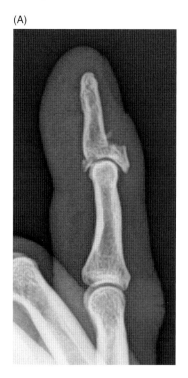

(B)

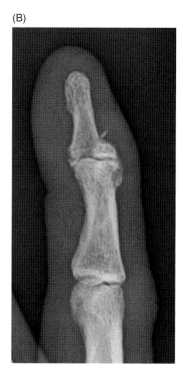

(C)

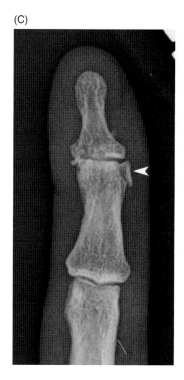

52-year-old man with crush injury to the small finger. Lateral (A), oblique (B), and PA (C) radiographs of the right small finger. There are comminuted intra-articular fractures involving the entire articular surface of the distal phalanx at the DIP joint. There is also a fracture involving the lateral condyle of the middle phalanx (arrowhead).

(D)

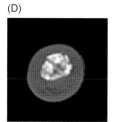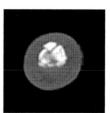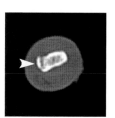

Axial CT through the DIP of the right small finger. There are comminuted fractures of the proximal end of the distal phalanx of the small finger. The lateral condylar middle phalanx fracture is also demonstrated (arrowhead).

Case 1–9
Dorsal DIP dislocation

(A)

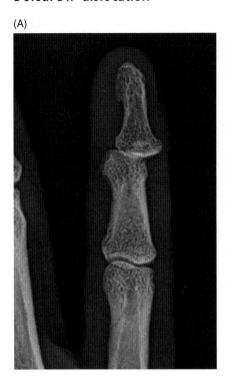

(B)

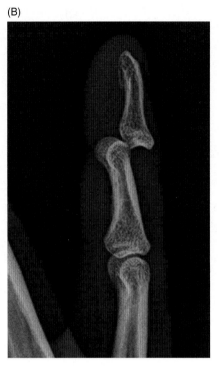

31-year-old woman who jammed her finger trying to catch a basketball pass. PA (A) and lateral (B) radiographs of the right small finger. There is dorsal dislocation of the distal phalanx. Dislocations in the fingers are usually dorsal and easily reducible, often by the patients themselves at the time of injury. The mechanism of injury is typically hyperextension [5–6].

Case 1–10
Volar DIP dislocation

(A)

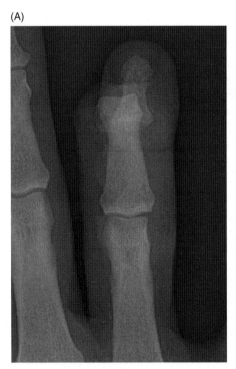

(B)

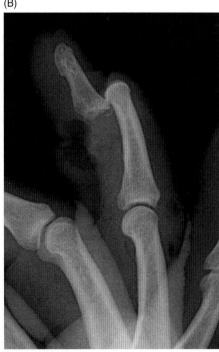

47-year-old man with a crush injury to the ring finger. PA (A) and lateral (B) radiographs of the right ring finger. There is volar dislocation of the distal phalanx with crush injuries of the soft tissues. Volar dislocations in the fingers are uncommon and often irreducible [5–6].

Case 1–11   Thumb dislocation

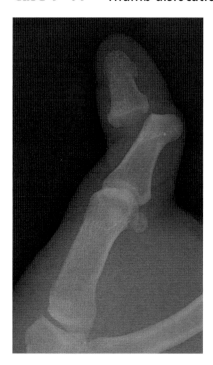

46-year-old man who injured his hand in an altercation. Oblique radiograph of the right thumb. There is dislocation of the thumb IP joint with dorsolateral dislocation of the distal phalanx. These are uncommon injuries. Hyperextension and rotation are the mechanism of injury. A ruptured palmar plate or tendon can become interposed into the joint preventing nonsurgical reduction [7].

Case 1–12   Medial condyle fracture of the middle phalanx

(A)

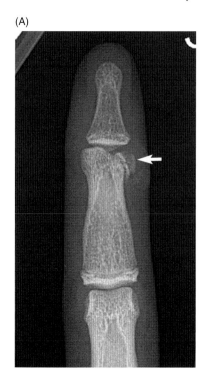

(B)

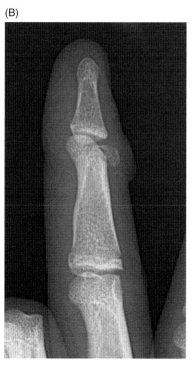

(C)

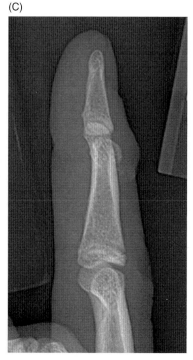

15-year-old male who injured his finger fighting with a dog. PA (A), oblique (B), and lateral (C) radiographs of the right middle finger. There is a fracture of the medial condyle of the middle phalanx at the DIP joint. This displaced, intra-articular fracture is best seen on oblique views, and may require open reduction and internal fixation. Bicondylar T- or Y-shaped fractures may occur. Intra-articular malunion may lead to posttraumatic osteoarthritis. Stable fixation of the small fragment can be technically challenging [1–2].

Case 1–13
Oblique phalanx fracture

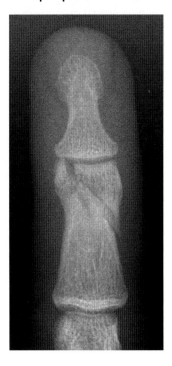

25-year-old man injured his hand playing football. PA radiograph of the right ring finger. There is an oblique fracture of middle phalanx extending to the joint surface. The mechanism of injury for oblique fractures is axial loading. Incongruity at the articular surface typically needs to be addressed surgically when it exceeds 2–3 mm.

Case 1–14
Crush injury of the thumb

(A)

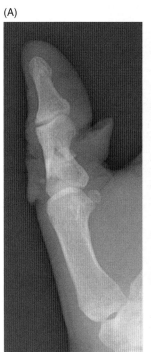

(B)

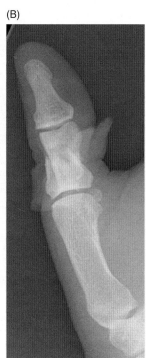

(C)

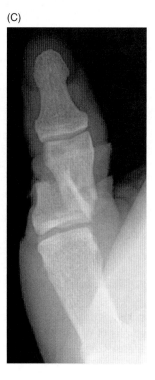

30-year-old man who sustained a crush injury to his thumb. Lateral (A), oblique (B), and PA (C) radiographs of the right thumb. There is a near amputation with fracture through the proximal phalanx. Circumferential soft tissue deformity and fracture deformity are at the same level; however, complete detachment has not occurred. Unfortunately, the digit was not replantable, and his hand was reconstructed by deepening the first web space.

Case 1–15
Dorsal PIP dislocation

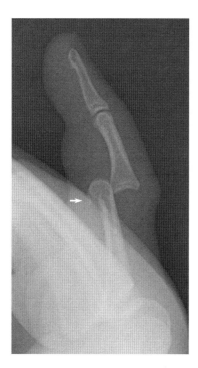

18-year-old man injured finger playing basketball. Lateral radiograph of the left small finger. There is dorsal dislocation of the middle phalanx. A small bone fragment (arrow) is seen at the volar aspect of the distal proximal phalanx, likely a displaced volar plate avulsion fracture from the volar aspect of the dislocated middle phalanx. PIP joint dislocations are the most frequent dislocations in the hand. Mechanism of injury for dorsal PIP dislocation is forced hyperextension with axial compression. Dislocations that may be easily reduced are considered simple; dislocations that are irreducible and require surgical treatment are considered complex [8]. These injuries are virtually always accompanied by volar plate fracture or soft tissue detachment and sometimes by collateral ligament injuries.

Case 1–16
Volar plate fracture

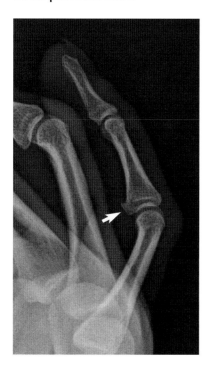

20-year-old woman who injured her finger in an altercation. Lateral radiograph of the right small finger. There is a mildly displaced volar plate fracture of the middle phalanx at the PIP joint of the small finger. The small triangular-shaped volar fragment comprises only a small fraction of the articular surface and the middle phalanx remains normally located at the PIP joint. When a large fragment is avulsed, the middle phalanx may dislocate dorsally and the injury is unstable [9].

Case 1–17
Volar plate fracture

(A)

(B)

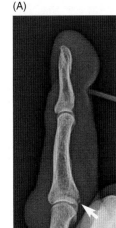
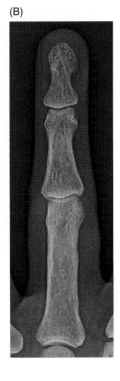

58-year-old man who jammed his ring finger when he fell on the stairs. Lateral (A) and PA (B) radiographs of the left ring finger. There is focal soft tissue swelling at the PIP joint (arrowhead). There is a very small, minimally displaced fracture of the middle phalanx at the volar margin at the PIP joint that corresponds to the attachment of the volar plate (arrow). Volar plate avulsion occurs from hyperextension injury that typically involves a small fragment of bone that is difficult to see. Small volar plate fractures may be easily overlooked if one does not specifically search for them.

Case 1–18
Volar plate fractures

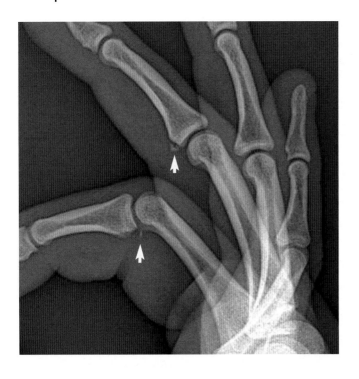

17-year-old man with finger injury, relocated in the field. Lateral radiograph of the fingers. There are tiny fracture fragments (arrows) at the volar aspect of the base of the middle phalanges of the index and middle fingers, indicative of volar plate injuries. The mechanism of injury is hyperextension injury to the volar plate. Volar plate mechanisms are present at the PIP and MCP joints, and avulsion injuries are typically manifested as fractures at the volar bases of the proximal or middle phalanges.

Case 1–19

Dorsal lip avulsion fracture

(A) (B) (C)

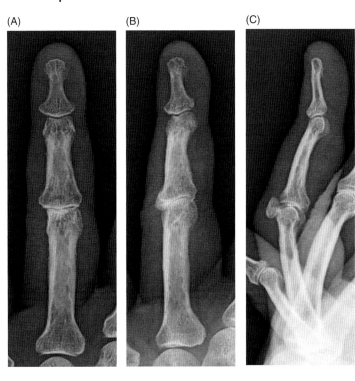

75-year-old man who jammed his ring finger playing basketball. PA (A), oblique (B), and lateral (C) radiographs of the left ring finger. The dorsal lip avulsion fracture of the base of the middle phalanx is best seen on the lateral radiograph (C). The fragment is retracted proximally and there is overlying soft tissue swelling. Dorsal lip avulsion fractures are usually the result of tensile loading of the central slip of the extensor tendon. Such loading may occur with forcible flexion of an actively extended finger or during volar dislocation of the PIP joint.

Case 1–20

Ulnar PIP dislocation

(A) (B)

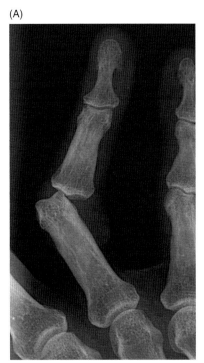
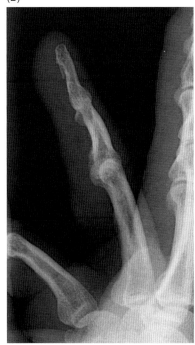

62-year-old man who fell down the stairs, injuring his hand. PA (A) and lateral (B) radiographs of the right ring finger. The PIP joint of the ring finger is dislocated toward the ulna (medially). The lateral view shows that, as all three phalanges of the ring finger are in the same coronal plane, there is no dorsal or volar component to the dislocation. Dislocations in the coronal plane are associated with collateral ligament injuries or avulsions. In this case, the radial (lateral) collateral ligament is disrupted. It is possible that the ulnar (medial) collateral ligament is also torn. There is no fracture.

Case 1–21

PIP collateral ligament avulsion fracture

(A)   (B)   (C)

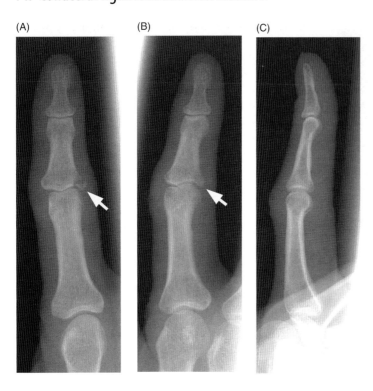

52-year-old woman who jammed her hand carrying a box through a doorway. PA (A), oblique (B), and lateral (C) radiographs of the right index finger. Soft tissue swelling surrounds the PIP joint. There is an avulsion fracture (arrow) of the medial margin of the middle phalanx of the index finger at the PIP joint, indicative of an ulnar (medial) collateral ligament avulsion. This injury may occur with forcible radial (lateral) deviation of the PIP joint. If the ligament tears without fracture, stress views may be necessary to demonstrate the lesion. (Source: Chew FS. Skeletal Radiology: The Bare Bones. 3rd Edition. Copyright © 2010 by Felix Chew.)

Case 1–22

Volar PIP dislocation

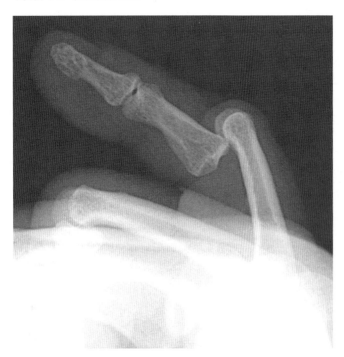

42-year-old man who injured his hand and has a history of recurrent dislocations. Lateral radiograph of the small finger. There is volar dislocation of the PIP joint. Volar dislocation is very unusual [8] and may be associated with an avulsion fracture of the dorsal lip of the base of the middle phalanx.

Case 1–23

Lateral condyle proximal phalanx fracture

(A)　　　　　(B)　　　　　(C)

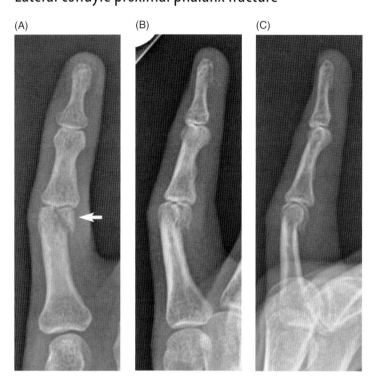

46-year-old woman who injured her hand playing water polo. The ball struck her extended finger. PA (A), oblique (B), and lateral (C) radiographs of the left small finger. There is a mildly displaced intra-articular fracture of the proximal phalanx of the small finger at the PIP joint that separates the lateral condyle. The fracture extends obliquely from the center of the articular surface to the lateral cortex. As a result, there is mild radial angulation of the finger distal to the fracture.

Case 1–24

Proximal phalanx fracture

(A)　　　　　(B)

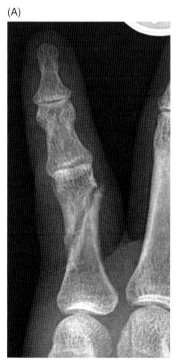
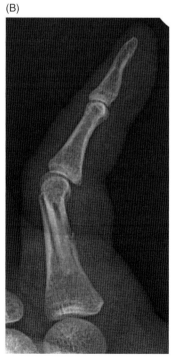

38-year-old man injured finger playing basketball. PA (A) and lateral (B) radiographs of the left small finger. There is an oblique fracture of the shaft proximal phalanx of the small finger with mild ulnar angulation of the distal phalanx and proximal distraction. The oblique fracture is characteristic of compressive loading along the long axis of the bone.

Case 1–25   Proximal phalanx fracture

(A)

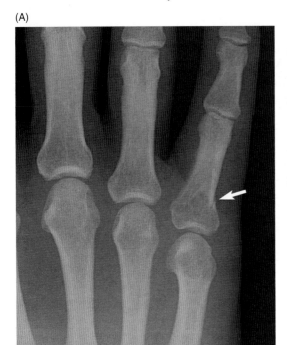

(B)

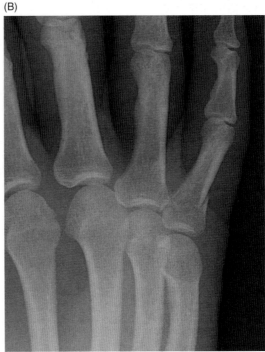

49-year-old man who caught his small finger in machinery. PA (A) and oblique (B) radiographs of the right hand. There is a mildly impacted and mildly angulated extra-articular fracture of the proximal shaft of the proximal phalanx of the small finger.

Case 1–26   Proximal phalanx fracture

(A)

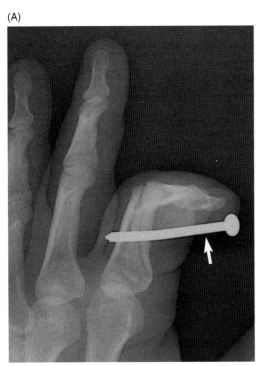

(B)

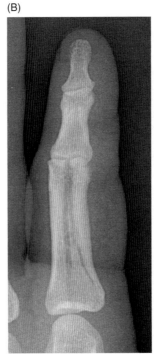

25-year-old man who accidentally drove a nail through his index finger with a pneumatic nail gun. PA radiographs of the left index finger before (A) and following (B) removal of the nail. The proximal phalanx of the index finger has been skewered by a common framing nail (arrow). There is a longitudinal fracture of the proximal phalanx extending into the PIP joint. When the nail entered the bone, the bone was split apart longitudinally. This case illustrates the penetrating form of direct loading, in which force is applied directly to the bone and the fracture propagates from the site of impact.

Case 1–27

Proximal phalanx fracture

(A)

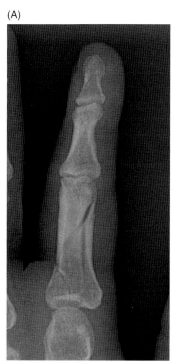

(B)

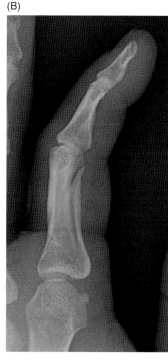

43-year-old woman whose hand was injured by the airbag in a motor vehicle crash. PA (A) and oblique (B) radiographs of the left index finger. There is a spiral fracture of the proximal phalanx extending into the MCP joint.

Case 1–28

Multiple crush injuries

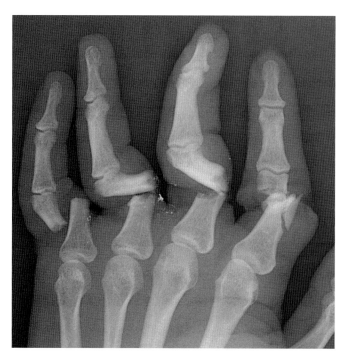

25-year-old man with hand injury caused by a mechanical press. Radiograph of the left hand. There are comminuted fractures of the proximal phalanges of all of the fingers, with near amputations. These injuries occurred in an industrial setting.

Case 1–29 Multiple finger amputations

(A)

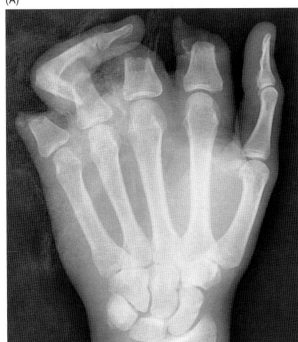

(B)

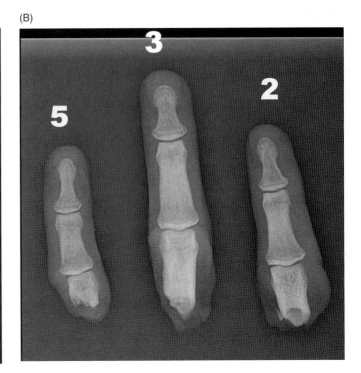

23-year-old man injured by a table saw. Radiograph of the left hand (A), radiograph of the amputated fingers (B). There are amputations of the index, middle, and little fingers through the proximal phalanges, with near amputation of the ring finger. The amputated parts should be retrieved and placed on ice for possible replantation.

Case 1–30 Gamekeeper fracture

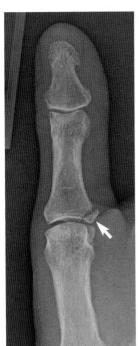

63-year-old woman who injured her thumb when she fell while walking in the woods. PA radiograph of the right thumb. There is a displaced avulsion fracture of the ulnar margin of the proximal phalanx of the thumb at the MCP joint (arrow), at the attachment of the ulnar collateral ligament. The injury is called the gamekeepers thumb. The mechanism of injury is valgus stress and hyperextension. Gamekeepers aside, this injury typically occurs during a fall on an outstretched hand in which the thumb is forced backward [10]. This causes injury to the ulnar collateral ligament (UCL), either an avulsion fracture or a sprain. In children, when the physis is open, this injury pattern results in a Salter type III fracture.

Case 1–31
Gamekeeper thumb

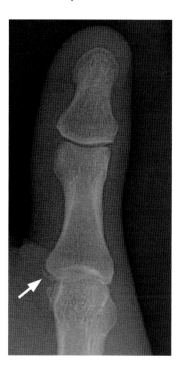

25-year-old man injured in an altercation. PA radiograph of the left thumb. There is an avulsion fracture (arrow) of the proximal phalanx of the thumb at the attachment of the ulnar collateral ligament. The fragment of bone is very thin, just the thickness of the cortex. The ulnar collateral ligament of thumb is the most frequently injured collateral ligament in the hand.

Case 1–32
Gamekeeper thumb

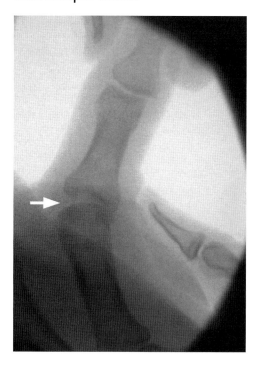

48-year-old man who injured his thumb in a skiing accident. PA radiograph of the thumb with radial stress obtained in the operating room under anesthesia. This case illustrates a pure ligamentous injury manifesting as widening of the joint space (arrow) on the stress view with no bony avulsion fragment. Without stress, the injury was radiographically occult. Complete tears may require surgery, in particular if there is displacement at the tear, with the torn ligament edges unopposed. Adductor aponeurosis can become interposed between the distal and proximal edges of the torn ligament, known as a Stener lesion, and is an indication for surgery [11].

Case 1–33

Index MCP ulnar collateral avulsion fracture

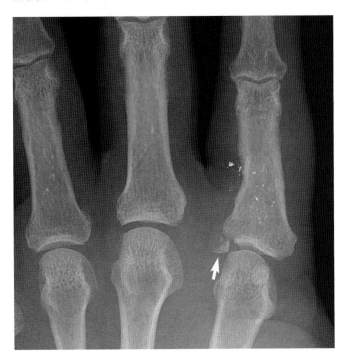

64-year-old man who jammed his finger playing football. It was dislocated and relocated in the field. PA radiograph of the left hand. There is a small avulsion fracture (arrow) of the ulnar margin of the proximal phalanx of the index finger, corresponding to the attachment of the MCP ulnar collateral ligament. The fragment is rotated approximately 90 degrees (counterclockwise on the radiograph). The arrow points to the attachment site of the ulnar collateral ligament. A gunshot wound to the proximal phalanx of the index finger occurred in the remote past, accounting for the metal fragments and deformity. Indications for surgery include more than 2-3mm of displacement of avulsed fragment and more than 20% of articular surface involvement of ulnar fragment [12].

References

1. Yoong P, Goodwin RW, Chojnowski A. Phalangeal fractures of the hand. *Clin Radiol.* 2010 Oct;65(10):773–80. doi: 10.1016/j.crad.2010.04.008. Epub 2010 Jun 11. PMID: 20797462.

2. Jones NF, Jupiter JB, Lalonde DH. Common fractures and dislocations of the hand. *Plast Reconstr Surg.* 2012 Nov;130(5):722e–736e. doi: 10.1097/PRS.0b013e318267d67a. PMID: 23096627.

3. Stark HH, Boyes JH, Wilson JN. Mallet finger. *J Bone Joint Surg Am.* 1962 Sep;44-A:1061–8. PMID: 14039487.

4. McMinn DJ. Mallet finger and fractures. *Injury.* 1981 May;12(6):477–9. PMID: 7275291.

5. Shah CM, Sommerkamp TG. Fracture dislocation of the finger joints. *J Hand Surg Am.* 2014 Apr;39(4):792–802. doi: 10.1016/j.jhsa.2013.10.001. PMID: 24679912.

6. Calfee RP, Sommerkamp TG. Fracture-dislocation about the finger joints. *J Hand Surg Am.* 2009 Jul-Aug;34(6):1140–7. doi: 10.1016/j.jhsa.2009.04.023. PMID: 19643295.

7. Naito K, Sugiyama Y, Igeta Y, Kaneko K, Obayashi O. Irreducible dislocation of the thumb interphalangeal joint due to displaced flexor pollicis longus tendon: Case report and new reduction technique. *Arch Orthop Trauma Surg.* 2014 Aug;134(8):1175–8. doi: 10.1007/s00402-014-2024-6. Epub 2014 Jun 6. PMID: 24902518.

8. Vicar AJ. Proximal interphalangeal joint dislocations without fractures. *Hand Clin.* 1988 Feb;4(1):5–13. PMID: 3277980.

9. Blazar PE, Steinberg DR. Fractures of the proximal interphalangeal joint. *J Am Acad Orthop Surg.* 2000 Nov–Dec;8(6):383–90. PMID: 11104402.

10. Madan SS, Pai DR, Kaur A, Dixit R. Injury to ulnar collateral ligament of thumb. *Orthop Surg.* 2014 Feb;6(1):1–7. doi: 10.1111/os.12084. PMID: 24590986.

11. Stener B. Displacement of the ruptured ulnar collateral ligament of the metacarpo-phalangeal joint of the thumb: A clinical and anatomical study. *J Bone Joint Surg Br* 1962; 44-B: 869–79.

12. Ishizuki M. Injury to collateral ligament of the metacarpophalangeal joint of a finger. *J Hand Surg Am.* 1988 May;13(3):444–8. PMID: 3379287.

Fractures and dislocations of the metacarpals

Felix S. Chew, M.D., and Catherine Maldjian, M.D.

Case 2–1
First MCP dislocation

(A)

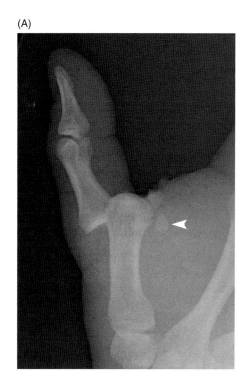

(B)

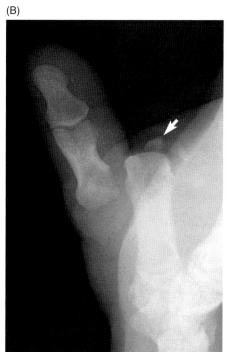

24-year-old man with blast injury from firework that exploded in his hand. Lateral (A) and PA (B) radiographs of the right thumb. There is dislocation of the first MCP joint with dorsolateral dislocation of the first proximal phalanx. There is an avulsion fracture of the proximal phalanx (arrow) at the insertion of the ulnar collateral ligament. The thumb sesamoid bones are not displaced (arrowhead), indicating that the volar plate has been disrupted distal to them. If there had been more proximal volar plate disruption, the sesamoid bones would have displaced with the proximal phalanx.

Case 2–2   Third MCP dislocation

(A)

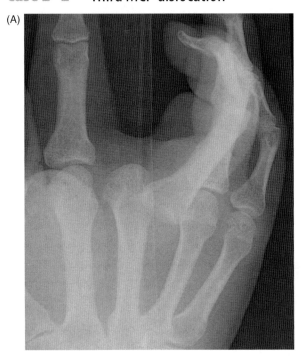

(B)

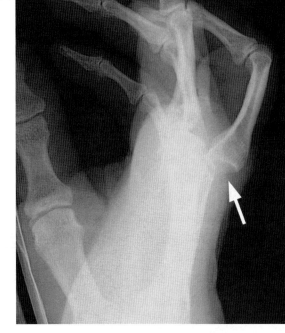

49-year-old man who fell 8 feet off a ladder. Oblique (A) and lateral (B) radiographs of the right hand. There is dislocation of the third MCP joint. The dorsal position of the middle finger is more evident on the lateral view (arrow). Simple MCP dislocations may be treated by closed reduction, but complex dislocations that are irreducible require surgical treatment [1].

Case 2–3   Second and third MCP dislocations

(A)

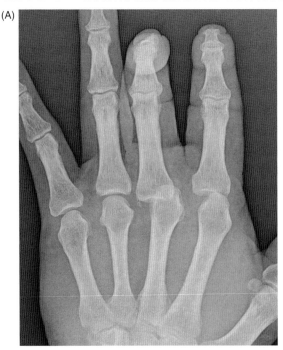

(B)

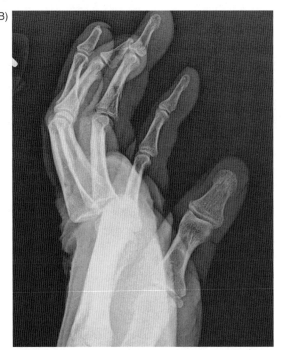

60-year-old man who fell on the sidewalk, landing on his hand. PA (A) and lateral (B) radiographs of the left hand. The PA radiograph shows overlap of the proximal phalanx of the middle finger with the third metacarpal head. The proximal phalanx of the index finger appears to be medially subluxated relative to the second metacarpal head and the MCP joint space appears narrowed (the fourth and fifth MCP joints are normal). However, the lateral radiograph shows dorsal dislocation of both the second and third MCP joints.

Case 2–4
Multiple MCP dislocations

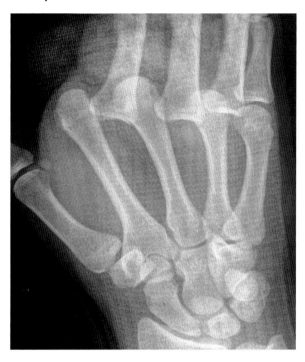

20-year-old man who fell from a height of 30 feet. Oblique radiograph of the right hand following placement of a fiberglass cast. There is dorsal dislocation of the second, third, and fourth MCP joints. The fiberglass cast obscures detail on the image.

Case 2–5
Sesamoid fracture

(A)

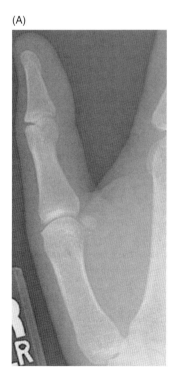

(B)

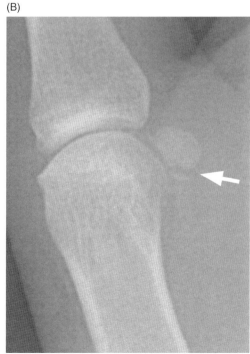

34-year-old man injured in altercation. Lateral radiograph of the right thumb (A) and photographic magnification (B). Magnified image shows sesamoid fracture (arrow) at the thumb MCP. A transverse fracture of the sesamoid results from direct impact or hyperextension injury [2–3]. Hyperextension injury would generally accompany other injuries such ulnar collateral ligament sprain. Differentiation of a sesamoid fracture from a developmental bipartite sesamoid can be made on the basis of non-corticated edges and absence of pain on clinical examination.

Case 2–6
Fifth metacarpal head fracture

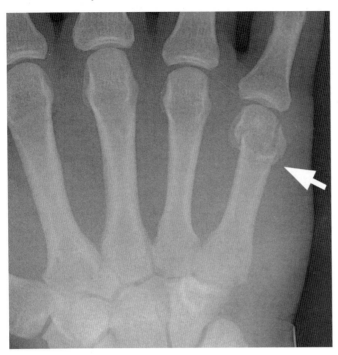

27-year-old man who injured his hand during an assault. Radiograph of the right hand. There is a comminuted intra-articular fracture (arrow) through the head and neck of the fifth metacarpal, with impaction.

Case 2–7
Boxer's fractures

(A)

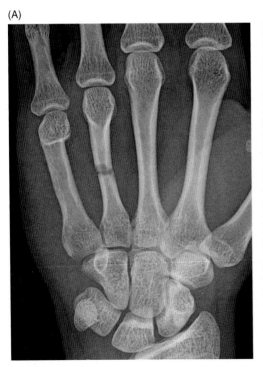

(B)

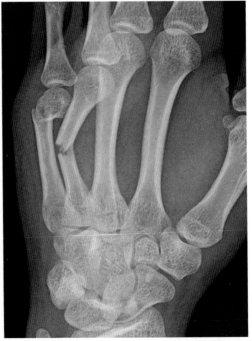

18-year-old man who punched a concrete wall. PA (A) and oblique (B) radiographs of the left hand. There are boxer's fractures of the fourth and fifth metacarpals, with volar angulation and soft tissue swelling. The fracture of the fifth metacarpal is through the neck and the fracture of the fourth metacarpal is through the mid-shaft. Boxer's fractures are metacarpal neck fractures with volar angulation that have been sustained by striking a blow with a closed fist. Treatment depends on the degree of angulation and whether the fracture is open.

Case 2–8 Third metacarpal neck fracture

(A)

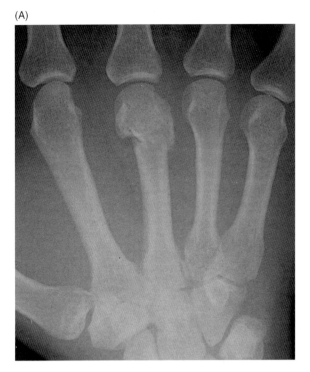

(B)

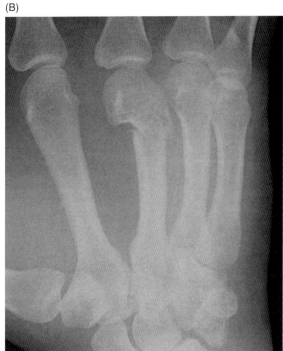

23-year-old man injured in an altercation. PA (A) and oblique (B) radiographs of the right hand. There is a transverse fracture of the third metacarpal neck with volar angulation. The mechanism of injury is axial loading and bending, similar to a boxer's fracture.

Case 2–9 Fourth metacarpal shaft fracture

(A)

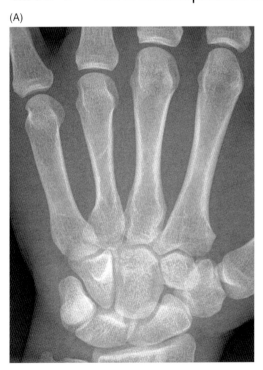

(B)

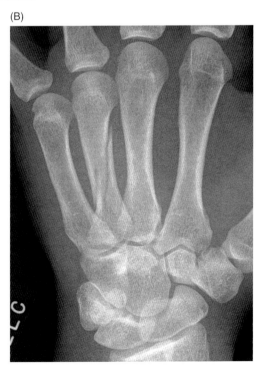

28-year-old man who was involved in a high-speed motor vehicle rollover crash. He was found thrown from the vehicle. PA (A) and oblique (B) radiographs of the left hand. There is a spiral fracture of the fourth metacarpal shaft. The fracture is challenging to see on the PA radiograph, but obvious on the oblique radiograph. Indirect rotational forces comprised of tensile, compressive, and shear components give rise to a spiral fracture.

Case 2–10
Extra-articular first metacarpal fracture

(A)

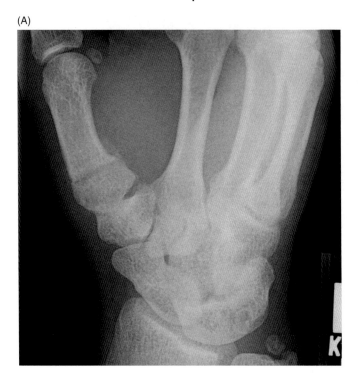

(B)

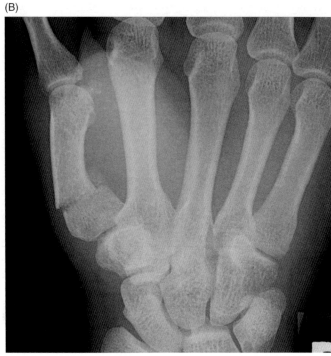

28-year-old man who complained of thumb pain after punching someone in the head. Oblique (A) and PA (B) radiographs of the right hand. There is a transverse fracture through the proximal shaft of the first metacarpal that does not involve the articular surface. Extra-articular first metacarpal fractures are typically treated without surgery.

Case 2–11
Bennett fracture

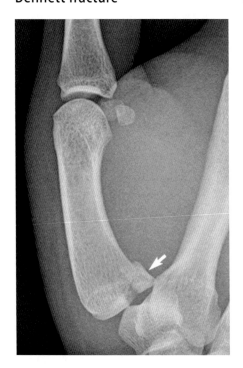

21-year-old man who injured his thumb playing basketball. PA radiograph centered over the base of the right thumb. There is an oblique fracture of the medial base of the first metacarpal with dorsal subluxation of the first CMC joint. The small, triangular-shaped medial fragment (arrow) remains in its normal anatomic location, attached by ligaments. This injury is a Bennett fracture [4], initially described by the surgeon for whom the fracture pattern is named [5]. A Bennett fracture is an oblique fracture incurred by mechanism of axial loading of a partially flexed first metacarpal. The dorsolateral pull of the abductor pollicis longus proximally and medial pull of the adductor pollicis on the metacarpal distally separate the two fragments in this injury. This injury is unstable and is treated surgically in many cases by percutaneous pinning; however, if there is an associated dorsal ligament complex tear, open reduction with internal fixation and repair of the ligament may become necessary [6].

Case 2–12
Bennett fracture

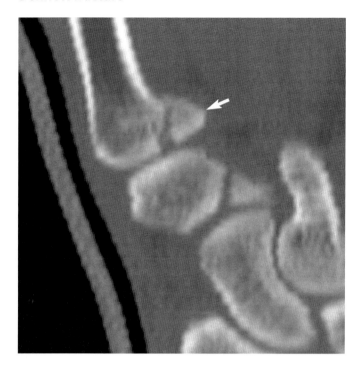

26-year-old man who injured his thumb in a football pileup. CT was obtained after closed reduction and casting. Coronal CT of the right wrist. There is a non-comminuted intra-articular fracture (arrow) at the base of the first metacarpal (Bennett fracture). These injuries constitute approximately one-third of all fractures of the first metacarpal.

Case 2–13
Bennett fracture-dislocation

(A)

(B)

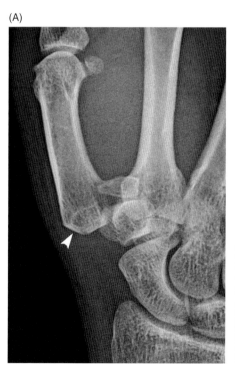
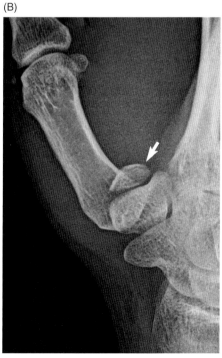

32-year-old man injured during an altercation. Lateral (A) and PA (B) radiographs of the right thumb. There is an oblique fracture of the medial base of the first metacarpal with dislocation of the first metacarpal. The small volar lip fragment (arrow) is rotated but remains attached at the CMC joint while the major metacarpal fragment is dislocated and displaced proximally, radially, and dorsally (arrowhead).

Case 2–14
Rolando fracture

(A)

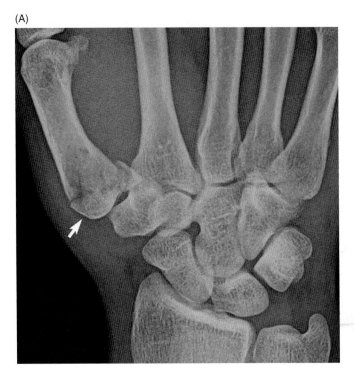

(B)

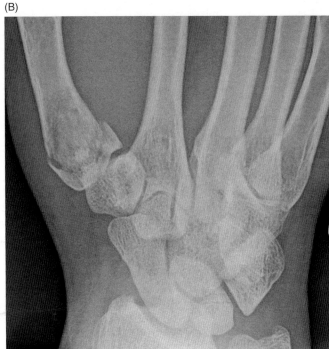

38-year-old man injured in an assault. PA (A) and oblique (B) radiographs of the right hand. There is a three-part Y-shaped fracture at the base of the first metacarpal (arrow). A Rolando fracture is a T- or Y-shaped intra-articular fracture of the base of the first metacarpal. Comminution and involvement of the entire articular surface distinguishes this fracture pattern from the more common Bennett fracture [7]. Rolando fractures are usually treated with internal fixation, but if highly comminuted, they might not be amenable to surgical correction and would then be treated conservatively [7].

Case 2–15
Rolando fracture

(A)

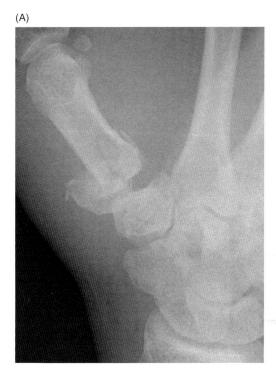

(B)

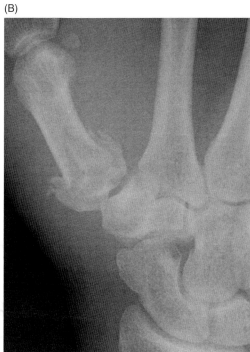

46-year-old man who was struck by a car while riding his bicycle. Lateral (A) and PA (B) radiographs of the right first metacarpal. There is a comminuted fracture of the base of the first metacarpal with displacement of the shaft fragment and subluxation at the CMC joint.

(C)

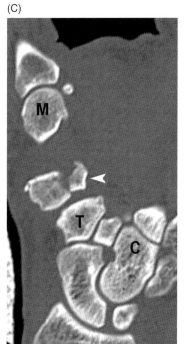

(D)

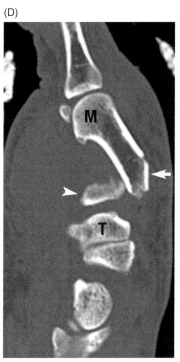

(E)

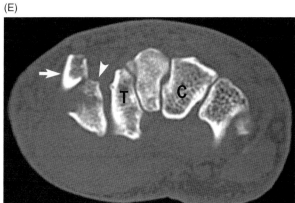

Multiplanar CT of the first metacarpal. (C) Coronal CT shows two major fragments the first metacarpal base, the smaller fragment (arrowhead) is displaced from the CMC joint. (D) The sagittal CT shows dorsal displacement of the shaft fragment (arrow). (E) The axial CT shows the smaller (arrowhead) and larger metacarpal base fragments as well as the displaced shaft fragment (arrow). M=first metacarpal head, T=trapezium, C=capitate.

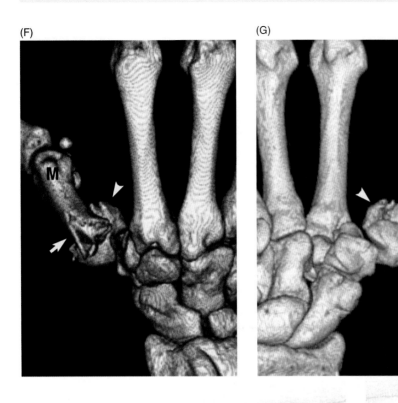

(F)

(G)

3D surface-rendered CT of the first metacarpal. Dorsal (F) and volar (G) views show the small (arrowhead) and large first metacarpal base fragments and the displaced first metacarpal shaft fragment (arrow). M=first metacarpal head.

Case 2–16
Dorsal first CMC dislocation

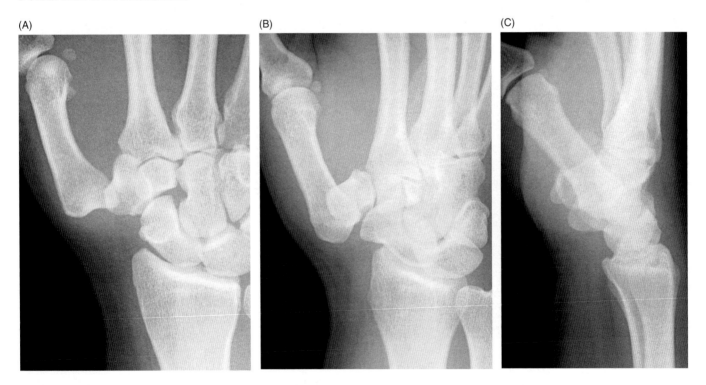

(A)

(B)

(C)

41-year-old woman who was hit by a truck while crossing the street. PA (A), oblique (B), and lateral (C) radiographs of the right wrist. There is dorsal and lateral dislocation of the first metacarpal at the CMC joint. Pure dislocation of the first CMC joint is rare. Longitudinal force along the long axis of the metacarpal during flexion of CMC joint results in tear of the dorsal capsule and necessitates open reduction with repair of the ligament [6].

Case 2–17
Dorsal second CMC dislocation

(A)

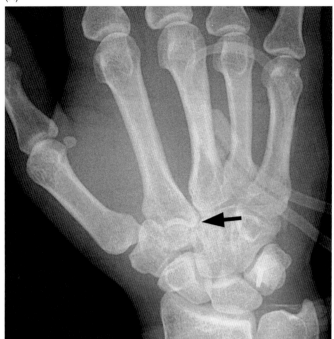

(B)

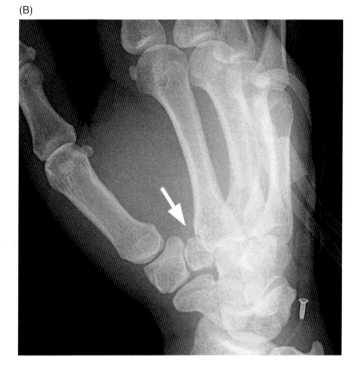

(C)

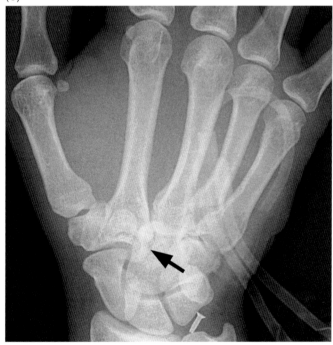

44-year-old woman in motorcycle crash. PA (A) and oblique (B-C) radiographs of the right hand. The base of the second metacarpal (black arrows) overlaps the trapezoid bone, indicating that their normal articulation has been disrupted. There is a normal articulation between the trapezium and the first metacarpal, but no articulation between the trapezoid and the second metacarpal. There is an empty space (white arrow) where the second metacarpal should articulate with the trapezoid. Isolated dislocation of the second CMC joint is uncommon.

Case 2–18   Multiple metacarpal base fractures

(A)   (B)   (C)

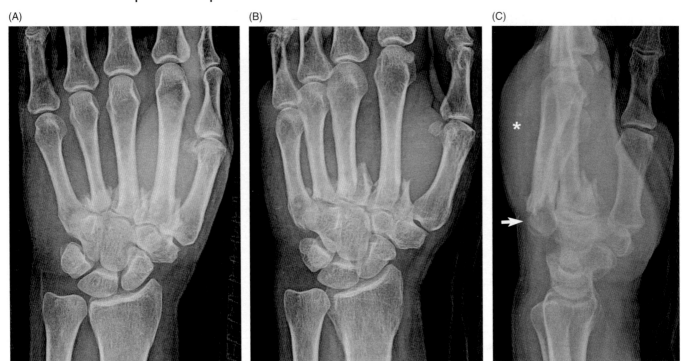

55-year-old woman injured in motorcycle crash. PA (A), oblique (B), and lateral (C) radiographs of the left hand. There are comminuted intra-articular fractures of the bases of the second through fifth metacarpals. There are dorsal dislocations of the third through fifth CMC joints (arrow). There is marked soft tissue swelling of the dorsal hand (*), raising concern for compartment syndrome.

Case 2–19   Fourth and fifth CMC fracture-dislocations

(A)   (B)

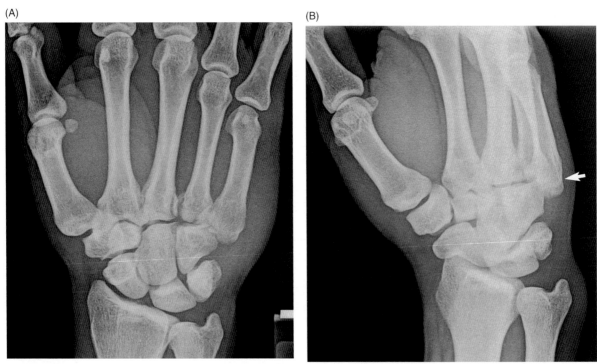

46-year-old man who punched a wall. PA (A) and oblique (B) radiographs of the right hand. There are intra-articular fractures of the bases of the fourth and fifth metacarpals. On the PA view, the fifth CMC joint space is obscured. On the oblique view, it is evident that there is dorsal dislocation of both the fourth and fifth CMC joints.

Case 2–20
Fourth and fifth CMC fracture-dislocations

(A)

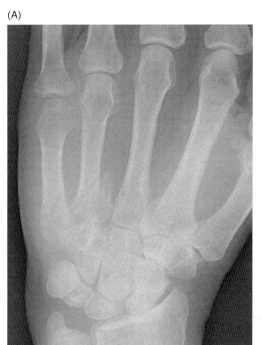

(B)

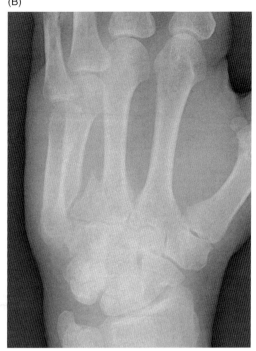

(C)

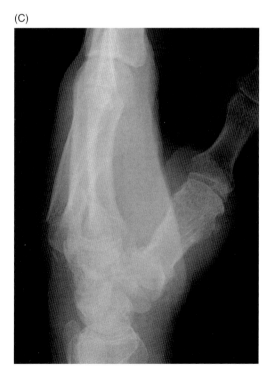

55-year-old man injured in a fall. PA (A), oblique (B), and lateral (C) radiographs of the left hand. There is dorsal dislocation of the fifth CMC joint and fracture at base of the fourth metacarpal. Fractures of fourth and fifth metacarpal bases may occur in conjunction with dislocation or subluxation, or with fractures of the hamate body [8].

Case 2–21
Volar fifth CMC dislocation with fourth metacarpal shaft fracture

(A)

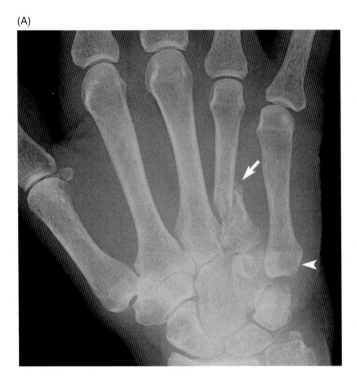

(B)

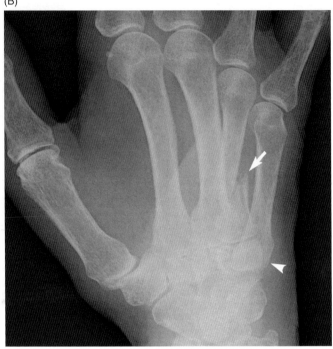

(C)

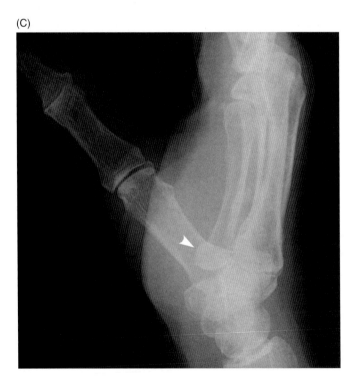

69-year-old woman injured in a fall. PA (A), oblique (B), and lateral (C) radiographs of the right hand. The base of the fifth metacarpal (arrowhead) appears to be floating and does not articulate with a carpal bone. It is also very anterior in position relative to the remaining metacarpals, consistent with fifth carpo-metacarpal volar dislocation. There is also a fracture of the fourth metacarpal (arrow). Metacarpal dislocations are typically dorsal [8]. Volar dislocation may be associated with volar plate entrapment and difficult to reduce. Of the CMC joints, the fifth CMC joint is the most prone to dislocation. Fractures of fourth and fifth metacarpal base often occur in conjunction with dislocations or subluxations. The most common dislocation of the CMC joints is the fifth CMC joint, constituting approximately 50% of all CMC dislocations. This injury is often accompanied by another metacarpal dislocation (80%). Two-thirds are dorsal dislocations. (Source: Chew FS et al. Musculoskeletal Imaging: A Teaching File. 3rd Edition. Copyright © 2012 by Felix Chew.)

Case 2–22 Multiple CMC dislocations

(A)

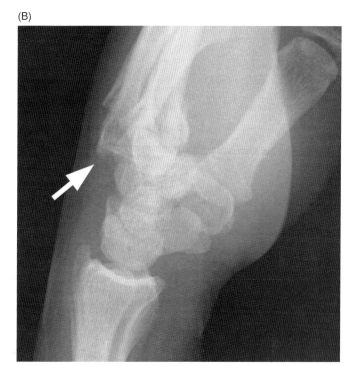

(B)

25-year-old woman struck by a car as a pedestrian. PA (A) and lateral (B) radiographs of the left hand. There are comminuted intra-articular fractures of the bases of the fourth and fifth metacarpals, with the fragments of the articular surfaces overlying the hamate. The bases of the second and third metacarpals overlie the distal carpal row on the AP and oblique views. On the lateral views, the dislocated second through fifth metacarpal bases (arrow) may be seen dorsal to the carpal bones.

Case 2–23 Partial CMC amputation

(A)

(B)

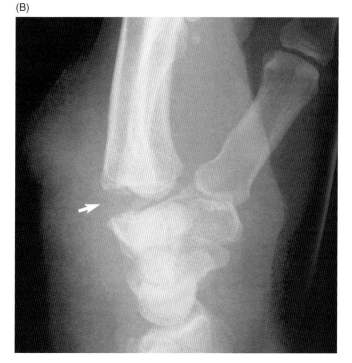

46-year-old man injured by a quilting saw. PA (A) and lateral (B) radiographs of the left hand. There is gross diastasis of the second through fifth CMC joints (arrows), with small sharply marginated fragments. The dorsal soft tissues are swollen. This injury was sustained in an industrial setting. All of the extensor tendons and neurovascular bundles to the fingers were severed in the accident.

References

1. Dinh P, Franklin A, Hutchinson B, Schnall SB, Fassola I. Metacarpophalangeal joint dislocation. *J Am Acad Orthop Surg.* 2009 May;17(5):318–24. PMID: 19411643.

2. Fotiadis E, Samoladas E, Akritopoulos P, Chatzisimeon A, Akritopoulou K. Ulnar sesamoid's fracture of the thumb: An unusual injury and review of the literature. *Hippokratia.* 2007 Jul;11(3):154–6. PMID: 19582212; PMCID: PMC2658801.

3. Mohler LR, Trumble TE. Disorders of the thumb sesamoids. *Hand Clin.* 2001 May;17(2):291–301, x. PMID: 11478051.

4. Pellegrini VD Jr. Fractures at the base of the thumb. *Hand Clin.* 1988 Feb;4(1):87–102. PMID: 327798.

5. Bennett EH. The classic: On fracture of the metacarpal bone of the thumb (1886). In: *Clin Orthop Rel Res.* 1987; 220: 3–6. PMID: 3297453.

6. Edmunds JO. Traumatic dislocations and instability of the trapeziometacarpal joint of the thumb. *Hand Clin.* 2006 Aug;22(3):365–92. PMID: 16843802.

7. Carlsen BT, Moran SL. Thumb trauma: Bennett fractures, Rolando fractures, and ulnar collateral ligament injuries. *J Hand Surg Am.* 2009 May–Jun;34(5):945–52. doi: 10.1016/j.jhsa.2009.03.017. PMID: 19411003.

8. Rawles JG Jr. Dislocations and fracture-dislocations at the carpometacarpal joints of the fingers. *Hand Clin.* 1988 Feb;4(1):103–12. PMID: 3277974.

Fractures and dislocations of the carpal bones

Felix S. Chew, M.D., and Catherine Maldjian, M.D.

Case 3–1
First CMC fractures

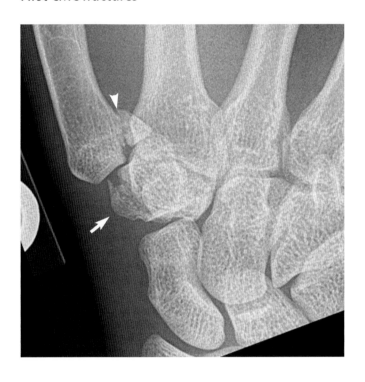

22-year-old man injured in motor vehicle crash. PA radiograph of the right wrist. There is an oblique intra-articular fracture (arrowhead) of the base of the first metacarpal at the ulnar aspect (Bennett fracture). There is a vertical intra-articular fracture of the trapezium extending through the body from the distal to proximal articular surfaces (arrow). An unstable fracture of the trapezium such as this is likely to be treated with internal fixation. This is the most common type of trapezium fracture and it often occurs in association with a Bennett fracture [1–2].

Case 3–2
Comminuted trapezium fracture

(A)

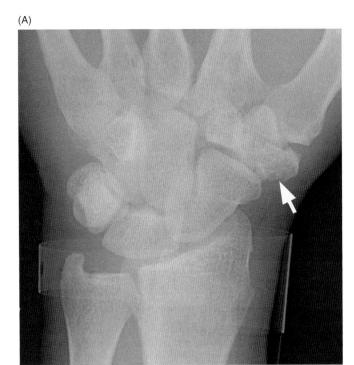

(B)

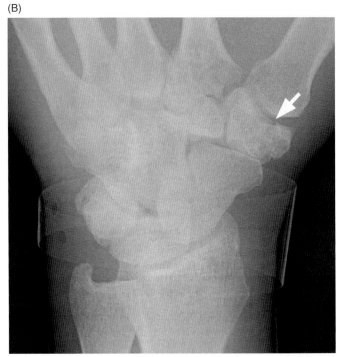

(C)

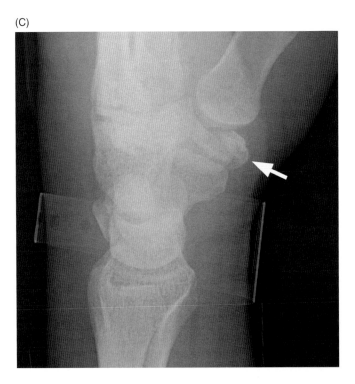

53-year-old man injured in motorcycle collision. PA (A), oblique (B), and lateral (C) radiographs of the left wrist. The trapezium has been compressed between the scaphoid and the first metacarpal base, resulting in comminuted fractures (arrows) that extend to its various articular surfaces.

Case 3–3
Trapezium avulsion fracture

(A)

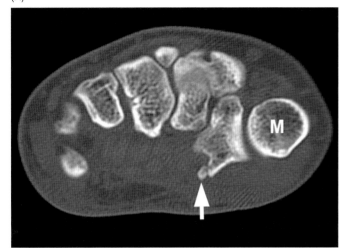

(B)

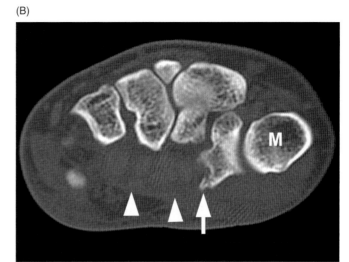

Adult who was injured in a fall on an outstretched hand. Axial CT through the right trapezium, distal (A) to proximal (B). The patient's doctor suspected a scaphoid fracture, but radiographs were normal, so CT was performed. There is an avulsion fracture of the volar ridge of the trapezium (arrows), the site of attachment of the transverse carpal ligament (arrowheads). The transverse carpal ligament forms the anterior floor of the carpal tunnel. M=first metacarpal.

Case 3–4
Scaphotrapezial dislocation

(A)

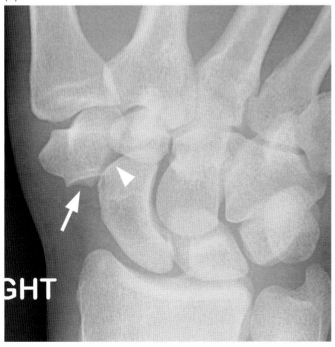

40-year-old man in motorcycle crash. Scaphoid radiograph of the right wrist. There is a laterally dislocated trapezium (arrow) relative to the scaphoid. The joint space between the trapezium and trapezoid is abnormally increased, and the lateral portion of the articular surface of the distal scaphoid is bare (arrowhead). These findings are indicative of dislocation of the trapezium from the scaphoid. This is an unusual high-energy injury that had a clinical presentation similar to the much more common scaphoid fracture.

(B)

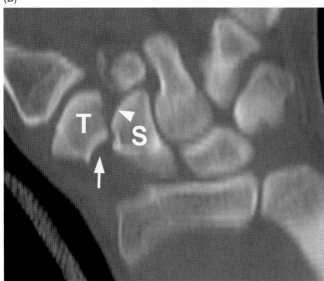

Coronal CT of the right wrist. The articular surfaces of the scaphoid (S, arrowhead) and trapezium (T, arrow) are dislocated from each other. The thumb has its normal articulation with the trapezium distally, but the trapezoid is separated from the trapezium medially.

(C)

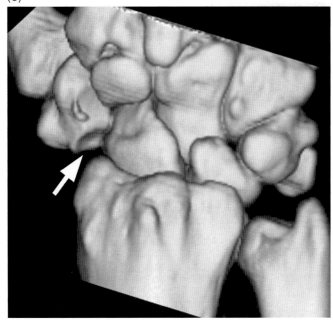

Surface-rendered 3D CT shows the bare articular surface of the trapezium (arrow), not articulating with the scaphoid. Scaphotrapezial dislocation is a rare injury that has been described only in case reports [3].

Case 3–5
Trapezoid fracture

(A)

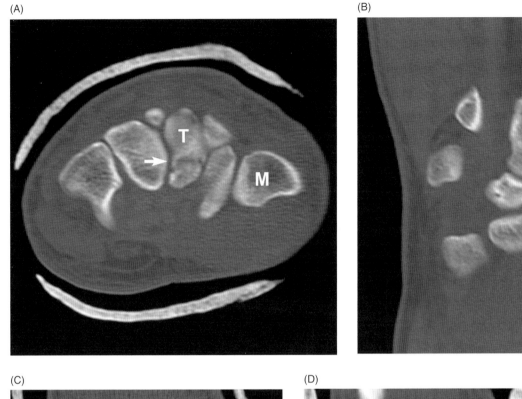

(B)

(C)

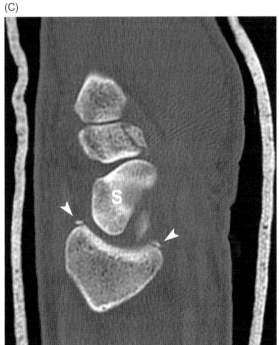

(D)

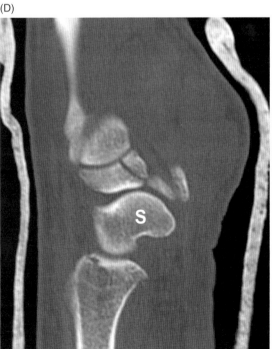

39-year-old man whose car struck a train. Multiplanar CT of the left wrist, axial (A), coronal (B), and sagittal (C-D). There is a fracture through the trapezoid (arrow) extending from the second CMC joint to the triscaphe joint. There are also avulsion fractures of the radial styloid and dorsal and volar rims (arrowheads). Trapezoid fractures are difficult to see on radiographs because of overlapping bones and generally require CT for diagnosis [4]. The trapezoid is the least commonly fractured carpal bone reported in the literature [2]. T=trapezoid, M=first metacarpal, S=scaphoid.

Case 3–6
Hamate body fracture

(A)

(B)

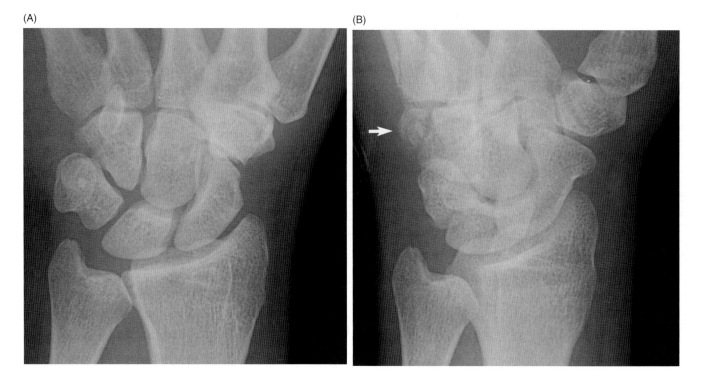

52-year-old man in motorcycle crash. PA (A) and oblique (B) radiographs of the left wrist. There is a mildly displaced fracture of the body of the hamate (arrow) at the fourth and fifth CMC joints. There is a small degree of comminution. The fourth and fifth CMC joints appear to be located. The overlying soft tissues are swollen.

Case 3–7   Hamate body fracture

(A)

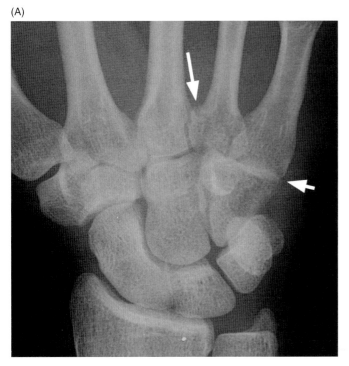

(B)

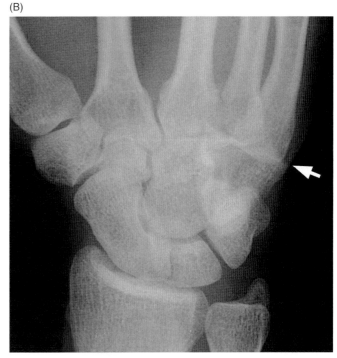

30-year-old man who punched a metal locker several times. PA (A) and oblique (B) radiographs of the right wrist. The joint spaces at the fourth and fifth CMC joints appear narrowed (short arrows). There may be a fracture (long arrow) at the base of the fourth metacarpal base. The overlying soft tissues are swollen (arrowheads). The fracture of the body of the hamate is difficult to identify on these radiographs, even in retrospect. Hamate fractures can be occult in 60% of cases by radiography alone, and may necessitate CT, if clinically warranted. Hamate body fractures are commonly associated with fourth and fifth metacarpal base fractures [5].

(C)   (D)   (E)

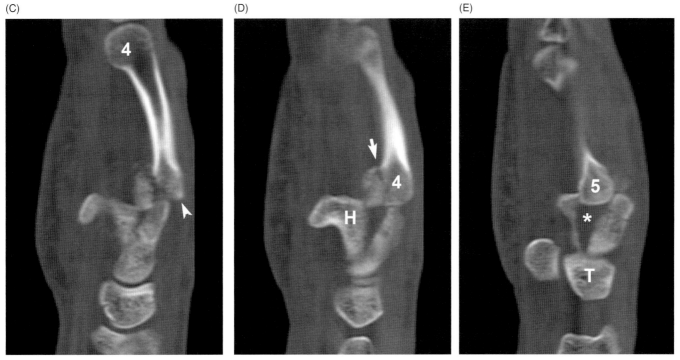

Sagittal CT through the right hamate, medial (C) to lateral (E). There is a fracture (arrow) at the base of the fourth metacarpal (4). There is dorsal subluxation of the fourth CMC joint (arrowhead). There is a fracture through the hamate body in the coronal plane. The hook of the hamate (H) is intact. The base of the fifth metacarpal (5) has displaced into the hamate fracture (*), separating the dorsal and volar fragments. T=triquetrum.

Case 3–8
Hook of hamate fracture

(A)

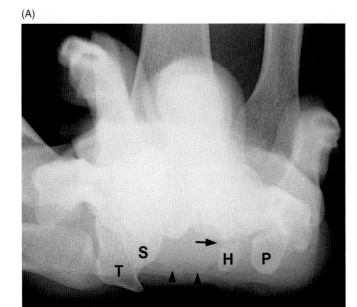

29-year-old man who developed pain in the palm of his hand after a mis-hit during batting practice. Carpal tunnel radiograph of the left wrist. There is a fracture (arrow) at the base of the hook of the hamate. The carpal tunnel view may show fractures at the hook of the hamate (H). The trapezium (T), scaphoid (S), and pisiform (P) bones should be identified. The carpal tunnel (arrowheads) is also demonstrated. The carpal tunnel view is obtained by dorsiflexing the wrist and aligning the x-ray beam tangentially along the volar aspect of the wrist.

(B)

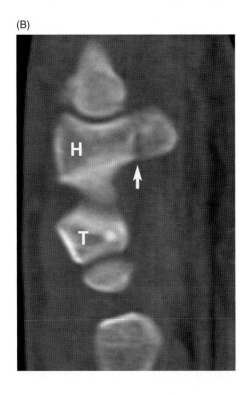

Sagittal CT of the left wrist. The fracture (arrow) at the base of the hook of the hamate is well-demonstrated. CT facilitates detection of fractures at the hook of the hamate [6]. Direct force incurred at the hypothenar eminence is a common mechanism of the injury. Such an injury might occur in golfers from the impact of the handle of the golf club, or in baseball players from the impact of the handle of the bat. Hamate fractures in general are uncommon. Symptomatic nonunion is a frequent complication of these fractures when treated conservatively. Nonunion can be treated with internal fixation or fragment excision [7]. H=hamate, T=triquetrum.

Case 3–9
Pisiform fracture

(A)

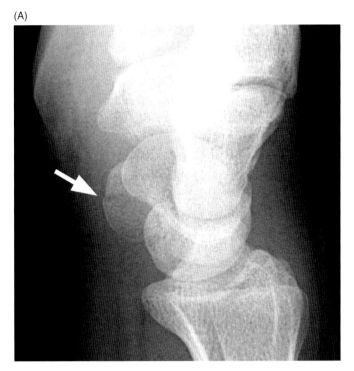

(B)

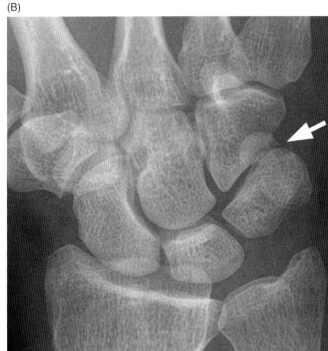

Construction worker who fell one story off of scaffolding, landing on his hands and knees. PA (A) and lateral (B) radiographs of the right wrist. There is a subtle fracture line through the

pisiform bone (arrows), visible only on two views but very difficult to see. The wrist is otherwise intact.

(C)

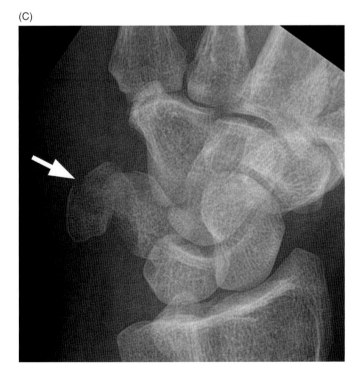

Oblique lateral radiograph of the right wrist, four weeks after injury. Bone resorption around the fracture site and displacement of fragments renders the fracture more evident (arrow). Fractures of the pisiform may occur in participants in sports where there is impaction stress on the ulnar aspect of the carpus, such as baseball, hockey, golf, and racquet sports. The pisiform may also be injured in falls on an outstretched hand, as in this case. Because it is a sesamoid bone, nonhealing pisiform fractures may be treated with simple excision [8].

Case 3–10
Triquetrum fracture

(A)

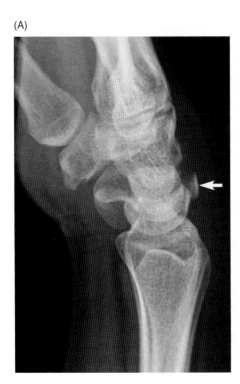

(B)

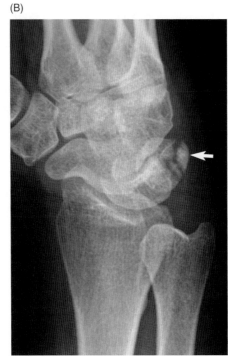

34-year-old woman who jumped from a second-story window to escape a fire. Lateral (A) and oblique (B) radiographs of the right wrist. There is an avulsion fragment of bone (arrow) at the dorsal aspect of the proximal carpal row seen on the lateral radiograph indicative of a triquetral avulsion fracture. The overlying soft tissues are swollen. The oblique radiograph shows the fracture is comminuted.

(C)

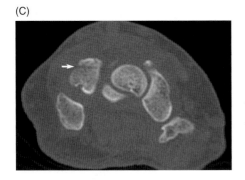

(D)

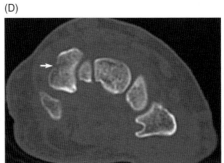

Axial CT through the triquetrum, proximal (C) and distal (D). There is a fracture through the triquetrum in the coronal plane (arrows). This is the second most common carpal bone fracture, after scaphoid fractures, comprising 7–20% of carpal bone fractures [2]. Radiotriquetral and ulnotriquetral ligament avulsion produces this injury, which often may be seen only on the lateral radiograph or CT.

Case 3–11   Scaphoid tubercle fracture

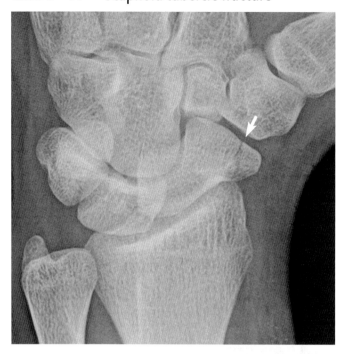

26-year-old man who fell on an outstretched hand. Oblique radiograph of the left wrist. The oblique view shows a fracture of the distal tubercle of the scaphoid (arrow) that extends to the articulation with the trapezium. The fracture is minimally displaced. According to the Herbert classification [9], this fracture is considered stable, and would generally not require operative treatment. Herbert classified stable scaphoid fractures as having displacement no greater than 1 mm and angulation between fragments no greater than 15 degrees. Non-displaced scaphoid waist fractures may be treated conservatively with good result [10].

Case 3–12   Scaphoid waist fracture

(A)

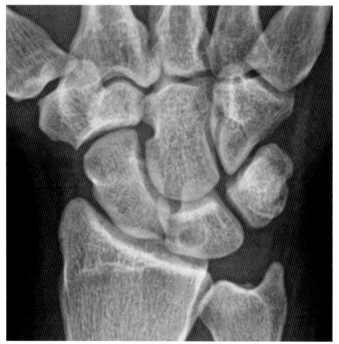

(B)

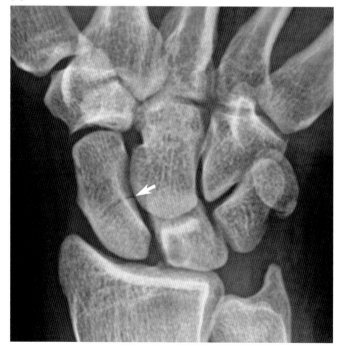

37-year-old man who was injured in a bicycle crash. Oblique (A) and scaphoid (B) radiographs of the right wrist. There is a minimally displaced fracture of the scaphoid waist (arrow), seen best on the angled scaphoid view. This view is obtained in the PA direction, centered on the snuff box, with ulnar deviation of the wrist and 20 to 30 degrees angulation of the tube toward the elbow, to produce an en face or even elongated view of the scaphoid. The scaphoid view is the best projection for scaphoid waist fractures [11]. Waist fractures constitute 70% of scaphoid fractures [12]. Falling on an outstretched hand with dorsiflexion is the mechanism of injury. Delayed union, nonunion and osteonecrosis of the proximal pole are potential complications and depend on how proximal the fracture site is relative to the entrance of the artery at the waist of the scaphoid. In general, more proximal fractures are more likely to develop complications [13–14].

Case 3–13
Scaphoid proximal pole fracture

(A)

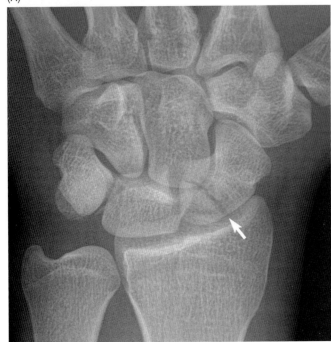

(B)

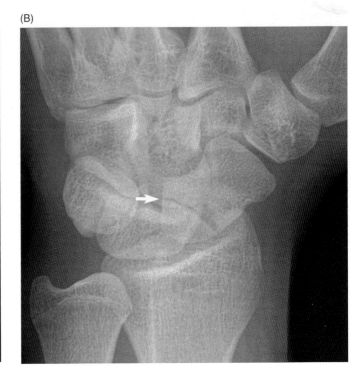

19-year-old man who fell on his outstretched hand. PA (A) and oblique (B) radiographs of the left wrist. There is a minimally displaced fracture through the proximal pole of the scaphoid (arrow), extending from the radiocarpal articular surface to the scaphocapitate articular surface. According to the Herbert classification [9], proximal pole scaphoid fractures are unstable, regardless of the amount of actual displacement or angulation, and likely to require operative fixation. There is a high risk for osteonecrosis of the proximal pole fragment.

Case 3–14

Scaphoid comminuted fracture

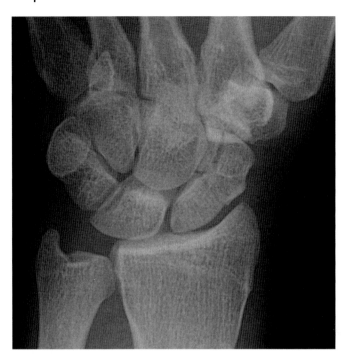

20-year-old man who fell on his outstretched hand. PA radiograph of the left wrist. There are minimally displaced fractures of the scaphoid extending transversely across the waist and then through the distal pole to the triscaphe joint. The peak incidence of scaphoid fractures is in the 10–19 age range, with much lower rates at age 40 and older [15]. Males are twice as likely as females to fracture their scaphoid [15], and the most common mechanism is a fall.

Case 3–15

Scaphoid fracture

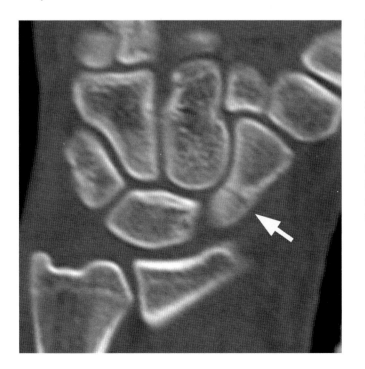

21-year-old man injured when a large stack of plywood sheets fell on him. Radiographs were suspicious for scaphoid fracture. Coronal CT of the left wrist. Coronal CT images through the dorsal cortex of the scaphoid at the waist definitively show a scaphoid fracture traversing the waist. When radiographs are normal or equivocal, and scaphoid fracture is still suspected, CT may be a useful next step. MRI is a reasonable alternative, particularly when soft tissue injuries are also suspected. Fractures of the proximal pole constitute 10% of all scaphoid fractures and have the highest complication rate of nonunion and proximal pole osteonecrosis. The scaphoid bone is the most commonly fractured of the carpal bones, and constitutes approximately two-thirds of all carpal fractures [16].

Case 3–16
Occult scaphoid fracture

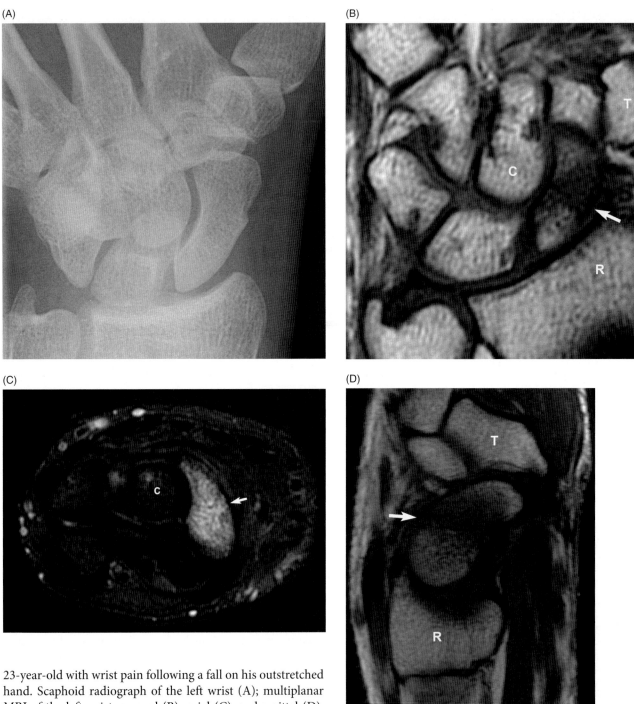

(A)

(B)

(C)

(D)

23-year-old with wrist pain following a fall on his outstretched hand. Scaphoid radiograph of the left wrist (A); multiplanar MRI of the left wrist, coronal (B), axial (C), and sagittal (D). The radiographs of the wrist are normal. Coronal T1 MR shows a fracture across the scaphoid waist (arrow). Axial T2 MR shows high signal in the scaphoid (arrow). Sagittal T1 MR shows the fracture through the waist (arrow) with surrounding edema displacing the normal fatty marrow. MRI is considered to be highly accurate for the detection of scaphoid fractures [17]. Radiography may miss up to 25% of scaphoid fractures on initial presentation [18]. C=capitate, T=trapezium, R=radius.

Case 3–17
Rotary subluxation of the scaphoid

(A)

(B)

(C)

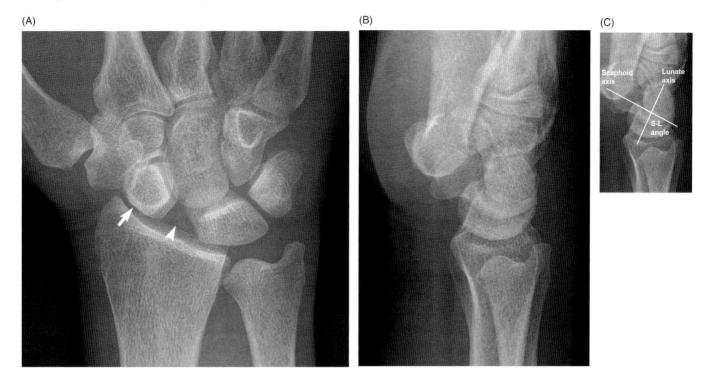

52-year-old man with wrist pain for two years after wrist injury. PA (A) and lateral (B) radiographs of the right wrist. The scaphoid appears almost round (arrow) on the PA view, and there is an abnormally wide gap (arrowhead) between the scaphoid and the lunate. On the annotated lateral view (C), the angle between the axis of the scaphoid and the axis of the lunate is approximately 90 degrees. These findings indicate that the scaphoid is abnormally rotated along its short axis, assuming a nearly vertical orientation relative to the coronal plane, rather than a 45 degree orientation. This condition is called rotary subluxation of the scaphoid. It is also called scapholunate dissociation, in reference to the cardinal anatomic abnormality, the loss of the scapholunate interosseous ligament, allowing the scaphoid and the lunate to move apart from each other. This injury is considered to be Stage I of the four stages of perilunate injury [19–21].

Case 3–18

Transsnaphoid perilunate dislocation

(A)

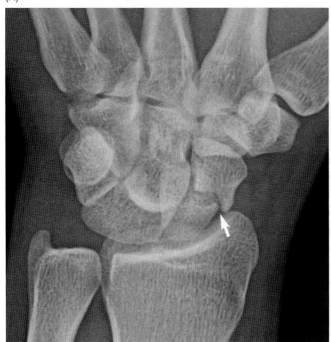

(B)

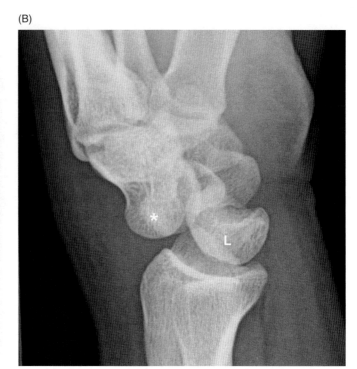

33-year-old man who fell on his arm playing basketball. PA (A) and lateral (B) radiographs of the left wrist. There is a displaced scaphoid waist fracture (arrow). The distal carpal row overlaps the proximal carpal row on the PA view. On the lateral view, the lunate (L) maintains its normal relationship with the radius, however, the capitate (*) is dorsally dislocated relative to the lunate. This injury is a perilunate dislocation, and in recognition of the associated scaphoid fracture, it is called a transscaphoid perilunate dislocation. The mechanism of injury is a

fall on an outstretched hand with dorsiflexion. Perilunate fractures are considered to be Stage II of the four stages of perilunate injury [19–21]. The characteristic feature is that the lunate maintains its normal relationship with the radius while the capitate dislocates around it. The carpus is open on the radial side, either through a soft tissue injury separating the scaphoid from the radius and lunate, or through a scaphoid waist fracture. The scaphoid, triquetrum, and other carpal bones dislocate from the lunate along with the capitate.

Case 3–19
Transsscaphoid midcarpal dislocation

(A)

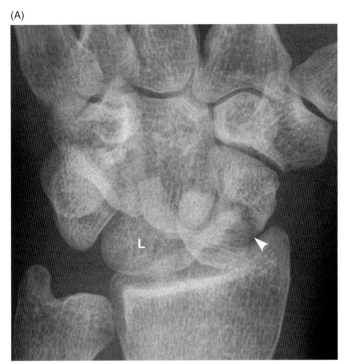

(B)

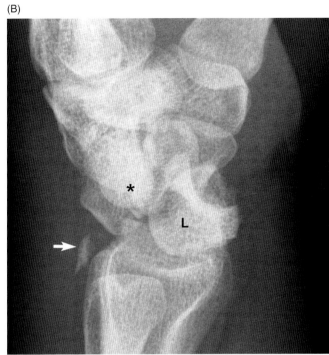

33-year-old man injured in a motorcycle crash. PA (A) and lateral (B) radiographs of the left wrist. There is a fracture through the waist of the scaphoid (arrowhead) and on the PA view, the lunate (L) has a triangular shape that overlaps the other carpal bones. On the lateral view, a small fragment of bone is seen at the dorsal lip of the radius (arrow). The lunate (L) is in the radial fossa, but it is rotated a few degrees in the volar direction. Because of the irregular shape of the lunate, this rotation causes it to assume a triangular rather than trapezoidal shape on the PA view [22]. The capitate (*) is dorsally dislocated from the lunate, along with the proximal fragment of the scaphoid and the other carpal bones. This injury is a transsscaphoid midcarpal dislocation, with avulsion fracture of the dorsal lip of the radius. Midcarpal dislocations are considered to be Stage III of the four stages of perilunate injury [19–21]. The defining characteristic is the rotary subluxation of the lunate combined with the dislocation of the capitate, like a perilunate dislocation with a rotated lunate.

Case 3–20
Lunate dislocation

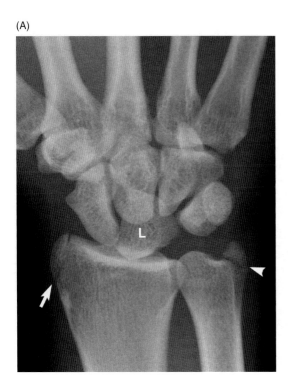

(A)

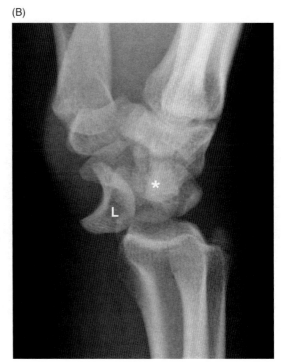

(B)

38-year-old man who fell while weight lifting. PA (A) and lateral (B) radiographs of the right wrist. The lunate (L) has a triangular shape on the PA view and overlaps the adjacent carpal bones, indicating that it is rotated and dislocated. There are minimally displaced fractures of the radial styloid process (arrow) and the ulnar styloid process (arrowhead). On the lateral view, the lunate (L) is rotated 90 degrees from its normal orientation and dislocated volarly from the radius. The capitate (*) is dorsally dislocated from the lunate with the other carpal bones attached. This is called a lunate dislocation and is considered the most severe stage, Stage IV, of the four stages of perilunate injury [19–21]. The defining characteristic is the rotation and dislocation of the lunate combined with the dislocation of the capitate, like a midcarpal dislocation with further rotation and dislocation of the lunate. The radius and ulna fractures are incidental.

Case 3–21

Transscaphoid trans-radial styloid perilunate dislocation

(A)

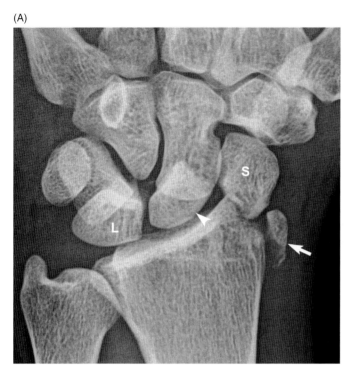

(B)

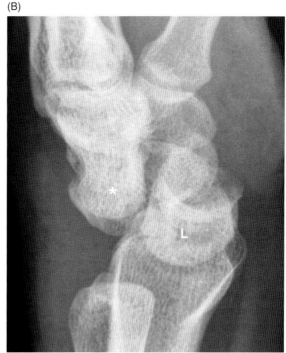

31-year-old man in motorcycle crash. PA (A) and lateral (B) radiographs of the left wrist. There is a displaced scaphoid waist fracture, with the proximal pole (arrowhead) remaining with the lunate (L) in the radial fossa, but the distal fragment (S) is displaced with the capitate and hand. There is a displaced radial styloid process fracture (arrow). There is perilunate dislocation, with the capitate (*) dorsally dislocated from the lunate (L). The distal carpus is translated somewhat in the radial direction. This is a variant of a perilunate dislocation with the plane of injury passing through the radial styloid and the scaphoid [23]. Note that the scaphoid and radial styloid fracture planes are aligned.

Case 3–22

Volar perilunate dislocation

(A)

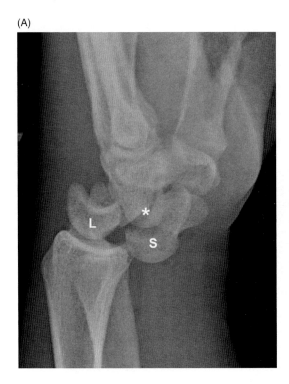

(B)

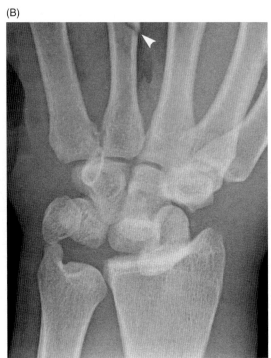

20-year-old man who was hit by a bus. Lateral (A) and PA (B) radiographs of the left wrist. There is volar dislocation of the capitate (*) from the lunate (L), with the hamate and scaphoid (S) still attached to the capitate, and the triquetrum still attached to the lunate. The distal carpal row and hand have come to rest volar to the lunate (L), which remains located in the radial fossa and normally aligned. On the PA view, the distal carpal row is misaligned and there is overlap of the lunate and capitate and the scaphoid and radius. There is also a degloving soft tissue injury of the medial hand, with fractures of the base of the fifth metacarpal and shaft of the fourth metacarpal (arrowhead). This is a variant of a perilunate dislocation. Volar perilunate dislocation is a rare injury, comprising fewer than 3% of all perilunate dislocations [24].

Case 3–23
Lateral perilunate dislocation

(A)

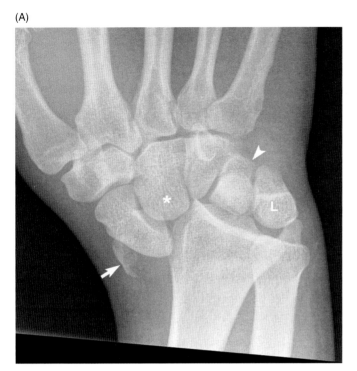

(B)

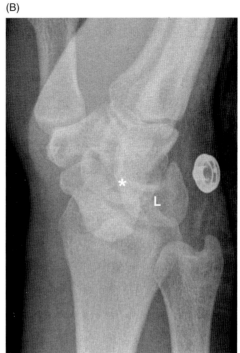

42-year-old fisherman who suffered torsional wrist injury while handling crab pots off Alaska. PA (A) and lateral (B) radiographs of the right wrist. On the PA view, there is a displaced radial styloid process fracture (arrow). There is a perilunate dislocation such that the hand and perilunate portion of the carpus are displaced over the radial styloid, and the triquetrum (arrowhead) has come to rest in the scaphoid fossa of the radius lateral to the lunate (L). On the lateral view, the lunate (L) appears to maintain articulation with the radius, although, understandably, the technologist was not able to provide a perfectly oriented lateral radiograph. This is a rare variant of a perilunate dislocation.

Case 3–24

Lunate dislocation, posterior

(A)

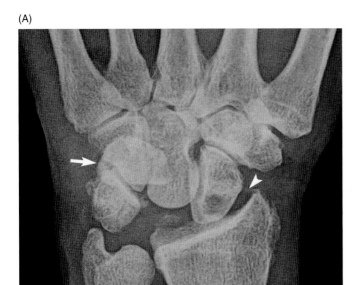

(B)

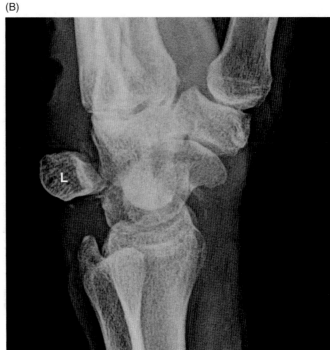

85-year-old woman in motor vehicle crash. PA (A) and lateral (B) radiographs of the left wrist. On the PA radiograph the lunate is absent from its normal location, and can be found overlapping the hamate and capitate (arrow). The lateral radiograph shows the lunate has been extruded posteriorly and rotated such that the proximal articular surface points posteriorly and the medial articular surface points distally. There are multiple small avulsion fractures involving the radial styloid, the triquetrum, the ulnar styloid, and the scaphoid. Each avulsion fracture represents the avulsion of a ligamentous attachment. The asymmetric width of the radioscaphoid joint space (arrowhead) indicates that the scaphoid is subluxated toward the ulna (ulnar translocation). There is an open wound over the dorsum of the wrist, and the lunate was visibly protruding into the wound. There is an incidental subchondral cyst in the scaphoid. The injury can be summarized as an open posterior lunate dislocation with gross radiocarpal instability. One can only speculate as to the mechanism of injury.

Case 3–25

Transsscaphoid transcapitate midcarpal dislocation

(A)

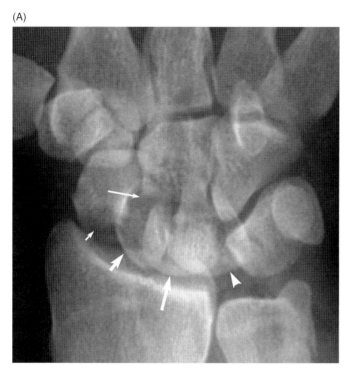

(B)

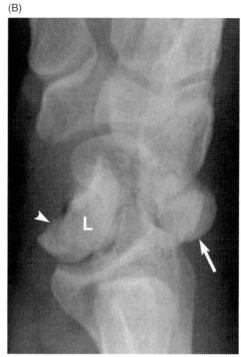

29-year-old man who fell from a height of 30 feet. PA (A) and lateral (B) radiographs of the right wrist. There are fractures of the scaphoid (short, small arrow) and capitate (long, small arrow). The proximal scaphoid fragment (short, large arrow), the lunate (arrowhead), and the proximal capitate fragment (long, large arrow) are difficult to identify on the PA radiograph and appear to be overlapping each other. The lateral radiograph shows there is dorsal midcarpal dislocation, with dorsal dislocation of the proximal capitate fragment (long, large arrow). The lunate (L) is still within the radial fossa but is rotated in the volar direction, and its volar rim is fractured (arrowhead).

(C)

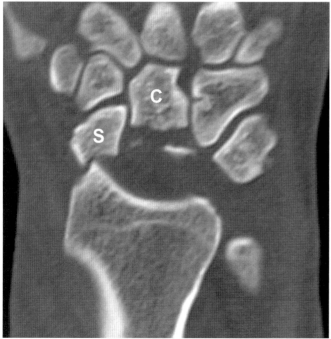

(D)

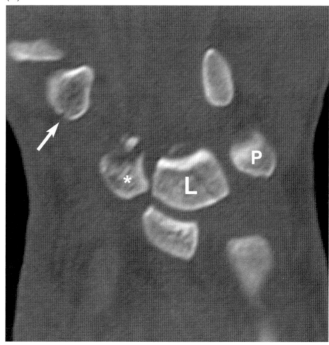

Coronal CT of the right wrist. The coronal CT slice (C) through the mid-radius shows the displaced distal scaphoid (S) and distal capitate (C) fragments, with absence of the lunate. A more volar slice (D) shows the lunate (L) perched on the volar margin of the radius, and the attached proximal pole fragment of the scaphoid (*). There is also a fracture of the trapezium (long arrow). The pisiform (P) is visible in the same plane as the lunate, indicating that the lunate has moved volar out of its normal position.

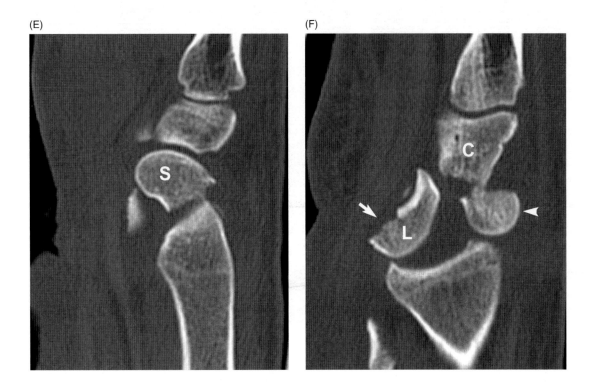

(E)   (F)

Sagittal CT of the right wrist. Sagittal CT (E) through the radial side of the wrist shows the distal scaphoid (S) fragment abutting the radial styloid. CT slice (F) through the middle of the wrist shows the distal capitate (C) fragment and the dorsally displaced and dislocated proximal capitate fragment (arrowhead). The rotated lunate (L) is perched on the volar lip of the radius, and the volar rim of the lunate (arrow) has been fractured and is absent from the image. This injury may be characterized as fracture-dislocation of the greater arc; the greater arc being an imaginary curve through the waists of the scaphoid, capitate, hamate, and triquetrum [25]. The lesser arc is a curve around the attachments of the lunate, and injuries of the lesser arc comprise the stages of perilunate injuries. One may also characterize this as a variant of the midcarpal dislocation. Many perilunate injuries, such as transscaphoid perilunate dislocations, involve both the greater and the lesser arcs.

Case 3–26

Complex carpal fracture-dislocation

(A)

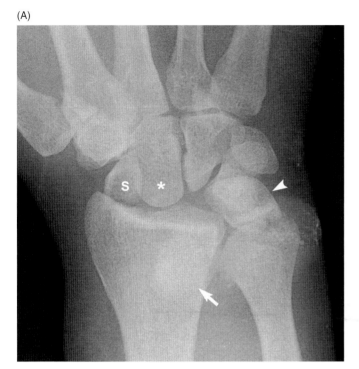

(B)

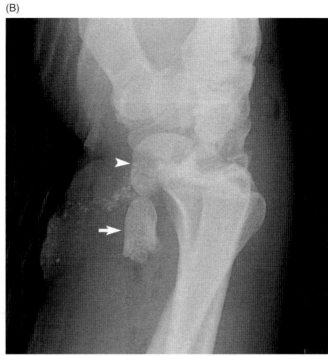

26-year-old man who was a pedestrian struck by a car. PA (A) and lateral (B) radiographs of the right wrist. There is a scaphoid waist fracture with the proximal pole (S) attached to the capitate. There has been perilunate dislocation of the capitate and hand from the lunate. The lunate (arrowhead) is volarly dislocated out of the radial fossa. The proximal pole of the scaphoid (arrow) is dislocated volarly from the radius and lunate, and displaced proximally. There is a Bennett fracture of the first metacarpal base.

Case 3–27
Complex carpal dislocation

(A)

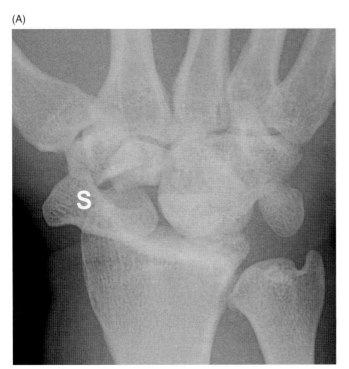

(B)

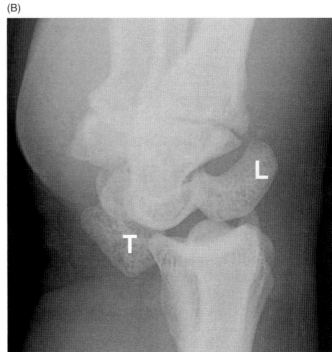

(C)

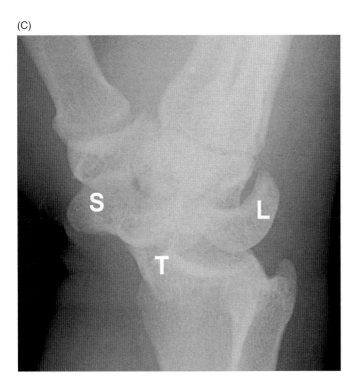

Worker whose hand was crushed between a wall and a truck backing up. PA (A), lateral (B), and oblique (C) radiographs of the right wrist. There has been individual dislocation of the bones of the proximal carpal row. There is radial and volar dislocation of the scaphoid (S). The lunate (L) is perched on the dorsal lip of the radius. The triquetrum (T) is dislocated volarly. There is scapholunate and lunotriquetral dissociation. There is volar dislocation of the capitate, and the capitate with attached hand has migrated into the radial fossa. The absence of fractures is consistent with the relatively slow application of force to the limb. Dislocation of the scaphoid itself is an unusual injury [26].

References

1. Edmunds JO. Traumatic dislocations and instability of the trapeziometacarpal joint of the thumb. *Hand Clin.* 2006 Aug;22(3):365–92. PMID: 16843802.

2. Suh N, Ek ET, Wolfe SW. Carpal fractures. *J Hand Surg Am.* 2014 Apr;39(4):785–91; quiz 791. doi: 10.1016/j. jhsa.2013.10.030. PMID: 24679911.

3. Ehara S, el-Khoury GY, Blair WF. Scaphotrapezial dislocation: A case report. *J Trauma.* 1988 Nov;28(11):1587–9. PMID: 3184223.

4. Kain N, Heras-Palou C. Trapezoid fractures: Report of 11 cases. *J Hand Surg Am.* 2012 Jun;37(6):1159–62. doi: 10.1016/j. jhsa.2012.02.046. Epub 2012 Apr 21. PMID: 22522106.

5. Welling RD, Jacobson JA, Jamadar DA, Chong S, Caoili EM, Jebson PJ. MDCT and radiography of wrist fractures: Radiographic sensitivity and fracture patterns. *AJR Am J Roentgenol.* 2008 Jan;190(1):10–6. PMID: 18094287.

6. Egawa M, Asai T. Fracture of the hook of the hamate: Report of six cases and the suitability of computerized tomography. *J Hand Surg Am.* 1983 Jul;8(4):393–8. PMID: 6886333.

7. Scheufler O, Radmer S, Erdmann D, Germann G, Pierer G, Andresen R. Therapeutic alternatives in nonunion of hamate hook fractures: Personal experience in 8 patients and review of literature. *Ann Plast Surg.* 2005 Aug;55(2):149–54. PMID: 16034244.

8. O'Shea K, Weiland AJ. Fractures of the hamate and pisiform bones. *Hand Clin.* 2012 Aug;28(3):287–300, viii. doi: 10.1016/j. hcl.2012.05.010. PMID: 22883867.

9. Herbert TJ, Fisher WE. Management of the fractured scaphoid using a new bone screw. *J Bone Joint Surg Br.* 1984 Jan;66(1):114–23. PMID: 6693468.

10. Modi CS, Nancoo T, Powers D, Ho K, Boer R, Turner SM. Operative versus nonoperative treatment of acute undisplaced and minimally displaced scaphoid waist fractures – A systematic review. *Injury.* 2009 Mar;40(3):268–73. Epub 2009 Feb 4. PMID: 19195652.

11. Russe O. Fracture of the carpal navicular. Diagnosis, non-operative treatment, and operative treatment. *J Bone Joint Surg Am.* 1960 Jul;42-A:759–68. PMID: 13854612.

12. Stewart MJ. Fractures of the carpal navicular (scaphoid): A report of 436 cases. *J Bone Joint Surg Am.* 1954 Oct;36-A(5):998–1006. PMID: 13211693.

13. Gelberman RH, Gross MS. The vascularity of the wrist. Identification of arterial patterns at risk. *Clin Orthop Relat Res.* 1986 Jan;(202):40–9. PMID: 3514029.

14. Razemon JP. Fractures of the carpal bones with the exception of fractures of the scaphoid. In: Razemon JP, Fisk GR, eds. *The wrist.* Edinburgh, Scotland: Churchill-Livingstone, 1988; 126–9.

15. Van Tassel DC, Owens BD, Wolf JM. Incidence estimates and demographics of scaphoid fracture in the U.S. population. *J Hand Surg Am.* 2010 Aug;35(8):1242–5. doi: 10.1016/j. jhsa.2010.05.017. PMID: 20684922.

16. Papp S. Carpal bone fractures. *Orthop Clin North Am.* 2007 Apr;38(2):251–60, vii. PMID: 17560407.

17. Murthy NS. The role of magnetic resonance imaging in scaphoid fractures. *J Hand Surg Am.* 2013 Oct;38(10):2047–54. doi: 10.1016/j. jhsa.2013.03.055. PMID: 24079527.

18. Brooks S, Wluka AE, Stuckey S, Cicuttini F. The management of scaphoid fractures. *J Sci Med Sport.* 2005 Jun;8(2):181–9. PMID: 16075778.

19. Lichtman DM, Wroten ES. Understanding midcarpal instability. *J Hand Surg Am.* 2006 Mar;31(3):491–8. PMID: 16516747.

20. Gelberman RH, Cooney WP III, Szabo RM. Carpal instability. *Instr Course Lect.* 2001;50:123–34. PMID: 11372306.

21. Schmitt R, Froehner S, Coblenz G, Christopoulos G. Carpal instability. *Eur Radiol.* 2006 Oct;16(10):2161–78. Epub 2006 Mar 1. PMID: 16508768.

22. Gilula LA. Carpal injuries: Analytic approach and case exercises. *AJR Am J Roentgenol.* 1979 Sep;133(3):503–17. PMID: 111512.

23. Scalcione LR, Gimber LH, Ho AM, Johnston SS, Sheppard JE, Taljanovic MS. Spectrum of carpal dislocations and fracture-dislocations: Imaging and management. *AJR Am J Roentgenol.* 2014 Sep;203(3):541–50. doi: 10.2214/AJR.13.11680. PMID: 25148156.

24. Youssef B, Deshmukh SC. Volar perilunate dislocation: A case report and review of the literature. *Open Orthop J.* 2008 Apr 11; 2: 57–8. doi: 10.2174/1874325 000802010057. PMID: 19478928; PMCID: PMC2687108.

25. Moneim MS. Management of greater arc carpal fractures. *Hand Clin.* 1988 Aug;4(3):457–67. PMID: 3049639.

26. Kolby L, Larsen S, Jorring S, Sorensen AI, Leicht P. Missed isolated volar dislocation of the scaphoid. *Scand J Plast Reconstr Surg Hand Surg.* 2007;41(5):264–6. PMID: 17886133.

Fractures and dislocations of the radius and ulna

Catherine Maldjian, M.D., and Felix S. Chew, M.D.

Case 4–1
Radial styloid fracture

(A)

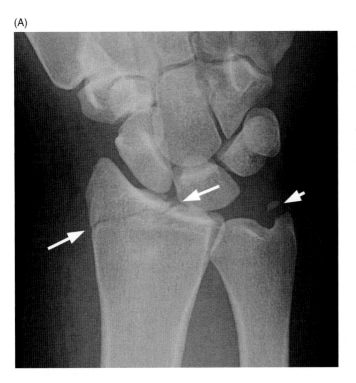

(B)

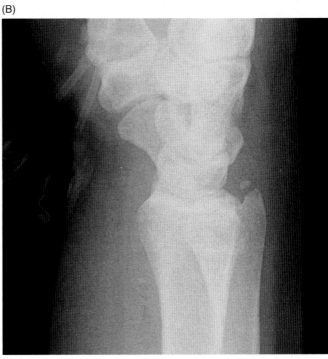

21-year-old man in motor vehicle crash. PA (A) and lateral (B) radiographs of the right wrist. There is a minimally displaced oblique fracture (long arrow) of the radial styloid extending to the joint surface at the scapholunate level. The so-called chauffeur fractures may manifest as small avulsion injuries of the radial styloid or oblique fractures of the radial styloid extending up to the articular surface of the scapholunate joint. The mechanism of injury is direct impaction of the radial styloid by the scaphoid. These are classically non-displaced as seen here, and best seen on the PA view [1]. Small ulnar styloid avulsion is also seen (short arrow). Ulnar styloid fractures are associated with distal radial fractures and when present, ulnar styloid avulsions bode a worse prognosis due to its impact on distal radioulnar function [2].

Radial styloid fracture

(A)

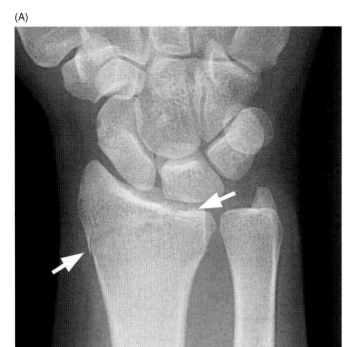

(B)

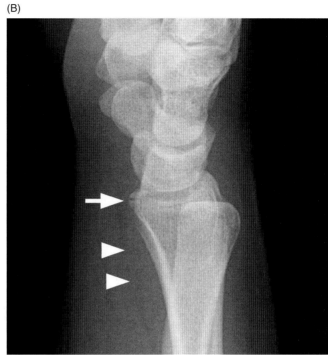

28-year-old woman with fall on outstretched hand. PA (A) and lateral (B) radiographs of the right wrist. The pronator fat pad is displaced (arrowheads). There is a subtle non-displaced oblique fracture of the radial styloid (arrows) extending to the joint surface at the scapholunate level.

Case 4–3

Radiocarpal fracture-dislocation

(A)

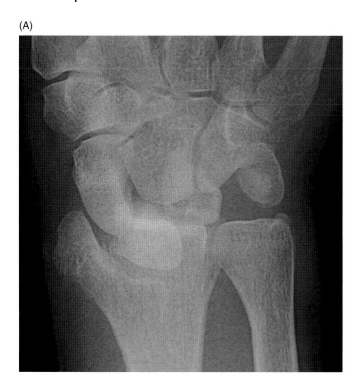

(B)

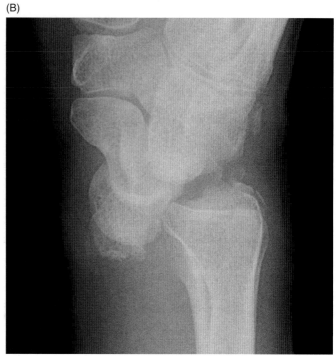

64-year-old man injured in motorcycle crash. PA (A) and lateral (B) radiographs of the right wrist. On the PA view, the lunate overlaps the distal radius, indicating dislocation; this is confirmed on the lateral view. The triquetrum overlaps the capitate and has flipped and rotated such that the radiocarpal articular surface faces towards the scaphoid and the lunotriquetral articular surface is parallel to the distal radial articular surface rather than the lunate. The triquetrum is within the radial fossa, while the remainder of the carpus has dislocated volarly. There is a radial styloid process fracture, with the fragment displaced with the scaphoid. There are small fragments about the dorsal aspect of the dislocated carpus that represent avulsion fractures from multiple carpal bones, including a hamate fracture at the fifth CMC joint. Radiocarpal dislocations result from high energy trauma and typically include a combination of injuries to the ligaments and bones that hold the wrist to the forearm [3]. In this case, the ligaments on the radial side are intact but attached to the displaced radial styloid fragment, while the other ligaments are torn.

Radiocarpal dislocation

(A)

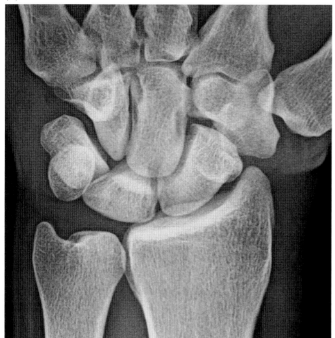

(B)

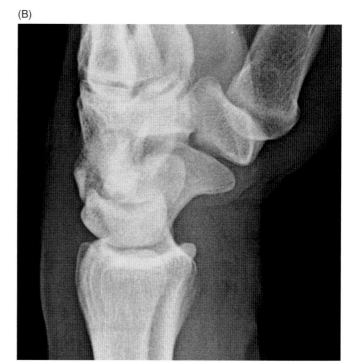

32-year-old man who fell from a 20-foot height, sustaining multiple injuries. PA (A) and lateral (B) radiographs of the left wrist. There are no fractures or dislocations. However, there is subtle ulnar translocation of the carpus; that is, the carpus, as a unit, is located more towards the ulna on the PA view than is normal. In the normal situation, the lunate articulates almost completely with the radius, with only a small portion of the articular surface extending over the ulna and the triangular fibrocartilage complex. In this case, almost all of the lunate is over the ulna, with only a small portion articulating with the radius. The scaphoid has also shifted from its normal articulation with the radial styloid process to articulate with the center of the radial fossa. The lateral view shows that the lunate and scaphoid are subluxated dorsally, so that their curved articular surfaces are not congruent with that of the distal radius. In this setting, there must have been transient radiocarpal dislocation with extensive injury of the radiocarpal ligaments.

(C)

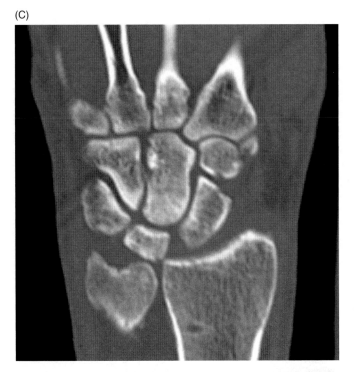

(D)

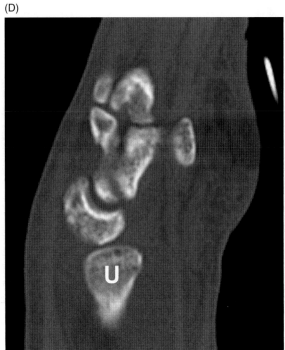

CT scan was obtained 6 weeks after the initial injury. Coronal (C) and sagittal (D) CT of the left wrist. Coronal CT shows the translocated position of the carpus relative to the forearm, with the lunate now completely off of the radius. The curvature of the articular surfaces of the proximal carpal row should be concentric with the curve of the radial fossa but is not. The scapholunate interval is abnormally widened. On the sagittal CT, the imaging plane passes through the ulna and lunate rather than the ulna and triquetrum. The lunate is dorsally subluxated and rotated in a volar direction. U=ulna.

Case 4–5
Comminuted intra-articular distal radius fracture

(A)

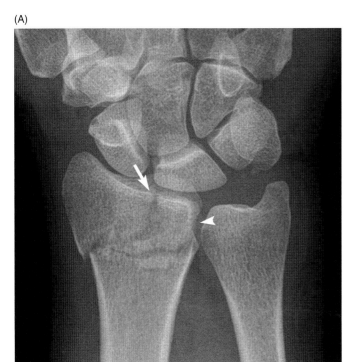

(B)

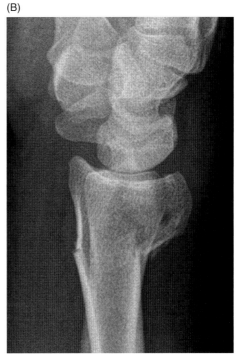

47-year-old man who slipped and fell on the ice. PA (A) and lateral (B) radiographs of the right wrist. There is a comminuted fracture of the distal radius with intra-articular component and some dorsal displacement. The fracture extends to both the radiocarpal joint (arrow) as well as the distal radioulnar joint (arrowhead), but the distal ulna is intact. The distal radial articular surface has assumed a dorsal tilt. Note the blurring of the pronator quadratus fat pad in the volar soft tissues. Distal radius fractures may have an intra-articular component in 70% of cases. The Frykman classification emphasizes the distinction between intra-articular fracture patterns and extra-articular fractures with and without involvement of the ulnar styloid [4]: Type I is extra-articular; Type II is like Type I with distal ulna fracture; Type III is intra-articular involving the radiocarpal joint; Type IV is like Type III with distal ulna fracture; Type V is intra-articular involving the distal radioulnar joint; Type VI is like Type V with distal ulna fracture, Type VII is intra-articular involving both radiocarpal and distal radioulnar joints; and Type VIII is like Type VII with distal ulna fracture. The pattern seen here is Frykman Type VII.

Case 4–6
Distal radius fracture

(A)

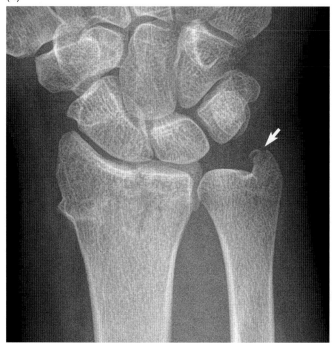

(B)

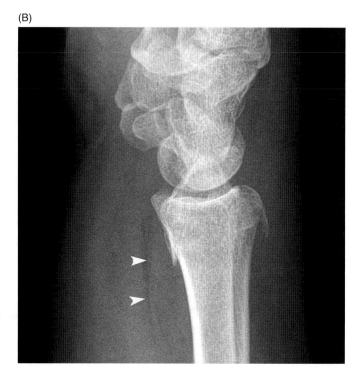

52-year-old woman who fell on an outstretched hand. PA (A) and lateral (B) radiographs of the wrist. There is a comminuted, impacted intra-articular fracture of the distal radius with fracture of the distal ulna (arrow). The pronator quadratus fat pad is bulging away from the volar aspect of the distal radius (arrowheads), a radiographic sign of soft tissue swelling associated with the fracture. There is also a mildly displaced avulsion fracture at the tip of the ulnar styloid process. The pronator quadratus fat pad sign is not considered a sensitive or specific indication for the presence or absence of radiographically occult fractures [5] but may be useful occasionally as a confirmatory finding.

Case 4–7
Die-punch distal radial fracture

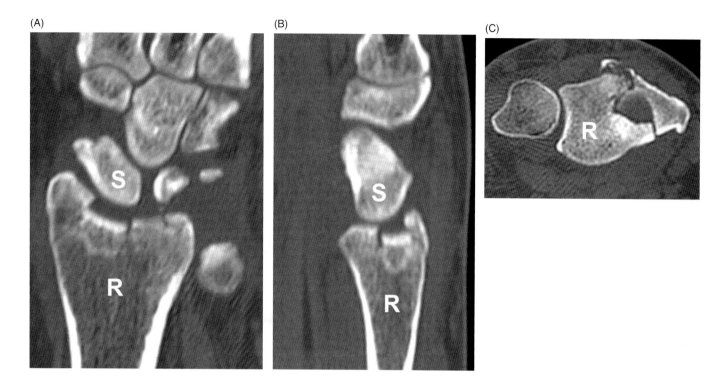

(A) (B) (C)

61-year-old woman fell backward onto her right wrist at the gym. Multiplanar CT of the right wrist, coronal (A), sagittal (B), and axial (C). Comminuted fracture of the distal radius demonstrates a discrete depressed segment characteristic of a die-punch fracture. This pattern occurs when a fracture fragment involving the articular surface is driven into the subchondral bone producing a depressed fracture. This is typically seen at the scaphoid or lunate fossa, when it occurs in the distal radius. Displaced articular fractures more commonly demonstrate osteoarthritis as a sequela. Some authors advocate surgical correction for intra-articular fractures of the radius with as little as 1 mm step-off at the articular surface [6]. S=scaphoid, R=radius.

Case 4–8
Extra-articular distal radius fracture (Colles fracture)

(A)

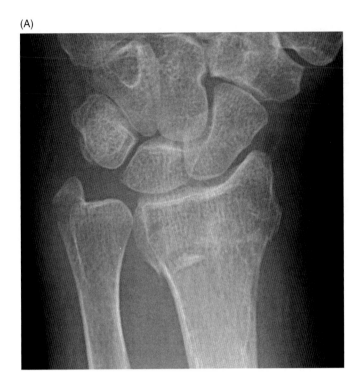

(B)

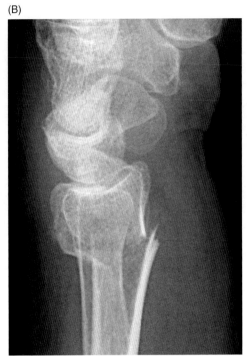

57-year-old woman who fell on outstretched hand. PA (A) and lateral (B) radiographs of the left wrist. The bones are demineralized. There is a fracture of the distal radial metaphysis with dorsal angulation but no involvement of the articular surfaces. The ulna appears too long because of the impaction and consequent shortening of the radius. Note the increased convexity of the pronator fat pad. The common mechanism of injury for a fracture such as this is falling on an outstretched hand, with volar tension and dorsal impaction. Traction forces transmitted through the triangular fibrocartilage complex may result in an ulnar styloid fracture, as seen here. This is one of the most commonly encountered extremity fractures in middle and older ages and is particularly associated with elderly women, with osteoporosis playing a role [7]. The original Colles fracture described an extra-articular distal radius fracture, but the eponym may be used refer to any distal radius fracture. Because of the potential for confusion, perhaps the term should be avoided.

Case 4–9   Distal radioulnar joint subluxation

(A)

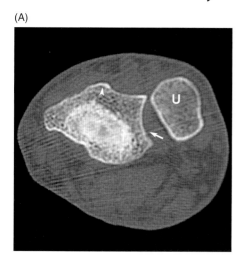

(B)

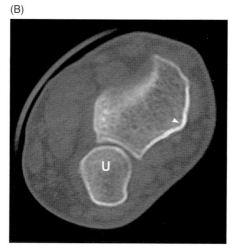

34-year-old man with chronic posttraumatic left distal radioulnar joint instability. He had previously suffered a crush injury of the left radius and ulna. Axial CT of the left distal radioulnar joint in pronation (A) and supination (B). In pronation, there dorsal displacement of the ulna (U) relative to the sigmoid notch of the radius (arrow), diagnostic of distal radioulnar joint subluxation. Lister's tubercle (arrowhead) is a landmark on the dorsal surface of the distal radius. In supination, the relationship of the ulna (U) to the sigmoid notch of the radius (articular surface of the radius at the distal radioulnar joint) is normal. Usually associated with distal radius fractures, isolated distal radioulnar joint disruption is unusual [8]. Axial CT to evaluate for distal radioulnar joint subluxation is typically performed in pronation, neutral, and supination, as the subluxation or dislocation may be reduced in certain positions and exaggerated in others.

Case 4–10   Galeazzi fracture-dislocation, type II

(A)

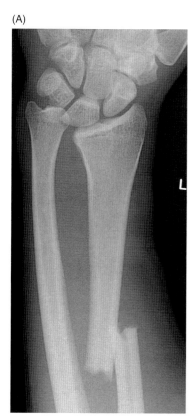

(B)

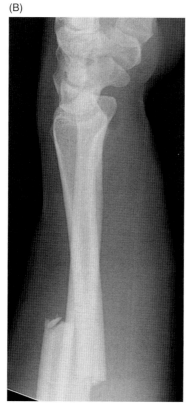

28-year-old man injured in a fall. PA (A) and lateral (B) radiographs of the left distal forearm. There is a fracture at the junction of the middle and distal thirds of the radial shaft with volar displacement and overriding of the fragments. There is widening of the distal radio-ulnar joint (DRUJ) with distal displacement of the ulnar head relative to the radius, consistent with DRUJ dissociation. This is a Galeazzi injury pattern, in which a distal radial shaft fracture is accompanied by DRUJ dislocation. The mechanism of injury is axial load from falling on an outstretched and hyperpronated forearm [9–10]. A complication of this injury may be chronic instability of the DRUJ. Radial fractures that are in closer proximity to the DRUJ are more often associated with instability so Galeazzi fracture-dislocations have been classified by the location of the radial fracture [11]. If the fracture is less than 7.5 cm from the distal radial articular surface then it is Type 1, and if it is more than 7.5 cm from the distal articular surface then it is Type 2. Treatment usually involves compression plating. The distal radioulnar instability may be occult and close inspection may be required to detect it at the time of surgery.

Case 4–11   Galeazzi fracture-dislocation, type I

(A)

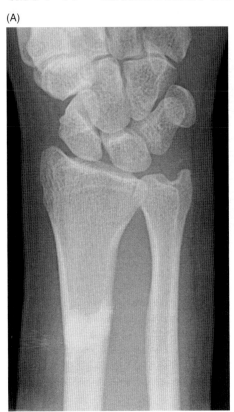

(B)

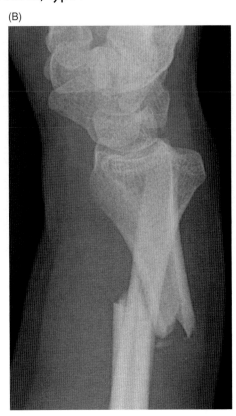

33-year-old woman injured in a go-kart crash. PA (A) and lateral (B) radiographs of the right distal forearm. There is a fracture of the distal radial shaft with dorsal displacement, shortening, and apex dorsal angulation. Dorsal dislocation of the DRUJ is evident on the lateral view. Galeazzi fracture-dislocations comprise approximately 7% of all adult forearm fractures.

Case 4–12   Nightstick fracture

(A)

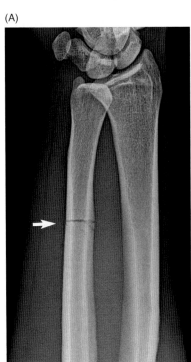

(B)

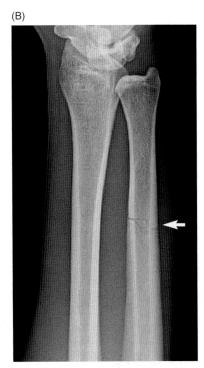

47-year-old man who was beaten with a stick. PA (A) and lateral (B) radiographs of the right distal forearm. There is an isolated non-displaced transverse fracture of the distal ulnar shaft (arrows), also called a nightstick fracture. The mechanism of injury is a direct blow such as from a stick or club, with the forearm raised in a protective posture. A fracture that results from the direct loading of a bone by a relatively low energy blow may be called a tapping fracture. Nightstick fractures are less often seen in the middle and proximal ulna than in the distal ulna and they are transverse or slightly oblique in morphology. Comminution, angulation exceeding 10 degrees, or displacement exceeding 50% are criteria for treatment by open reduction and internal fixation.

Case 4–13   Both bones forearm fractures

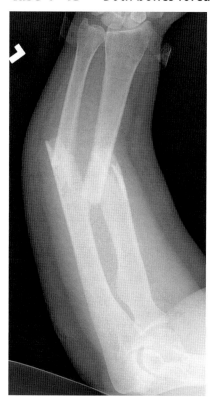

30-year-old woman injured in a rollover motor vehicle crash. PA radiograph of the left distal forearm. There are fractures of the ulnar and radial shafts, a situation called both bones fractures of the forearm. The majority of forearm fractures involve both bones and occur as the result of falls. Most of these occur in the middle thirds. Separation of the forearm bones and proper alignment is important to preserve supination and pronation. These fractures are typically treated with open reduction and internal fixation. Synostosis is a possible complication that would require additional surgery.

Case 4–14   Segmental both bones forearm fractures

(A)

(B)

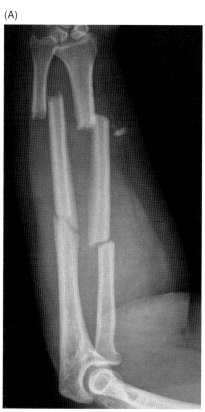
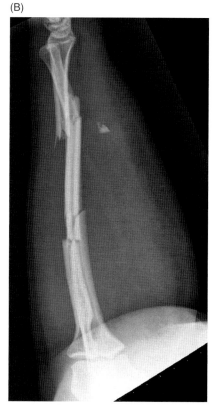

37-year-old woman who injured her left arm in an industrial accident. PA (A) and lateral (B) radiographs of the left forearm. Multilevel transverse fractures of both bones is consistent with segmental fractures. These fractures were treated with internal fixation to restore normal alignment.

Case 4–15   Open both bones forearm fractures

(A)

(B)

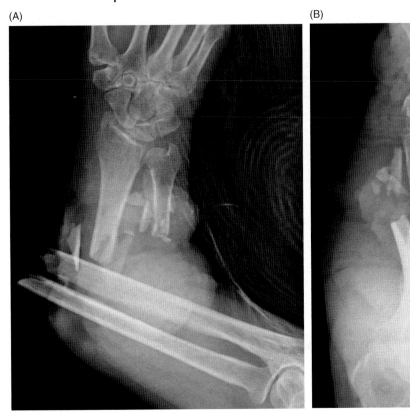

63-year-old woman who was bitten in the forearm by a dog (pit bull terrier). PA (A) and lateral (B) radiographs of the right forearm. There is a mangling injury of the forearm with open comminuted fractures of the radius and ulna. Multiple operations were required, but the limb was saved.

Case 4–16   Forearm amputation

(A)

(B)

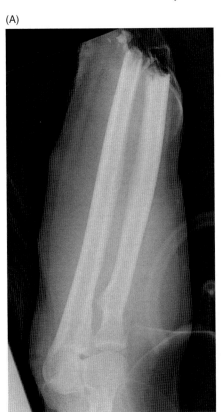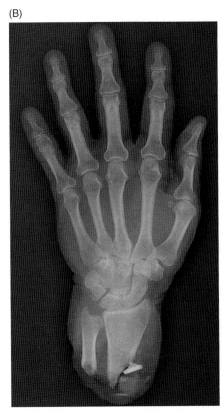

57-year-woman injured by circular power saw. PA radiographs of the left forearm (A) and severed wrist and hand (B). There are transverse fractures of the distal forearm with complete amputation. The severed part should always be retrieved for possible replantation.

Case 4–17
Monteggia fracture-dislocation, type I

(A)

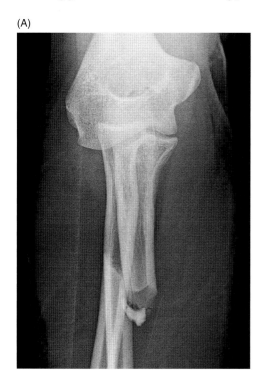

(B)

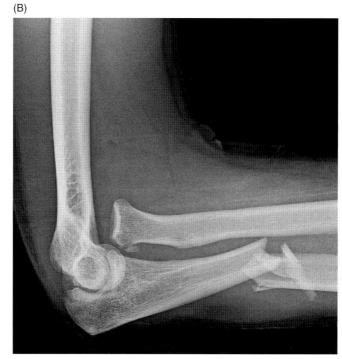

29-year-old man who was struck in the right forearm. AP (A) and lateral (B) radiographs of the right proximal forearm. There is a fracture of the proximal third of the ulna (arrow) with apex anterior angulation, and anterior radial head dislocation (arrowhead). There is also a small bone fragment that was probably fractured off the margin of radial head. Fractures of the ulnar shaft with radial head dislocation are called Monteggia fracture-dislocations [12]. About 90% of ulnar fractures are proximal, with 10% mid and 1% distal in location [13]. The Bado classification can be used to describe these injuries: Type I is an ulnar shaft fracture with apex anterior angulation and anterior radial head dislocation; Type II is an ulnar shaft fracture with apex posterior angulation and posterior dislocation of the radial head; Type III is an ulnar shaft fracture with apex lateral angulation and lateral dislocation of the radial head; and Type IV is any of the other types combined with a comminuted radial head or neck fracture. In all of these types, the radial head dislocation includes dislocation of both the radiocapitellar and the proximal radioulnar joints. Type I, as seen in this case, is the most common (65% of Monteggia fracture-dislocations) and was the pattern originally described by Monteggia [14].

Case 4–18

Monteggia fracture-dislocation, type II

(A)

(B)

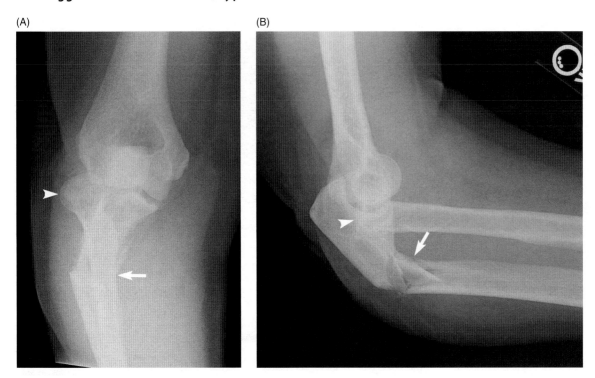

67-year-old woman who fell on her outstretched hand. AP (A) and lateral (B) radiographs of the right proximal forearm. Posterolateral dislocation of the radial head (arrowhead) is seen with an ulnar fracture with apex posterior angulation (arrow). This is a Monteggia fracture-dislocation, Type II. This is the second most common type of Monteggia fracture-dislocation [14].

Case 4–19

Monteggia fracture-dislocation, type III

(A)

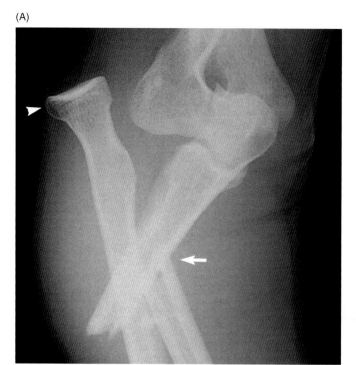

(B)

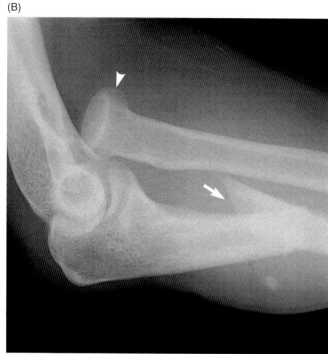

39-year-old man injured in a fall. AP (A) and lateral (B) radiographs of the right proximal forearm. There is fracture of the ulna with apex lateral angulation (arrow) and lateral radial head dislocation (arrowhead), making this a Monteggia fracture-dislocation, Type III. In Monteggia injuries, the orientation of the ulnar angulation (apex of the fracture angle) points to the direction of radial head dislocation. As in this case, the apparent angulation of a fracture on radiographs can be changed by altering the spatial relationship of the fracture site to the x-ray beam and detector. While the lateral view alone may suggest a Type I injury, correlation of both views gives the correct information.

Case 4–20   Monteggia fracture-dislocation, type IV

(A)

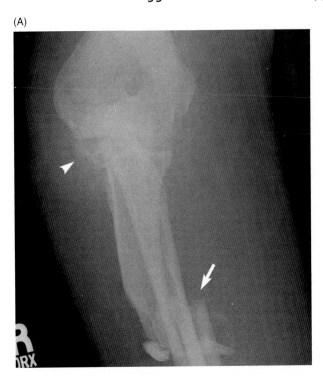

(B)

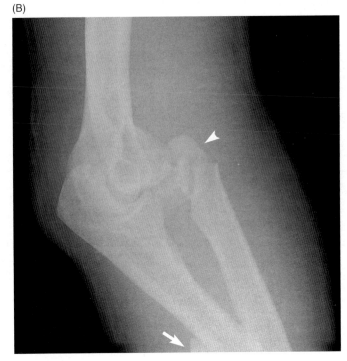

36-year-old man injured in a logging accident. AP (A) and lateral (B) radiographs of the right proximal forearm. There is a fracture of the ulna (arrow) with apex anterior angulation and anterior radial head dislocation. There is also a comminuted fracture (arrowhead) of the radial head and neck, consistent with a Monteggia fracture-dislocation, Type IV. The severity of the radial head fracture may necessitate reconstruction with a prosthesis.

Case 4–21   Essex-Lopresti fracture-dislocation

(A)

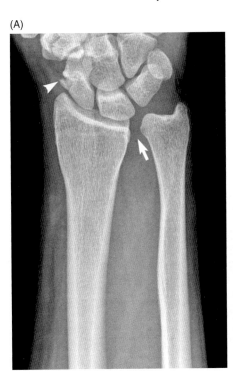

(B)

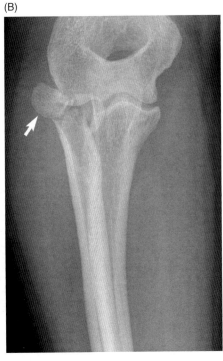

36-year-old woman who was injured when she fell off her mountain bike and landed on her left arm. AP radiograph of the left wrist (A) and AP radiograph of the left elbow (B). There is scaphoid waist fracture (arrowhead) and dislocation of the DRUJ (arrow). There is a comminuted radial head fracture with dislocation of the fragments (arrow). Radial head fracture with DRUJ dislocation, with or without radial head dislocation is called an Essex-Lopresti injury [15–16]. The scaphoid waist fracture, while present in this case, is not part of the Essex-Lopresti injury. The mechanism of injury is longitudinal compression of the forearm with forces transmitted down the interosseous membrane, which is torn along its entire length. This injury is unstable and needs to be corrected at both ends for a proper outcome.

References

1. Cautilli RA, Joyce MF, Gordon E, Juarez R. Classification of fractures of the distal radius. *Clin Orthop Relat Res.* 1974;(103):163–6. PMID: 4412455.

2. Stoffelen D, De Smet L, Broos P. The importance of the distal radioulnar joint in distal radial fractures. *J Hand Surg Br.* 1998 Aug;23(4):507–11. PMID: 9726556.

3. Ilyas AM, Mudgal CS. Radiocarpal fracture-dislocations. *J Am Acad Orthop Surg.* 2008 Nov;16(11):647–55. PMID: 18978287.

4. Altissimi M, Antenucci R, Fiacca C, Mancini GB. Long-term results of conservative treatment of fractures of the distal radius. *Clin Orthop Relat Res.* 1986 May;(206):202–10. PMID: 3708976.

5. Fallahi F, Jafari H, Jefferson G, Jennings P, Read R. Explorative study of the sensitivity and specificity of the pronator quadratus fat pad sign as a predictor of subtle wrist fractures. *Skeletal Radiol.* 2013 Feb;42(2):249–53. doi: 10.1007/s00256-012-1451-0. Epub 2012 Jun 9. PMID: 22684408; Central PMCID: PMC3539072.

6. Trumble TE, Culp RW, Hanel DP, Geissler WB, Berger RA. Intra-articular fractures of the distal aspect of the radius. *Instr Course Lect.* 1999;48:465–80. PMID: 10098077.

7. Alffram P, Bauer GC. Epidemiology of fractures of the forearm. A biomechanical investigation of bone strength. *J Bone Joint Surg Am.* 1962 Jan;44-A:105–14. PMID: 14036674.

8. Head RW. Anterior dislocation of the ulna without accompanying fracture of the ulnar styloid. *Br J Radiol.* 1971 Jun;44(522):468. PMID: 5579177.

9. Miki ZD. Galeazzi fracture-dislocations. *J Bone Joint Surg Am.* 1975 Dec;57(8):1071–80. PMID: 1201989.

10. Walsh HP, McLaren CA, Owen R. Galeazzi fractures in children. *J Bone Joint Surg Br.* 1987 Nov;69(5):730–3. PMID: 3680332.

11. Rettig ME, Raskin KB. Galeazzi fracture-dislocation: A new treatment-oriented classification. *J Hand Surg Am.* 2001 Mar;26(2):228–35. PMID: 11279568.

12. Bado JL. The Monteggia lesion. *Clin Orthop Relat Res.* 1967 Jan–Feb;50:71–86. PMID: 6029027.

13. Boyd HB, Boals JC. The Monteggia lesion. A review of 159 cases. *Clin Orthop Relat Res.* 1969 Sep–Oct;66:94–100. PMID: 5348909.

14. Bruce HE, Harvey JP, Wilson JC Jr. Monteggia fractures. *J Bone Joint Surg Am.* 1974 Dec;56(8):1563–76. PMID: 4434024.

15. Essex-Lopresti P. Fractures of the radial head with distal radio-ulnar dislocation; Report of two cases. *J Bone Joint Surg Br.* 1951 May;33B(2):244–7. PMID: 14832324.

16. Funk DA, Wood MB. Concurrent fractures of the ipsilateral scaphoid and radial head. Report of four cases. *J Bone Joint Surg Am.* 1988 Jan;70(1):134–6. PMID: 3335563.

Fractures and dislocations of the elbow and arm

Catherine Maldjian, M.D., and Felix S. Chew, M.D.

Case 5–1   Radial neck fracture

(A)

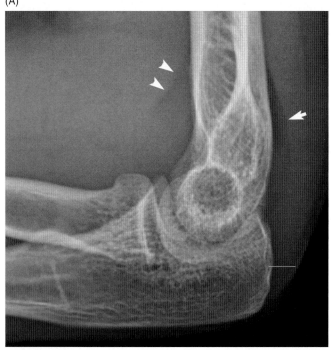

(B)

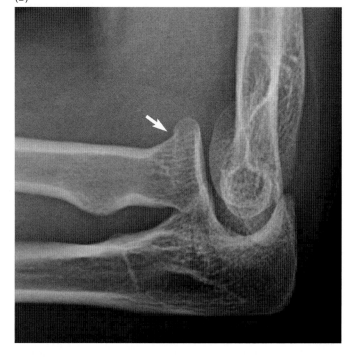

(C)

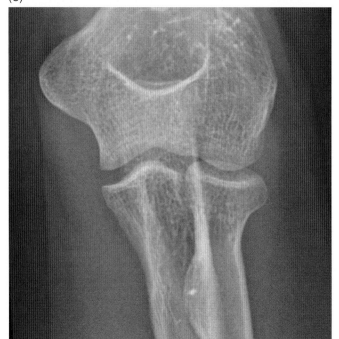

31-year-old woman injured in a fall on an outstretched hand. Lateral (A), radial head-capitellum view (B), and AP (C) radiographs of the left elbow. The lateral view demonstrates a posterior fat pad sign (short arrow) and an anterior fat pad sign (spinnaker sail sign) (arrowheads). The radial head-capitellum view shows a minimally impacted fracture of the radial neck (long arrow). The anterior and posterior fat pads are displaced away from the humerus when an elbow joint effusion is present, an indirect sign of fracture. The presence of either fat pad sign should raise suspicion for fracture; oblique views or even cross-sectional imaging may be required to identify the fracture. One study of adults who had radiographs showing only a fat pad sign but no fracture following elbow trauma found that 75% of the adults had a fracture that could be subsequently demonstrated on MRI [1].

Case 5–2 Radial head fracture

(A)

(B)

(C)

(D)

39-year-old woman who fell backward onto her arm. AP (E), lateral (F), radial head (C), and radial head-capitellum (D) radiographs of the left elbow. A single fracture line is present through the radial head (arrow), with no displacement, seen only on the radial head and capitellar views. There is an elbow effusion, indicated by anterior (arrow) and posterior (arrowhead) fat pad signs on the lateral view. The radial head-capitellum view is a lateral view with 45 degrees cephalad angulation, and displays the capitellum and radial head,

projecting it away from the ulna. Radial head (and neck) fractures may be categorized according to the Mason classification [2–3]: Type I is non-displaced head fracture (or minimally impacted neck fracture); Type II is a displaced fracture of the margin of the head (or an impacted, angulated, or depressed neck fracture); Type III is a comminuted fracture of the entire head; and Type IV is a head or neck fracture that is associated with elbow dislocation.

(E)

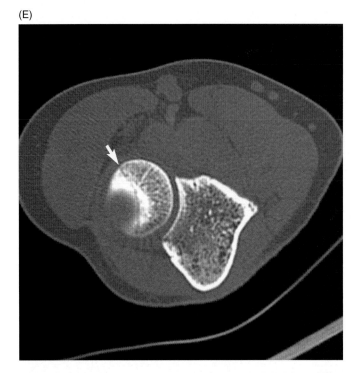

(F)

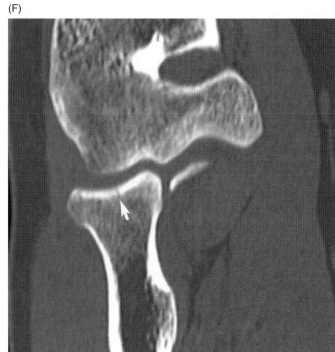

Axial (E) and coronal (F) CT of the left elbow. The axial image shows the minimally displaced fracture. The coronal view confirms that there is no offset in the articular surface. This is a

Mason Type I fracture (non-displaced radial head or neck fracture). Radial head and neck fractures are the most frequent adult injuries to the elbow and constitute 50% of elbow injuries [2–3].

Case 5–3   Radial head fracture

(A)

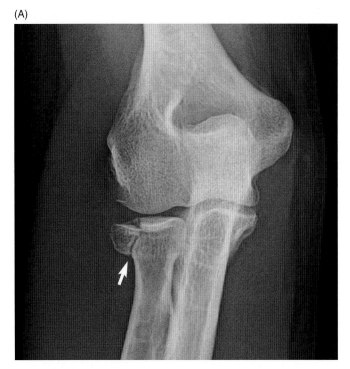

(B)

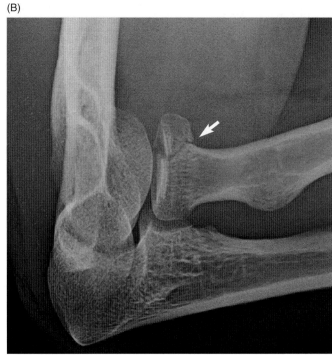

44-year-old man injured in bicycle crash. AP (A) and radial head-capitellum (B) radiographs of the right elbow. There is a mildly depressed fracture of the margin of the radial head,

involving approximately 25% of the articular surface. This is a Mason Type II fracture (marginal radial head fracture with displacement).

Case 5–4
Olecranon fracture

(A)

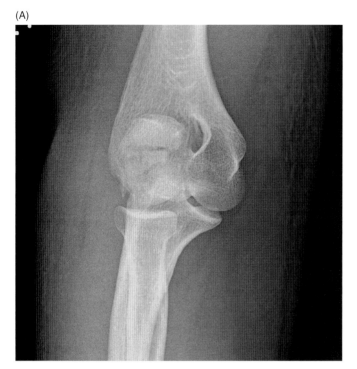

(B)

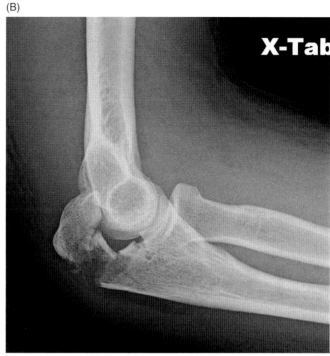

32-year-old man who fell from a two-story height. AP (A) and lateral (B) radiographs of the right elbow. There is a comminuted olecranon fracture with proximal retraction by the triceps mechanism. Inability to extend the elbow occurs with olecranon fractures and may result in suboptimal AP radiographs. Most olecranon fractures are transverse and occur at the trochlear notch [4]. Olecranon fractures are the second most common injury in the adult after proximal radial fractures and are responsible for 20% of elbow injuries. Olecranon fractures may be categorized according to the Mayo classification: Type I is non-displaced (subtype I-A is non-comminuted, subtype I-B is comminuted); Type II is displaced-stable (subtype II-A is non-comminuted, subtype II-B is comminuted); Type III is unstable (subtype III-A is non-comminuted, subtype III-B is comminuted). This fracture would be Mayo Type II-B, stable comminuted.

Case 5–5

Posterior elbow dislocation

(A)

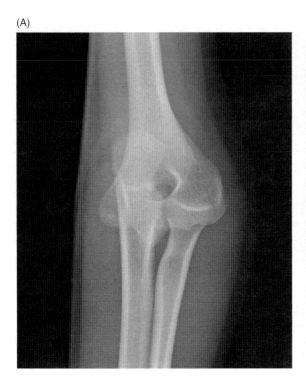

(B)

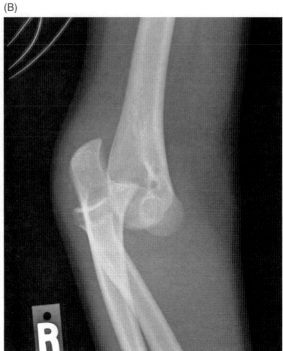

18-year-old woman injured in a fall from a 25-foot forest watch tower. AP (A) and lateral (B) radiographs of the right elbow. There is posterior elbow dislocation. Elbow dislocation generally refers to dislocation of the ulna from the humerus. Most elbow dislocations (80–90%) are posterior or posterolateral. The radius and ulna typically dislocate from the humerus together in the same direction. Elbow dislocations may be classified as simple (no fracture) or complex (associated with fracture), and as to the direction of the displacement of the ulna relative to the humerus (posterior, posterolateral, posteromedial, lateral, medial, or anterior). This case is a simple posterior elbow dislocation.

Case 5–6

Complex posterior elbow dislocation

(A)

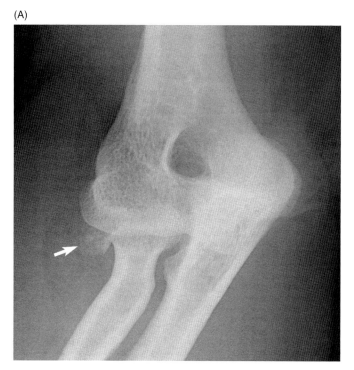

(B)

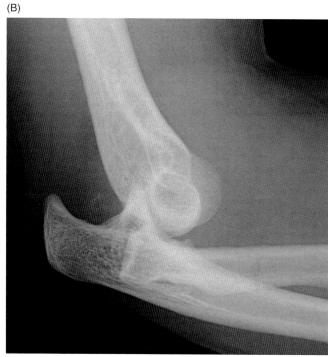

40-year-old woman injured in a ground-level fall. AP (A) and lateral (B) radiographs of the right elbow. There is a posterior dislocation with a displaced fracture of the radial head. The radial head fragment is dislocated and displaced laterally (arrow). Small bone fragments are present in the olecranon notch. Nearly half of elbow dislocations occur in conjunction with fractures, including the distal humerus, the proximal radius, and the proximal ulna. The radial head fracture in the case presented here is a Mason Type IV.

Case 5–7

Trans-olecranon anterior elbow fracture-dislocation

(A)

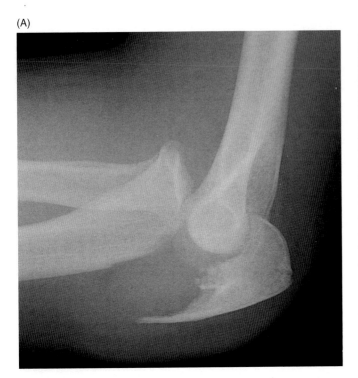

(B)

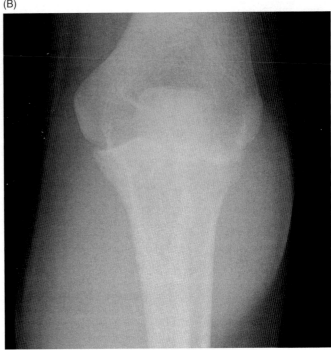

(C)

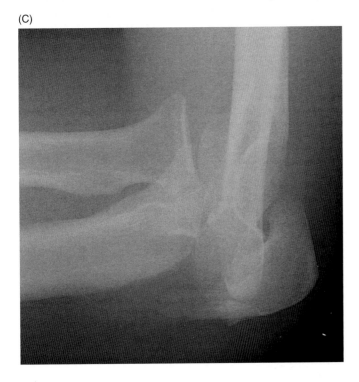

16-year-old male who was struck by a car as a pedestrian. Lateral (A), AP (B), and radial head-capitellum (C) radiographs of the left elbow. There is an oblique fracture through the olecranon with anterior dislocation of the radius and distal ulna as a unit, leaving the proximal olecranon fragment still articulating with the trochlea. Soft tissue swelling over the olecranon is present. This is a trans-olecranon anterior fracture-dislocation of the elbow. The olecranon fracture could be classified as Mayo III-A, unstable non-comminuted. It resembles the Monteggia fracture-dislocation in mechanism, but unlike the Monteggia injury, this ulnar fracture involves the olecranon rather than the proximal ulnar shaft and the proximal radioulnar joint remains intact rather than dislocating.

Case 5–8   Elbow fracture-dislocation

(A)

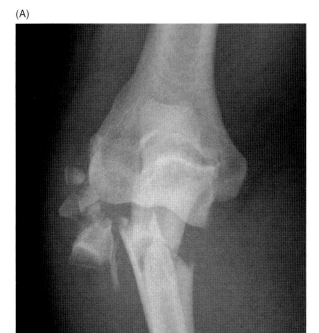

(B)

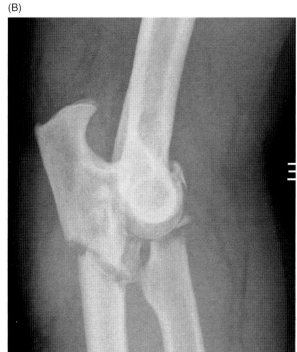

58-year-old man who fell off a ladder. AP (A) and lateral (B) radiographs of the right elbow. There is a severe elbow injury consisting of a fracture of the proximal ulnar shaft, highly comminuted and displaced fracture-dislocation of the proximal radius, and posterior dislocation of the proximal ulnar fragment. Reconstruction is likely to involve a radial head replacement [5], and heterotopic ossification of the injured soft tissues is a common complication.

Case 5–9   Capitellum fracture

(A)

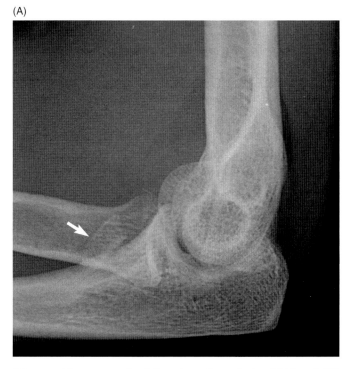

(B)

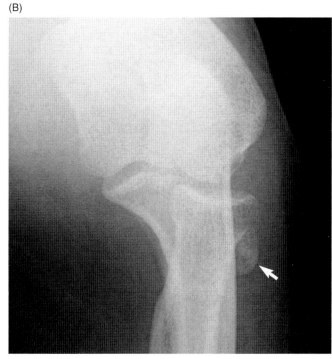

36-year-old woman who fell on her elbow. Lateral (A) and AP (B) radiographs of the left elbow. There is a joint effusion and displaced capitellum fracture. Shearing forces from radial head or lateral trochlear groove may produce this fracture pattern. Distal humerus fractures are relatively uncommon in adults, seen most frequently in young men and the elderly.

Case 5–10
Capitellum fracture

(A)

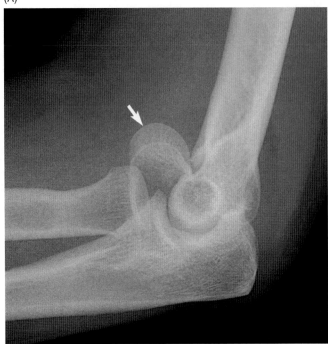

(B)

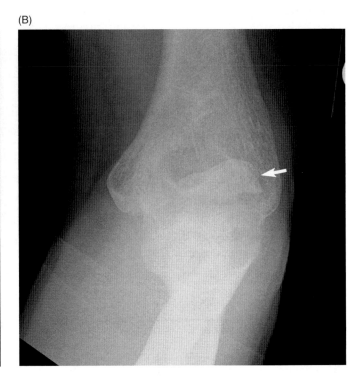

45-year-old woman in a bicycle accident. Lateral (A) and AP (B) radiographs of the left elbow. There is a large joint effusion and a displaced capitellum fracture. The fragment (arrow) typically lies above the radial head, as seen here. Rotation of the fragment may occur. Lateral projections are essential as the frontal view may not show this fracture well.

(C)

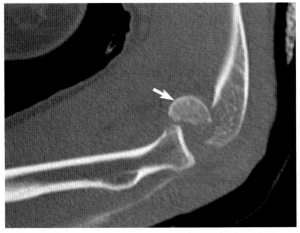

Sagittal CT of the left elbow through the radiocapitellar joint. The capitellum fragment includes the articular surface. The fragment is displaced, rotated 90 degrees, and anteriorly dislocated, relative to the radial head. Less commonly, the capitellum fragment may be displaced laterally or posteriorly [6]. Most capitellum fractures have complex involvement of the articular surfaces of not only the capitellum itself but also the trochlea [7].

Case 5–11

Intercondylar distal humerus fracture

(A)

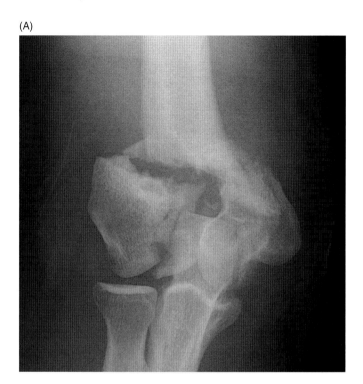

(B)

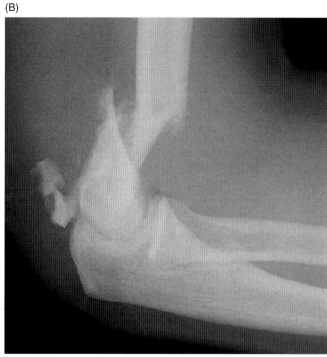

62-year-old man who fell from roof. AP (A) and lateral (B) radiographs of the right elbow. There is a T-shaped distal humerus fracture. The mechanism of injury is falling on a flexed elbow. The articular part of the fracture typically lies between the trochlear groove and the capitellotrochlear sulcus. This fracture then extends into horizontal (T) or oblique (Y) components into the condyles, which are displaced by their respective muscle attachments. Distal humerus fractures have been divided into three groups according to the OTA/AO system, which is one of many imperfect classification systems [8]. Type A fractures are extra-articular; Type B fractures are intra-articular and unicondylar (partial articular); and Type C fractures are intra-articular and bicondylar (complete articular). Type A fractures are subdivided into A1, which is medial epicondylar, A2, which is supracondylar, and A3, which is comminuted supracondylar. Type B fractures are subdivided into B1, which is lateral condylar, B2, which is medial condylar, and B3, which is capitellar. Type C fractures are subdivided into C1, which is Y- or T-shaped intercondylar, C2, which is intercondylar with a distal shaft comminution, and C3, which is intercondylar with comminution of the articular surfaces [9].

Case 5–12

Transcondylar humerus fracture

(A)

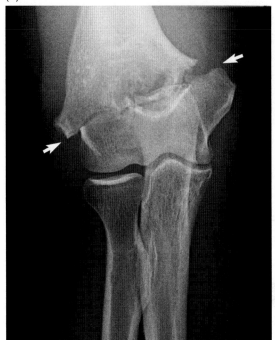

(B)

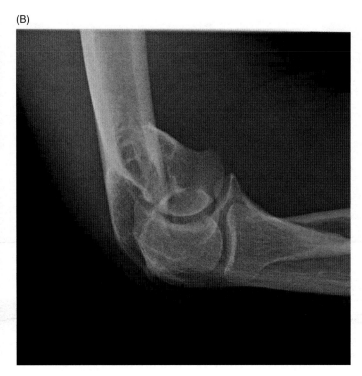

55-year-old man injured when he hit a pole while riding his bicycle. AP (A) and lateral (B) radiographs of the right elbow. There is a fracture (arrows) that extends transversely across the distal humerus at the level of the condyles. The condyles and olecranon fossa are disrupted, but the fracture does not extend distally to separate the condyles from each other or involve the articular surfaces. These are the uncommon adult counterparts of supracondylar fractures in children. Non-displaced fractures are treated with immobilization and displaced fractures are treated with open reduction and internal fixation [10].

Case 5–13
Humeral shaft fracture

(A)

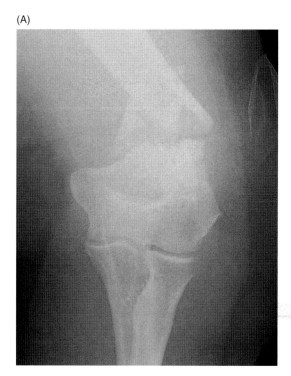

(B)

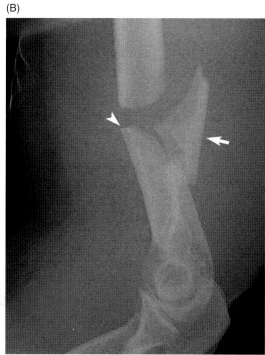

50-year-old woman injured in motorcycle crash. AP (A) and lateral (B) radiographs of the left elbow. There is a transverse distal humeral fracture (arrowhead) with a posterior butterfly fragment (arrow). The transverse with butterfly fragment fracture pattern can be reproduced by bending the bone. Bending produces tensile stress on the convex side of the bend, leading to a transverse fracture. At the same time, bending produces compressive stress on the concave side of the bend, leading to oblique fractures. These all meet in the center, producing the transverse fracture and the butterfly fragment. The butterfly fragment is produced by two oblique fractures converging and will always be on the concave side of the bend.

Case 5–14
Humeral shaft fracture

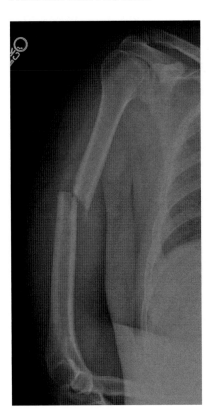

33-year-old man who fell on the dock while attempting to board his boat. AP radiograph of the right humerus. There is a transverse mid-humeral shaft fracture with apex posterior and lateral. Most humeral fractures are transverse or spiral and most involve the middle third of the shaft as seen in this case. Mechanisms of injury include direct blow, fall, motor vehicle crash, and torsional stress from athletic activities. Up to 17% of these patients may also sustain radial nerve injuries, which may manifest clinically as wrist drop [11]. Fractures causing separation of the humeral shaft proximal to the deltoid tuberosity result in medial displacement of the proximal fragment by the pectoralis muscles, but separation distal to the deltoid tuberosity leads to abduction of the proximal fragment by the deltoid muscle, as seen here. Humeral shaft fractures are usually treated with a hanging cast or external brace. Because of the normal high degree of mobility of the ball-and-socket glenohumeral joint, rotational and angular deformities from fractures of the humerus are better tolerated than similar deformities about joints with more constrained motion.

Case 5–15
Humeral shaft fracture

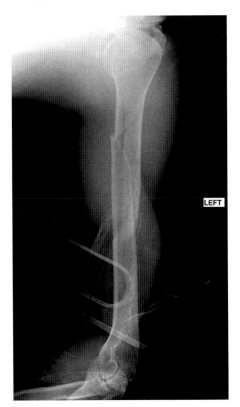

70-year-old woman who sustained a ground-level fall. AP radiograph of the left humerus. There is a spiral fracture of the humeral shaft with minimal displacement. Spiral fractures are caused by loading under torsion (twisting). The fracture line extends around the entire circumference of the bone in a spiral with a straight component connecting the two ends. Spiral fractures may be left-handed or right-handed, depending on the direction of the spiral.

Case 5–16
Open distal humerus fracture-dislocation with extrusion

(A)

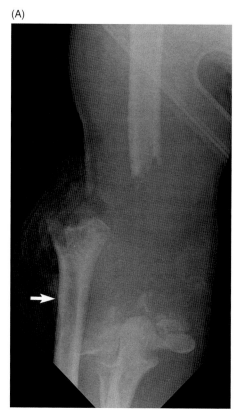

(B)

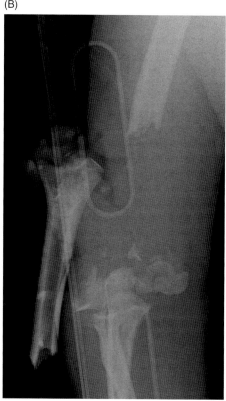

19-year-old man whose car crashed into a tree. AP radiographs of the right humerus (A) and elbow (B). There is an open humeral fracture with a segment of the bone (arrow) extruded beyond the soft tissues onto the surface of the body. There is severe comminution of the distal humerus. This is a high energy injury and requires surgical treatment. Nerve palsies are more common [12]. Wound treatment includes debridement, irrigation, and prophylactic IV antibiotic therapy. Distal humeral defects may be treated with bone graft, such as from the fibula [13]. Amputation may be required.

Case 5–17

Surgical neck of humerus fracture

(A)

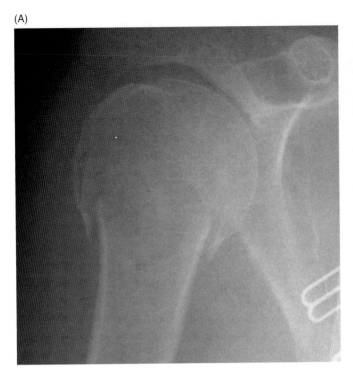

(B)

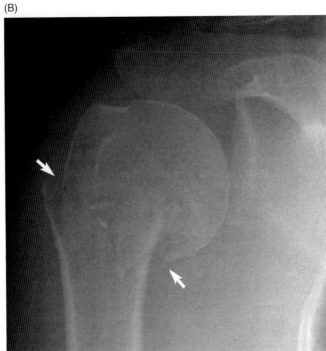

54-year-old woman with a ground-level fall while playing soccer, falling onto her elbow. Internal (A) and external (B) rotation radiographs of the right shoulder. There is a surgical neck fracture (arrows) with medial impaction, comminution, and displacement. The surgical neck is the portion of the proximal humerus that extends transversely across the metaphysis just inferior to the humeral head and separating it from the shaft. The anatomic neck is more vertical in orientation and separates the articular surface of the humeral head from the greater and lesser tuberosities. These four parts are used in the Neer classification, in which each part is evaluated for fracture, displacement, and angulation. In the Neer classification, one-part fractures are minimally displaced, regardless of comminution. Surgical neck fractures are the most commonly encountered fractures of the humerus, the vast majority of which are minimally displaced or angulated, or one-part Neer fractures [14].

Case 5–18

Surgical neck of humerus fracture

(A)

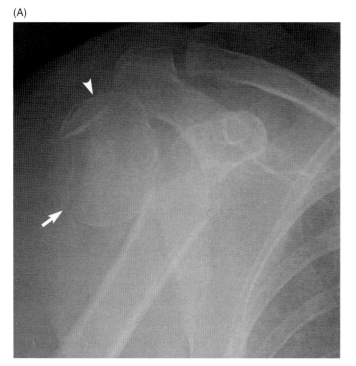

(B)

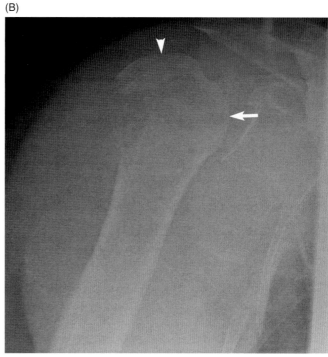

(C)

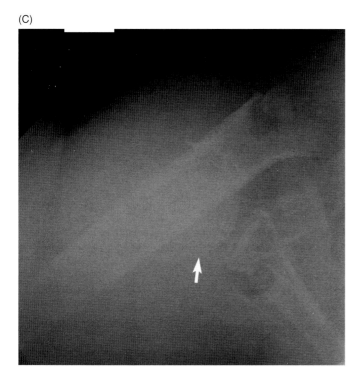

63-year-old woman who was a pedestrian struck by a car from behind, ending up on the hood and roof of the car. AP (A), Grashey (B), and axillary (C) radiographs of the right shoulder. A widely displaced fracture of the surgical neck is present, with separate, displaced humeral head (arrow) and greater tuberosity (arrowhead) fragments. Including the humeral shaft, this could then be called a Neer three-part fracture. The humeral shaft is anteromedially displaced, which is the most common direction of displacement with these fractures. CT may be useful to identify all the fragments and delineate their spatial relationships with each other.

Case 5–19   Glenohumeral fracture-dislocation

(A)

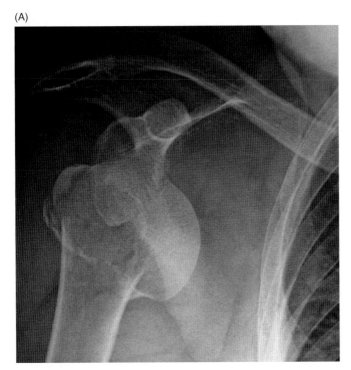

(B)

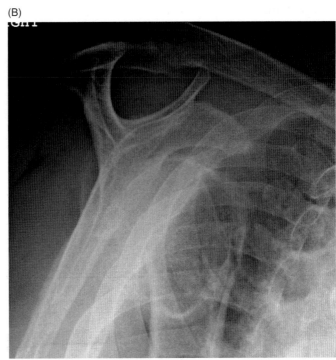

53-year-old man who stumbled and fell down the stairs carrying an old, heavy television set. AP (A) and Y-view (B) radiographs of the right shoulder. There are comminuted humeral head and surgical neck fractures with anterior dislocation of the major humeral head fragment.

(C)   (D)   (E)

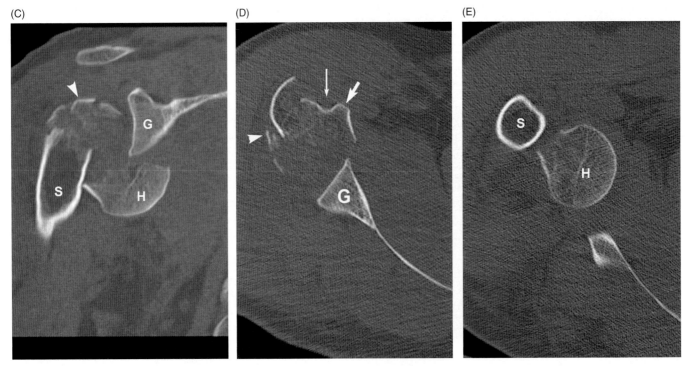

Multiplanar CT of the right shoulder. (C) The coronal CT shows a comminuted surgical neck and humeral head fracture with inferior dislocation of the major head (H) fragment. There is a comminuted greater tuberosity fragment (arrowhead). (D) Axial CT at the level of the glenoid (G) shows absence of an articulating humeral head, and comminution of the proximal humerus with greater tuberosity fragments (arrowhead) and a lesser tuberosity fragment (arrow) that includes the bicipetal groove (long arrow). (E) Axial CT below the glenoid shows the humeral head fragment (H) and the humeral shaft (S), side-by-side.

Case 5–20
Bony humeral avulsion of the glenohumeral ligaments (BHAGL)

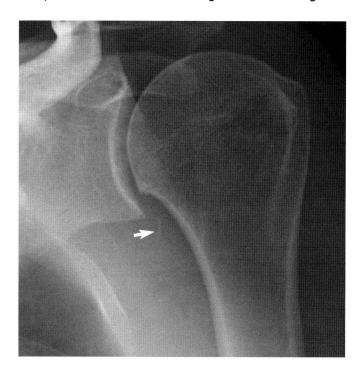

39-year-old woman with repeated left shoulder dislocations. AP radiograph of the left shoulder. The shoulder is normally located. There is a thin fragment of bone (arrow) at the inferior glenohumeral joint consistent with a bony humeral avulsion of the glenohumeral ligaments (BHAGL lesion). This lesion may be associated with muitidirectional glenohumeral instability [15]. More common than the BHAGL is the soft tissue counterpart, the humeral avulsion of the glenohumeral ligaments (HAGL).

Case 5–21
Greater tuberosity of the humerus fracture

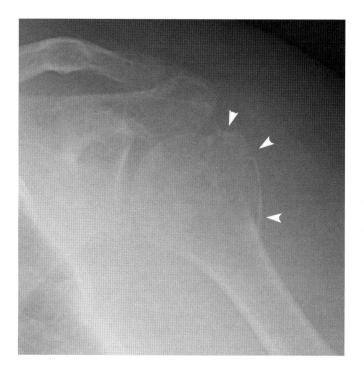

63-year-old woman injured in a ground-level fall. Previous dual energy x-ray absorptiometry (DXA) showed osteoporosis. Grashey view of the left shoulder. There is a minimally displaced, comminuted fracture of the greater tuberosity (arrowheads). Greater tuberosity fractures usually occur in conjunction with surgical neck fractures, and isolated greater tuberosity fractures are relatively uncommon. The fracture seen here is an eggshell type non-displaced greater tuberosity fracture. Surrounding supporting structures including periosteum, tendinous, and joint capsule maintain the fracture fragment in near-anatomic alignment. Anterior dislocations may be associated with greater tuberosity fractures in approximately 15% of cases. Lesser tuberosity fractures occur at a similar rate with posterior dislocation. Displaced tuberosity fractures imply that the rotator cuff is injured and typically leads to open reduction, internal fixation, and cuff repair.

Case 5–22
Greater tuberosity of the humerus fracture

(A)

(B)

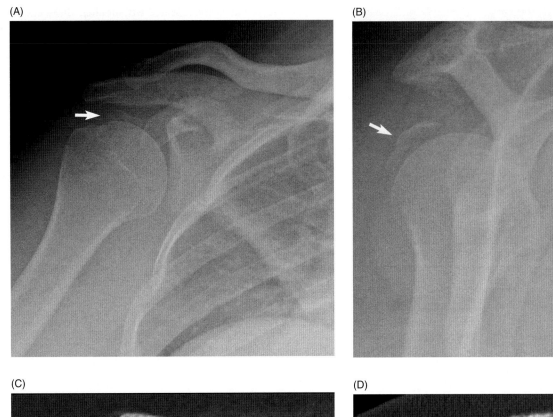

(C)

(D)

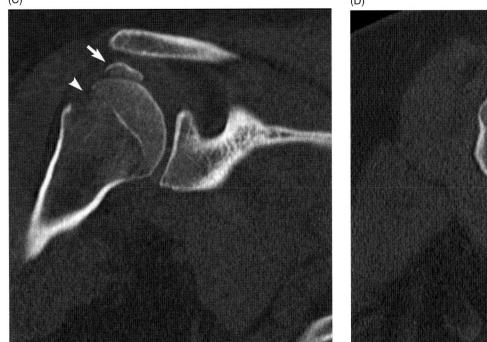

48-year-old woman with ground-level fall. AP (A) and Y-view (B) radiographs and CT of the right shoulder, oblique coronal (C), and oblique sagittal (D). There is a greater tuberosity avulsion fracture at the insertion of the supraspinatus tendon. The fragment of bone (arrows) is superiorly displaced and proximally retracted by the supraspinatus. The CT scan shows the donor site of the fracture (arrowhead). Displaced greater tuberosity fractures imply a longitudinal rotator cuff tear. Labral tears may also be associated.

Case 5–23
Lesser tuberosity of the humerus fracture

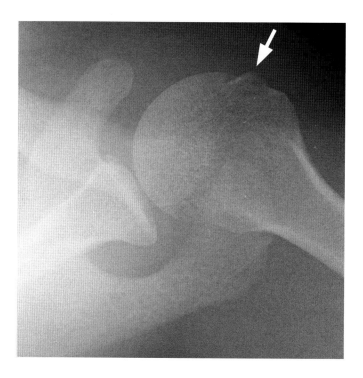

23-year-old man in motor vehicle crash. Axillary radiograph of the left shoulder. Lesser tuberosity avulsion fracture (arrow) at the site of the subscapularis tendon. There is no significant displacement and this fracture was treated conservatively. This is a rare injury and when the fragment is small may be seen only on the axillary view, as in this case, or on CT. External force when positioned at 60 degrees abduction and maximal external rotation is the described mechanism [16]. Lesser tuberosity fractures may also be associated with posterior glenohumeral dislocation [17].

References

1. O'Dwyer H, O'Sullivan P, Fitzgerald D, Lee MJ, McGrath F, Logan PM. The fat pad sign following elbow trauma in adults: Its usefulness and reliability in suspecting occult fracture. *J Comput Assist Tomogr.* 2004 Jul–Aug;28(4):562–5. PMID: 15232392.

2. Ruchelsman DE, Christoforou D, Jupiter JB. Fractures of the radial head and neck. *J Bone Joint Surg Am.* 2013 Mar 6;95(5):469–78. doi: 10.2106/JBJS.J.01989. PMID: 23467871.

3. Duckworth AD, McQueen MM, Ring D. Fractures of the radial head. *Bone Joint J.* 2013 Feb;95-B(2):151–9. doi: 10.1302/0301-620X.95B2. 29877. PMID: 23365021.

4. Kiviluoto O, Santavirta S. Fractures of the olecranon. Analysis of 37 consecutive cases. *Acta Orthop Scand.* 1978 Feb;49(1):28–31. PMID: 654892.

5. Fowler JR, Goitz RJ. Radial head fractures: Indications and outcomes for radial head arthroplasty. *Orthop Clin North Am.* 2013 Jul;44(3):425–31, x. doi: 10.1016/j. ocl.2013.03.013. Epub 2013 Apr 17. PMID: 23827844.

6. Lindem MC. Fractures of the capitellum and trochlea. *Ann Surg* 1922 July; 76(1): 78–82. PMCID: PMC1400075. PMID: 17864670.

7. Guitton TG, Doornberg JN, Raaymakers EL, Ring D, Kloen P. Fractures of the capitellum and trochlea. *J Bone Joint Surg Am.* 2009 Feb;91(2):390–7. PMID: 19181983.

8. Henley MB. Intra-articular distal humeral fractures in adults. *Orthop Clin North Am.* 1987 Jan;18(1):11–23. PMID: 3796956.

9. Nauth A, McKee MD, Ristevski B, Hall J, Schemitsch EH. Distal humeral fractures in adults. *J Bone Joint Surg Am.*

2011 Apr 6;93(7):686-700. doi: 10.2106/JBJS.J.00845. PMID: 21471423.

10. Perry CR, Gibson CT, Kowalski MF. Transcondylar fractures of the distal humerus. *J Orthop Trauma.* 1989;3(2):98–106. PMID: 2661784.

11. Mast JW, Spiegel PG, Harvey JP Jr, Harrison C. Fractures of the humeral shaft. A retrospective study of 240 adult fractures. *Clin Orthop Relat Res.* 1975 Oct;(112):254–62. PMID: 1192642.

12. Marsh JL, Mahoney CR, Steinbronn D. External fixation of open humerus fractures. *Iowa Orthop J.* 1999;19:35–42. PMCID: PMC1888611 PMID: 10847515.

13. Kouvidis GK, Chalidis BE, Liddington MI, Giannoudis PV. Reconstruction of a severe open distal humerus fracture with complete loss of medial column by using a free fibular osteocutaneous graft.

Eplasty. 2008 Apr 29;8:e24. PMCID: PMC2374498; PMID: 18509480.

14. Sandstrom CK, Kennedy SA, Gross JA. Acute shoulder trauma: What the surgeon wants to know. *Radiographics.* 2015 Mar–Apr;35(2):475–92. doi: 10.1148/rg.352140113. PMID: 25763730.

15. Oberlander MA, Morgan BE, Visotsky JL. The BHAGL lesion: A new variant of anterior shoulder instability. *Arthroscopy.* 1996 Oct;12(5):627–33. PMID: 8902140.

16. Ross GJ, Love MB. Isolated avulsion fracture of the lesser tuberosity of the humerus: Report of two cases. *Radiology.* 1989 Sep;172(3):833–4. PMID: 2772197.

17. Pace A, Ribbans W, Kim JH. Isolated lesser tuberosity fracture of the humerus. *Orthopedics.* 2008 Jan;31(1):94. PMID: 19292144.

Fractures and dislocations of the shoulder and thoracic cage

Felix S. Chew, M.D., Catherine Maldjian, M.D., and Eira Roth, M.D.

Case 6–1
Anterior shoulder dislocation

(A)

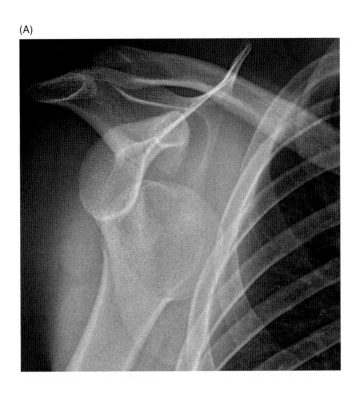

(B)

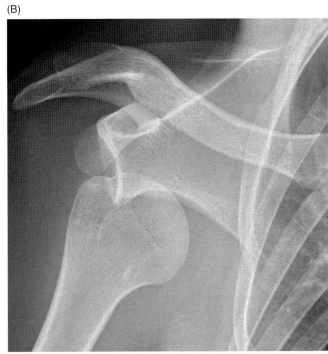

20-year-old man who fell off his longboard while going downhill, reportedly at 20 MPH, landing on his right shoulder and buttocks. AP (A) and Grashey (B) radiographs of the right shoulder. The AP radiographs show that the humeral head is dislocated and projects in a subcoracoid location. The glenoid fossa is empty. The Grashey view, a 45-degree oblique view that shows the glenoid articular surface in profile, shows that the inferior margin of the glenoid overlies the superolateral portion of the humeral articular surface.

(C)

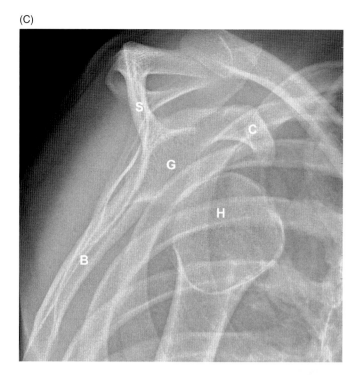

(D)

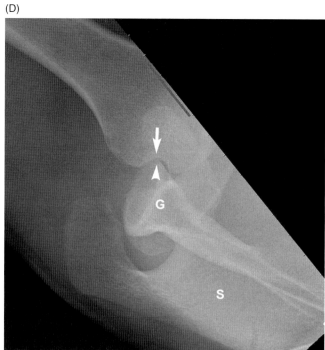

Y-view (C) and axillary (D) lateral radiographs of the right shoulder. The Y-view, a lateral view of the scapula that projects the scapular body (B) in profile with the scapular spine (S) and the coracoid process (C) providing the limbs of the Y, shows that the humeral head (H) is located anterior and inferior to the glenoid process (G). The axillary lateral view shows the anterior location of the humeral head, and impaction of the anterior bony margin of the glenoid rim (arrowhead) into the humeral head, causing an impaction fracture.

Case 6–2
Anterior shoulder dislocation with coracoid fracture

(A)

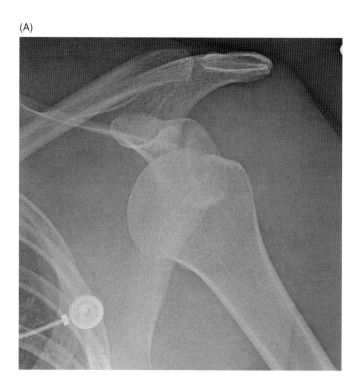

(B)

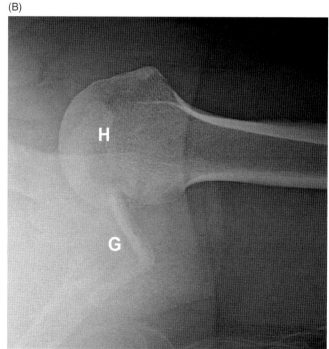

18-year-old man in motor vehicle crash. AP (A) and axillary (B) lateral radiographs of the left shoulder. The humeral head has dislocated from the glenoid fossa into a subcoracoid position on the AP radiograph. The axillary lateral shows that the head (H) is anterior to the glenoid process (G), and that the glenoid is impacted into the head. Approximately 95% of shoulder dislocations occur anteriorly, with the head in a subcoracoid position, as in this case. External rotation and abduction is the common mechanism.

(C)

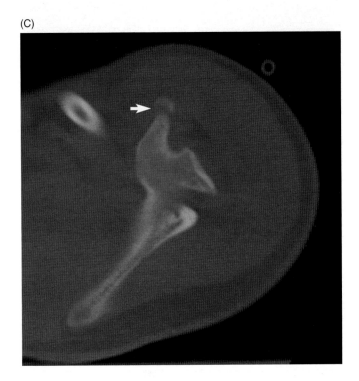

(D)

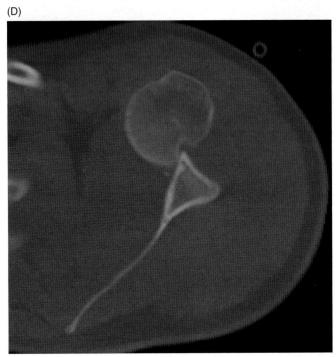

Axial CT of the left shoulder, superior (C) to inferior (D). Axial CT through the level of the coracoid shows a mildly displaced avulsion fracture of the tip of the coracoid process (arrow) and an empty glenoid fossa. CT at a slightly inferior level shows the anteriorly dislocated humeral head and the impaction of the anterior margin of the glenoid into the humeral head. This is a Hill-Sachs lesion, the compression fracture of the humeral head that was described by Hill and Sachs [1]. This occurs in more than 50% of anterior dislocations.

Case 6–3

Anterior shoulder dislocation

(A)

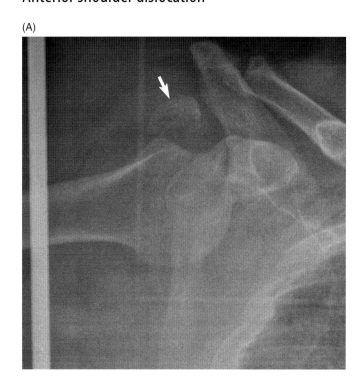

61-year-old man in high-speed rollover motor vehicle crash. AP radiograph of the right shoulder. Initial trauma radiograph shows anterior dislocation of the glenohumeral joint. Greater tuberosity avulsion fracture (arrow) at the insertion of the supraspinatus is also present.

(B)

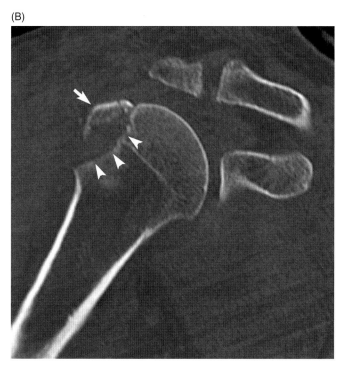

(C)

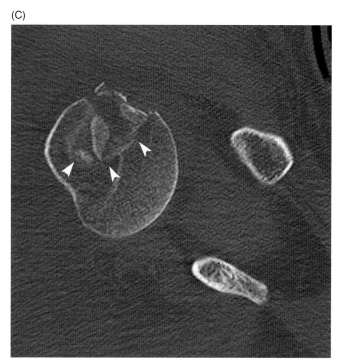

Coronal (B) and axial (C) CT of the right shoulder following closed reduction of the dislocation. The greater tuberosity fracture (arrow) involves the insertion of the supraspinatus tendon. There is a large, complex impaction fracture of the humeral head (arrowheads). Persistent pain after healed greater tuberosity fracture may be a sign of rotator cuff tear or labral injury, which are associated with greater tuberosity fractures. Isolated greater tuberosity fractures can occur in the setting of anterior dislocation, impaction injury with the acromion or superior glenoid [2]. Greater tuberosity fractures are seen in approximately 15% of anterior dislocations.

Case 6–4
Hill-sachs lesion

(A)

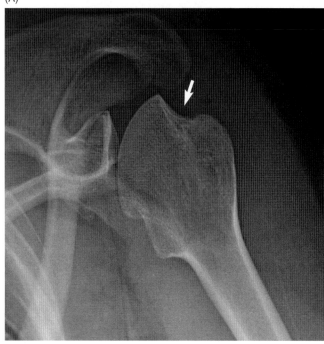

30-year-old man with intractable left shoulder instability and recurrent dislocations. Apical oblique radiograph of the left shoulder. Oblique radiograph of the shoulder shows a large depression (arrow) in the posterior humeral head, corresponding to an impaction fracture caused by repeated anterior shoulder dislocations. This depression is a Hill-Sachs lesion.

(B)

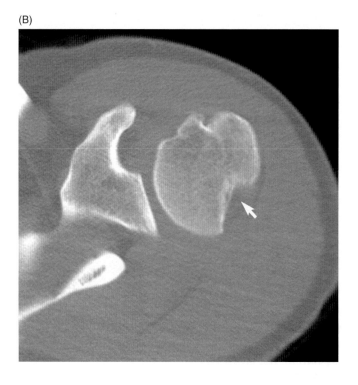

Axial CT of the left shoulder through the humeral head. There is a large defect (arrow) in the posterolateral humeral head. In the neutral position, as the patient was positioned for the CT scan, the Hill-Sachs lesion is safely in the posterolateral position away from the glenoid.

(C)

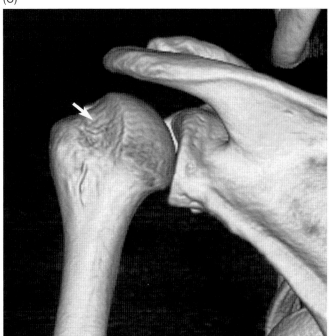

3D surface-rendered CT, posterior view of the left shoulder. The size of the Hill-Sachs lesion can be appreciated on the posterior surface-rendered view. With external rotation of the humerus, the defect is large enough that it may catch the anterior glenoid rim, resulting in anterior dislocation of the humeral head when it returns to neutral rotation.

Case 6–5

Bankart fracture

(A)

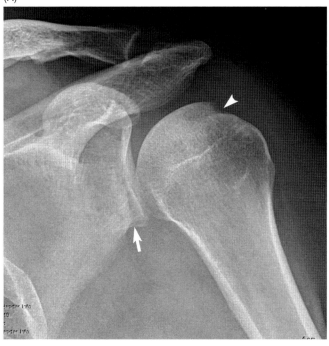

37-year-old man who landed on his left shoulder when he crashed his bicycle. He presents for follow-up after reduction of an anterior shoulder dislocation. AP radiograph of the left shoulder. A bony fragment of the anterior inferior portion of the glenoid rim (arrow) is displaced medially, parallel to the articular surface. There is also a Hill-Sachs lesion (arrowhead). Fractures of the inferior glenoid rim may be difficult to identify on radiographs and may require CT or MRI for diagnosis [3]. These fractures occur in 8% of anterior dislocations [4], and can predispose to instability and further episodes of dislocation [5].

(B)

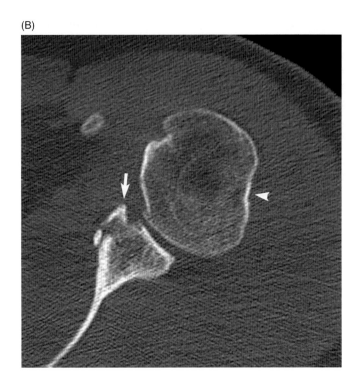

Axial CT of the left shoulder at the level of the inferior glenoid process. The glenoid fracture is comminuted and the major articular fragment (arrow) is mildly depressed from the articular surface. The Hill-Sachs lesion is evident as the flattening of the posterolateral side of the humeral head (arrowhead).

Case 6–6

Bankart fracture

(A)

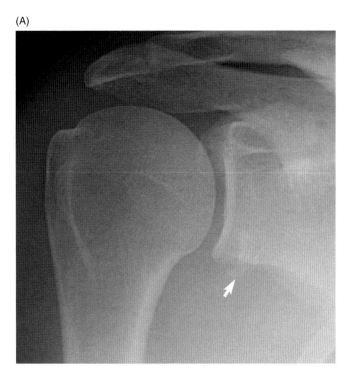

(B)

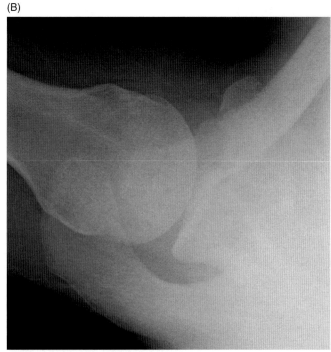

43-year-old man with previously reduced right anterior shoulder dislocation. Grashey (A) and axillary (B) lateral radiographs of the right shoulder. There is an osteochondral fragment (arrow) at the anterior inferior margin of the glenoid process. The fragment is difficult to see on the axillary lateral radiograph.

(C)

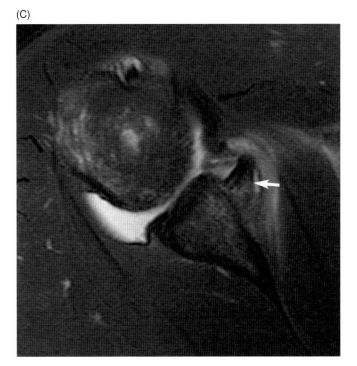

(D)

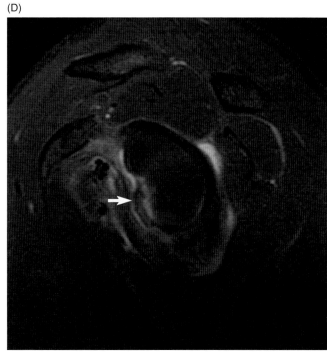

(E)

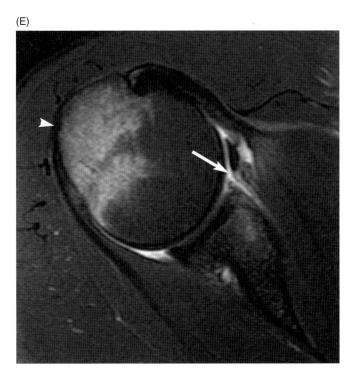

Multiplanar MRI of the right shoulder. (C) The axial MRI through the inferior glenoid shows a depressed fracture of the anterior-inferior glenoid rim (arrow). (D) The sagittal MRI shows that the fracture fragment involves the anterior-inferior quadrant of the glenoid process (arrow). (E) Axial MRI through the humeral head shows there is a bone bruise in the humeral head (arrowhead), which is the biomechanical equivalent of a Hill-Sachs lesion, but no actual depressed impaction fracture is present. An anterior labral tear (long arrow) extends superiorly from the fracture. This injury of the anterior-inferior glenoid-labral complex is called a Bankart lesion; when there is a fracture, it is called a bony Bankart lesion. An MRI is often necessary for accurate preoperative evaluation of both bony and non-bony Bankart lesions [6].

Case 6–7
Posterior shoulder dislocation

(A)

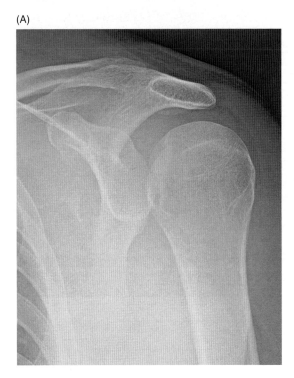

(B)

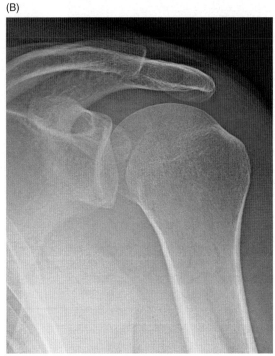

(C)

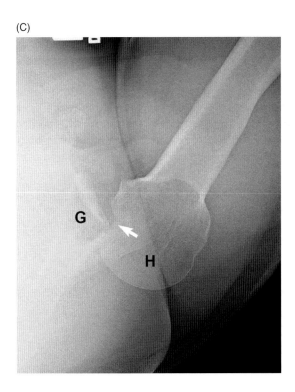

43-year-old man in motorcycle crash. Internal rotation (A), Grashey (B), and axillary lateral (C) radiographs of the left shoulder. On the AP view, the humerus is internally rotated. The AP view demonstrates loss of the normal half-moon overlap of the humeral head and glenoid. The articular surface of the humerus is not concentric with that of the glenoid process. The Grashey view, which is angled medio-laterally to obtain a true AP of the glenohumeral joint, should normally show no overlap between the glenoid process and the humeral head; in this case, some overlap is present. The axillary lateral shows the posterior displacement and impaction of the posterior bony rim of the glenoid process into the anterior aspect of the humeral head, resulting in an impaction fracture (arrow). Posterior shoulder dislocation is much less common than anterior shoulder dislocation. H=humeral head, G=glenoid process.

(D)

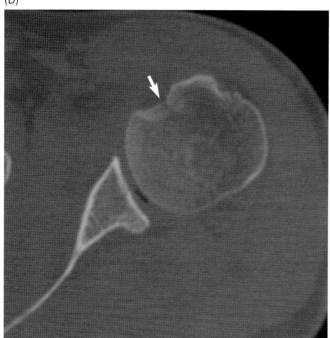

Axial CT of the left shoulder following reduction of the dislocation. There is an impaction fracture (arrow) along the anterior aspect of the humeral head, just medial to the lesser tuberosity. Because it is analogous to the Hill-Sachs lesion that occurs in anterior shoulder dislocation, this anterior humeral head impaction fracture may be called a reverse Hill-Sachs lesion or, when referring to the appearance on radiographs, a trough line [7]. The reverse Hill-Sachs lesion may be accompanied by a posterior glenoid rim fracture, sometimes called a reverse Bankart fracture.

Case 6–8
Reverse Hill-Sachs and reverse Bankart fractures

(A)

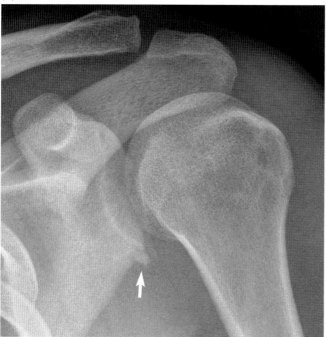

(B)

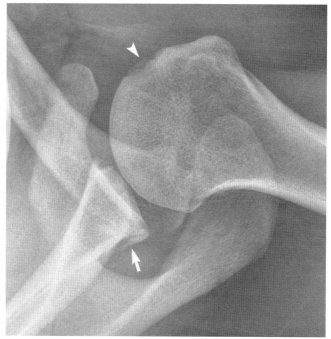

33-year-old woman with seizure disorder and recurrent posterior shoulder dislocations. AP (A) and axillary lateral (B) radiographs of the left shoulder. There are small bone fragments at the posterior-inferior margin of the glenoid process (arrows). The glenohumeral joint is normally located. There is an impaction fracture of the anterior humeral head (arrowhead).

Case 6–9
Posterior shoulder fracture-dislocation

(A)

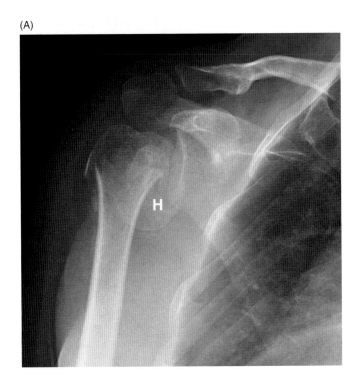

(B)

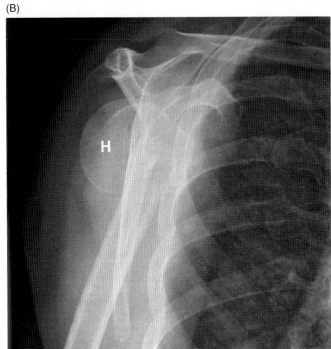

(C)

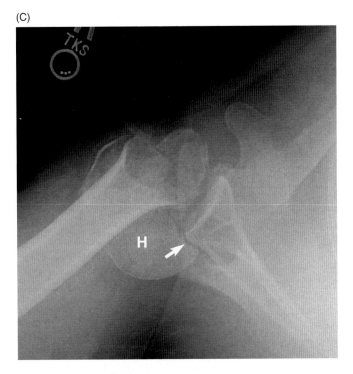

46-year-old man who fell off the top step of his porch, landing on his adducted shoulder. AP (A), Y-view (B), and axillary lateral (C) radiographs of the right shoulder. There is a displaced surgical neck fracture with greater tuberosity fragment and posterior dislocation of the humeral head (H). This is a posterior fracture-dislocation. There is an impaction fracture (arrow) at the anteromedial aspect of the humeral head (reverse Hill-Sachs lesion).

Case 6–10   Luxatio erecta

(A)

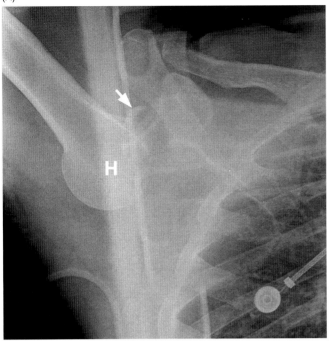

(B)

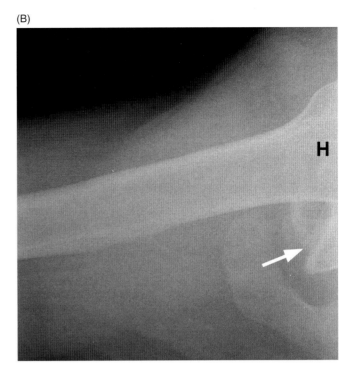

Adult with multiple blunt trauma. AP (A) and axillary lateral (B) radiographs of the right shoulder. The initial radiograph is a detail from a chest radiograph obtained on the trauma board, subsequently followed by AP and axillary views of the right shoulder. The arm is hyperabducted, and the humeral head

(H) is dislocated anteriorly and inferiorly. On the axillary view, the humeral head (H) may be seen anterior to the empty glenoid fossa (long arrow). This is a rare form of shoulder dislocation that is commonly associated with fractures of the greater tuberosity (short arrow) or tears of the rotator cuff [8].

Case 6–11   Luxatio erecta

(A)

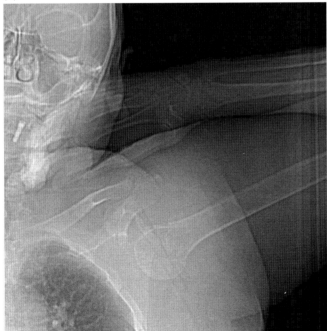

(B)

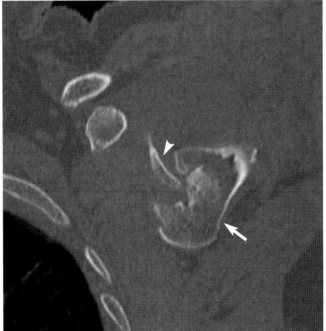

81-year-old woman injured in ground-level fall. CT of the left shoulder. (A) The scout image shows inferior dislocation of the humeral head with the arm elevated above the horizontal and the hand folded behind the neck. The patient was unable to

bring the arm down. (B) Coronal CT images shows the glenoid (arrowhead) deeply impacted into the humeral head (arrow), locking it into its dislocated position.

Case 6–12
Intrathoracic shoulder fracture-dislocation

(A)

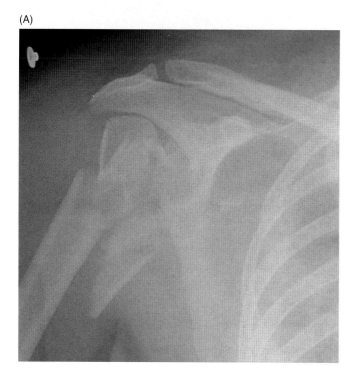

(B)

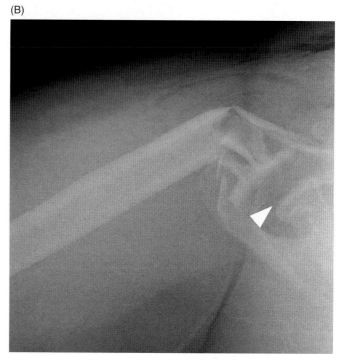

Woman injured in a fall while horseback riding. AP (A) and axillary lateral (B) radiographs of the right shoulder. There is a severely comminuted fracture of the proximal humerus. The glenoid fossa (arrowhead) is empty, indicative of dislocation of the humeral head, but the humeral head is not evident on these radiographs.

Detail of AP radiograph of the chest. The humeral head fragment (H) overlies the lateral margin of the right upper ribs.

(C)

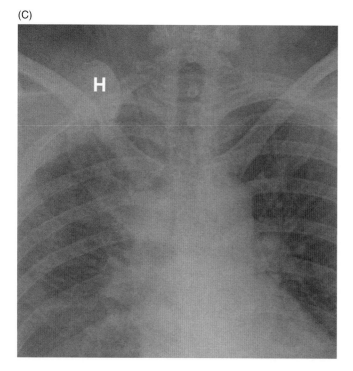

(D)

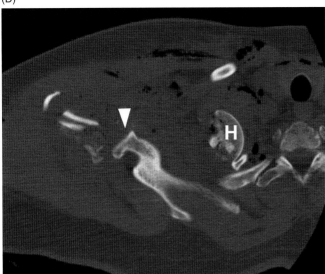

Axial CT of the right shoulder. The glenoid fossa is empty (arrowhead). The humeral head fragment (H) is displaced medially into the rib cage, posterior to the clavicle, anterior to the scapula. Gas may be seen dissecting through the soft tissues.

(E)

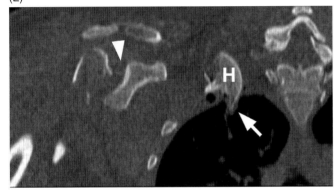

Coronal CT of the right shoulder. There is an empty glenoid fossa (arrowhead) and a medially displaced humeral head fragment (H). The humeral head fragment has pierced the pleura, and protrudes into the lung (arrow). Intrathoracic humeral head dislocation is an unusual phenomenon that requires immediate surgical attention [9–10].

113

Case 6–13

Acromioclavicular joint injury, Type I

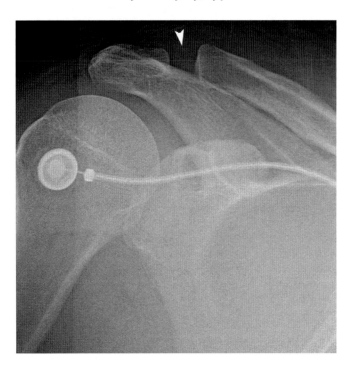

33-year-old man in a motor vehicle crash. AP radiograph of the right shoulder. The space between the acromion and the distal clavicle is abnormally wide (arrow), but there is no superior subluxation of the clavicle relative to the acromion. There are no fractures. The horizontal stability of the acromioclavicular (AC) joint is maintained by the AC ligaments that surround the joint capsule. A simple sprain of these ligaments allows the AC joint to widen. AC joint injuries (also called AC separations) may be classified into six types [11–12]. Type I corresponds to an isolated sprain of the AC ligament, and can be recognized radiographically as widening of the AC joint without vertical displacement from the acromion or the coracoid process. This case is an AC joint injury, Type I.

Case 6–14

Acromioclavicular joint injury, Type II

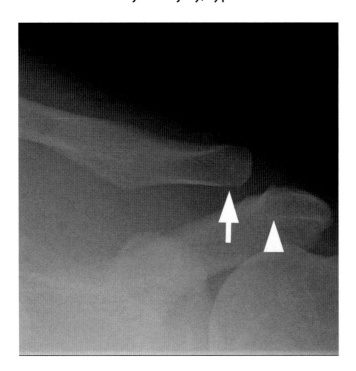

21-year-old man in motor vehicle crash. Standing AP radiograph of the left acromioclavicular (AC) joint. There is subluxation of the left AC joint. The inferior surface of the distal clavicle (arrow) is superior to the inferior surface of the acromion (arrowhead). These findings are indicative of AC separation, Type II. The vertical stability of the AC joint is maintained by the two coracoclavicular ligaments, the conoid ligament on the medial side and the trapezoid ligament on the lateral side. Sprain of the coracoclavicular ligaments combined with a tear of the AC ligaments allows the clavicle and the acromion to displace vertically. When the displacement is manifested on radiographs as subluxation of the AC joint, as in this case, it corresponds to an AC joint injury, Type II.

Case 6–15 Acromioclavicular joint injury, Type III

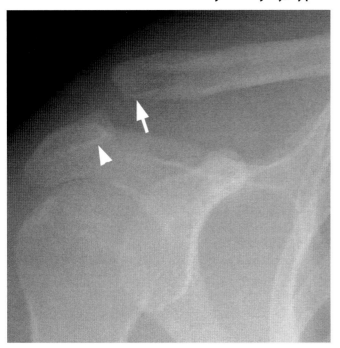

26-year-old man who injured his shoulder playing soccer. AP radiograph of the right shoulder. There is superior dislocation of the distal clavicle relative to the acromion by approximately one shaft width. The undersurface of the distal clavicle (arrow) should be aligned with the undersurface of the acromion (arrowhead). Complete tears of the coracoclavicular ligaments allow the clavicle to separate completely from the acromion, also widening the distance between the clavicle and coracoid. This corresponds with an AC joint injury, Type III.

Case 6–16 Acromioclavicular joint injury, Type IV

(A)

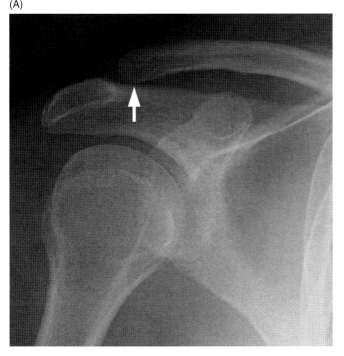

(B)

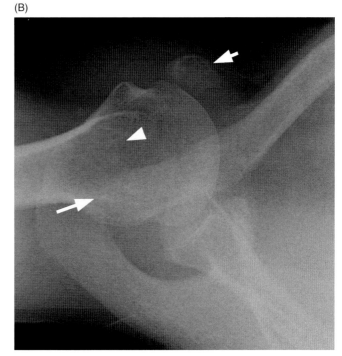

38-year-old man with multiple previous shoulder dislocations. Internal rotation (A) and axillary lateral (B) radiographs of the right shoulder. On the AP view, the AC joint appears subluxated, with mild elevation of the distal clavicle (arrow) relative to the acromion, suggesting an AC separation, Type II. However, on the axillary lateral view, the articular surface of the distal clavicle (long arrow) is posterior to the articular surface of the acromion (arrowhead), indicative of posterior AC separation. The distal clavicle displaces into or through the trapezius muscle. This AC joint injury is classified as Type IV. The tip of the coracoid process has also been avulsed (short arrow). The pectoralis minor, coracobrachialis, and short head of the biceps muscles attach to the tip of the coracoid; because the coracoclavicular ligaments attach closer to the base of the coracoid, the coracoid fracture is not part of the Type IV AC injury.

Case 6–17
Acromioclavicular joint injury, Type V

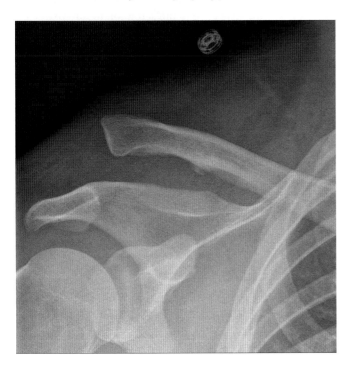

35-year-old man who crashed his motorcycle into a fire hydrant. AP radiograph of the right shoulder. There is right AC separation, with the distal clavicle located approximately three shaft widths above its anatomic position relative to the acromion. With this injury, AC joint injury, Type V, in addition to the tears of the AC and coracoclavicular ligaments, there is a disruption of the deltotrapezial fascia, allowing further displacement of the clavicle away from the acromion than on the Type III injury. Distinguishing Type III from Type V may be unreliable with imaging, as the AC joint is unstable and may change during the radiologic examination. There is also an AC joint injury, Type VI, that has been described, but only rarely seen, in which the clavicle is displaced below the acromion (subacromial supracoracoid dislocation) or below the coracoid (subcoracoid dislocation). This may occur in association with fractures of the ipsilateral clavicular shaft or other injuries [13].

Case 6–18
Distal clavicle fracture

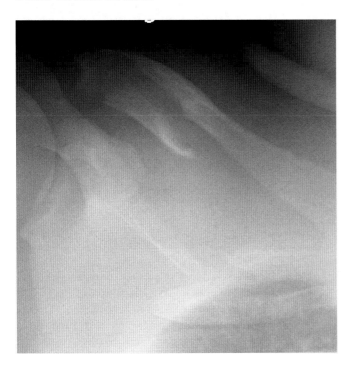

16-year-old male involved in high-speed rollover motor vehicle crash. 30-degree cephalic angulation AP radiograph of the right clavicle. There is an oblique distal clavicle fracture seen best on the angulated view. This view displaces the clavicle away from the ribs and affords improved visualization. 15% of clavicular fractures occur in the distal third. Middle third fractures are Class A, distal fractures are Class B, and medial third fractures are Class C. Class B fractures are subdivided into Type I (non-displaced), Type II (CC ligament tear with superior displacement of the proximal segment from the sternocleidomastoid, and Type III (articular fractures at the AC joint). Articular fractures of the distal clavicle may result in degenerative arthritis.

Case 6–19

Distal clavicle fracture

(A)

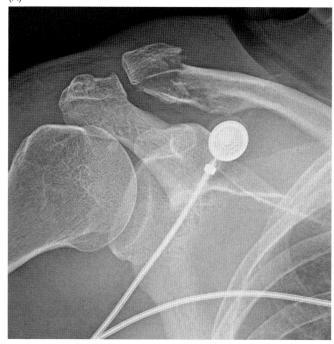

45-year-old woman struck by a car as a pedestrian. AP radiograph of the right shoulder. There is a comminuted fracture of the distal clavicle, with superior displacement of the distal fragment. The acromioclavicular joint is subluxated. There is an avulsion fragment of the inferior aspect of the distal shaft that corresponds with the attachments of the lateral coracoclavicular ligaments. The medial clavicular segment is not displaced and the coracoclavicular distance appears normal, suggesting the medial coracoclavicular ligaments are intact.

(B)

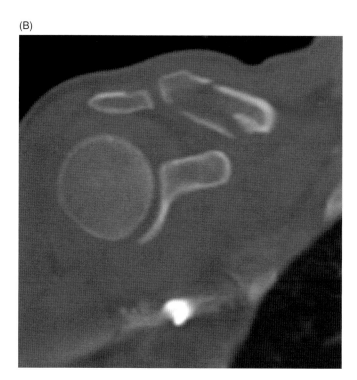

(C)

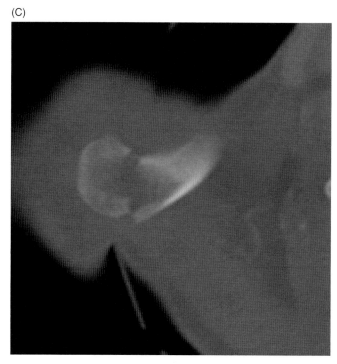

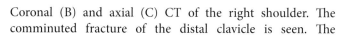

Coronal (B) and axial (C) CT of the right shoulder. The comminuted fracture of the distal clavicle is seen. The acromioclavicular and glenohumeral joints are intact. Axial CT through the clavicle shows mild displacement.

Case 6–20
Clavicle shaft fracture

(A)

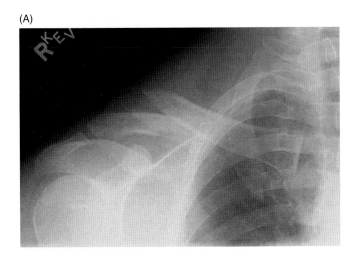

(B)

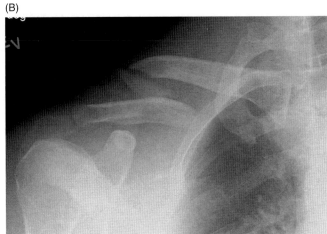

43-year-old man injured in bicycle accident. AP radiograph of the right shoulder without (A) and with cephalic angulation (B). There is a comminuted mid-shaft fracture. Elevation of the medial fragment results from the pull of the sternocleidomastoid while the weight of the arm keeps the lateral segment down. Overriding of the fragments as seen here is common. The majority, up to 80%, of clavicular fractures are sustained in the midclavicle. Midclavicular fractures at the junction of the mid and lateral thirds occurs with birth trauma.

Case 6–21
Medial clavicle fracture

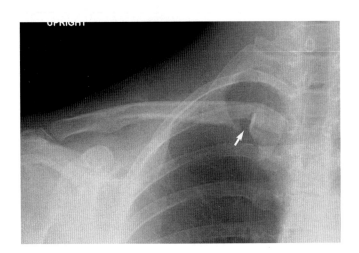

39-year-old woman in fall from bicycle. AP radiograph of the right clavicle. There is a fracture of the medial clavicle (arrow). These fractures comprise only 5% of all clavicular fractures. Overlapping bones and their tendency to be non-displaced contribute to the difficulty in identifying them. This is the least common variety of clavicular fracture. 80% of fractures are midclavicular, 10–15% are distal clavicular, and only 5% are medial. This location of fracture is highly associated with multisystem trauma, and for this reason there is a high associated mortality rate [14].

Case 6–22

Posterior sternoclavicular dislocation

(A)

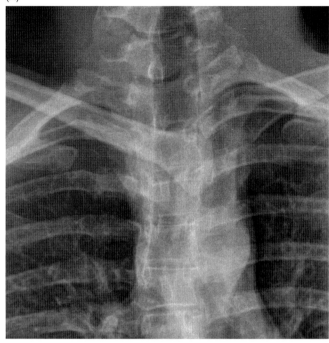

29-year-old man injured in an altercation; he was slammed forward against a parked car. AP radiograph of the chest (detail). AP radiograph shows asymmetry of the medial clavicles; the sternomanubrium joints themselves are difficult to visualize on radiographs. The medial head of the right clavicle projects inferior to that of the left and more medial than normal.

(B)

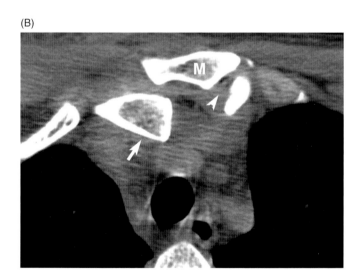

Axial CT of the sternoclavicular joints. The right head of the clavicle (arrow) has been dislocated to a position posterior to the manubrium (M). The left sternoclavicular joint (arrowhead) is normally located.

(C)

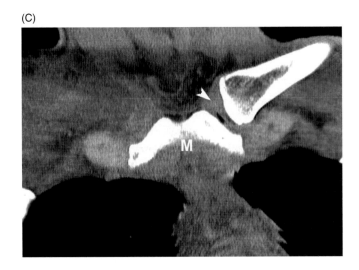

(D)

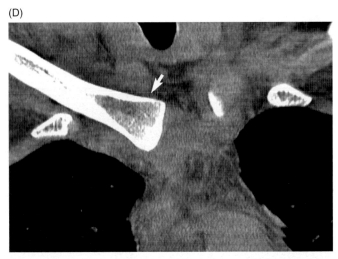

Coronal CT of the sternoclavicular joints, anterior (C) to posterior (D). Coronal image through the manubrium shows the normally located left sternoclavicular joint (arrowhead).

A more posterior slice shows the dislocated right clavicular head (arrow).

(E)

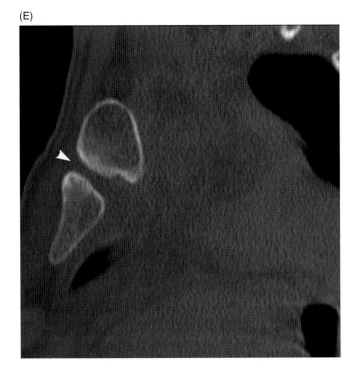

(F)

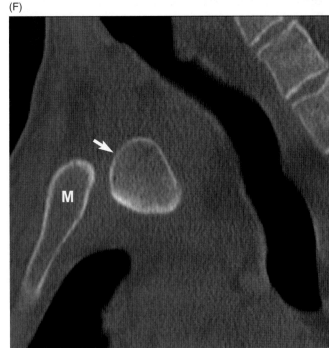

Sagittal CT of the sternoclavicular joints, left (E) to right (F). Sagittal image through the left sternoclavicular joint (arrowhead) shows it to be normally located. The slice through the

right sternoclavicular joint shows the right clavicular head (arrow) posteriorly dislocated from the manubrium (M).

Case 6–23
Acromion fracture

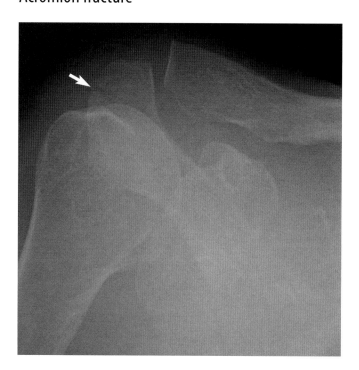

44-year-old man who fell from the top of a tree. AP radiograph of the right shoulder with cephalic angulation. There is a transverse fracture of the acromion process (arrow). Fracture of the acromion was occult on the straight AP view. Acromial fractures are rare and usually treated conservatively. Anterior and lateral fractures with inferior displacement have a propensity to encroach on the subacromial space and lead to rotator cuff impingement. ORIF is considered in these cases.

Scapula fracture

(A)

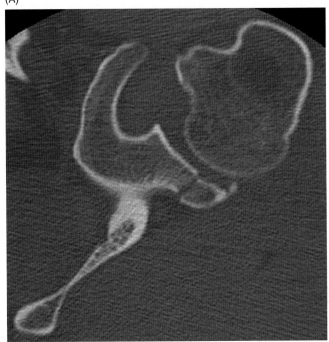

Patient was injured in a high-speed motor vehicle crash. Axial CT of the left scapula, through the glenoid process. There is a fracture through the glenoid process. The glenohumeral joint is normally located. The fractures extend through the scapular spine. The glenoid, acromion, and coracoid processes are attached to the same fragment. Fractures like these are generally treated without surgery. However, open reduction and internal fixation may be required in cases of coracoid, scapular neck, and articular fractures of the scapula. Most scapular fractures occur in the body or spine, and the next most common is in the neck of the scapula. Scapular fractures tend to occur in the setting of high energy trauma usually from direct forces. 80 to 90% of cases of scapular fractures sustain other injuries including rib fracture, clavicular fracture, shoulder dislocation, brachial plexus injury, axillary artery injury, and pneumothorax (23%) [15].

(B)

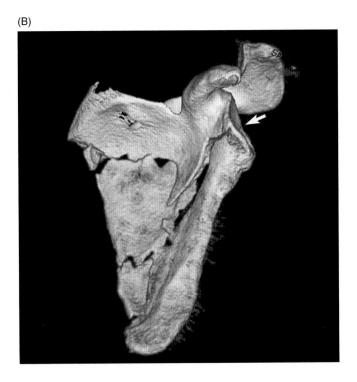

3D surface-rendered CT of the left scapula, anterior view. There are comminuted fractures of the scapular body that extend from the medial margin across to the glenoid fossa (arrow). The lateral margin of the scapular body is intact.

Case 6–25
Scapulothoracic dissociation

(A)

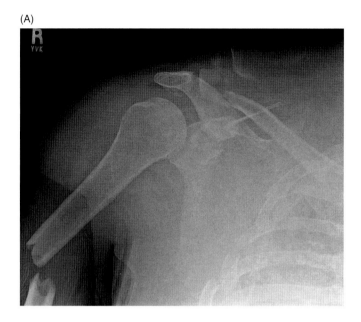

(B)

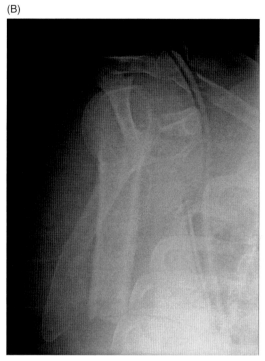

55-year-old man who crashed his motorcycle into a stationary pole. AP (A) and Y-view (B) of the right shoulder. There are fractures of the distal clavicle, coracoid, ribs, and humeral shaft. Scapular fractures are highly associated with other injuries and tend to occur in the setting of high-velocity trauma. Clavicular fractures occur in 23% of scapular fractures and may produce a "floating shoulder." The superior shoulder suspensory complex maintains the attachments of the upper extremity to the axial skeleton and is comprised of the mid- to distal clavicle, CC and AC ligaments, acromion and coracoid process, and glenoid. The clavicle serves as the main stabilizer of the upper extremity to the axial skeleton in this construct. When the ring is disrupted in two places, a floating shoulder results, which is unstable. These two fractures usually involve the scapula and the clavicle. The coracoid is important as an attachment for the coracoclavicular ligaments between the clavicle and scapula. The fracture through the base of the coracoid implies that these connections to the clavicle are no longer functioning. The distal clavicle fracture severs the connection to the scapula near the AC joint. This also can result in a floating shoulder. The term floating shoulder was initially described in scapular neck fractures in conjunction with ipsilateral clavicular fractures [16].

(C)

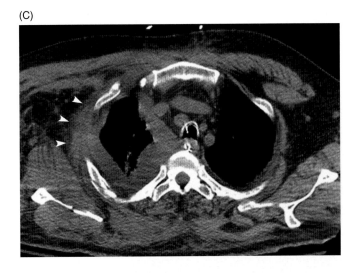

(D)

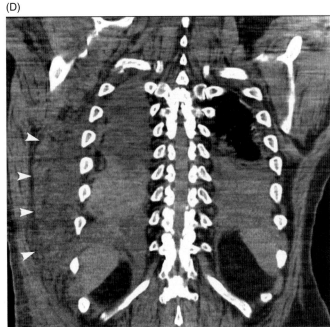

Multiplanar CT of the thorax. Axial (C) and coronal (D) CT images show soft tissue thickening along the expected course of the right serratus anterior muscles (arrowheads). There are also multiple right rib fractures, and abnormally increased separation of the scapula (arrows) from the thoracic cage. For comparison, the left side is normal.

Case 6–26
Body of sternum fracture

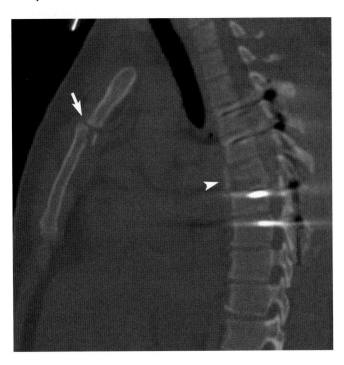

27-year-old man at a worksite who was crushed from above by a falling object. Sagittal CT of the thorax in the midline. There is a mildly displaced fracture through the posterior aspect of the sternum at the sternomanubrial junction (arrow). There is slight anterior subluxation of the body of the sternum relative to the manubrium, with retrosternal hematoma. The patient also had a burst fracture of the thoracic spine at the same level (arrowhead), already reduced and fixed at the time of the CT scan. Sternal injuries are usually attributed to direct blunt force trauma, such as an impact with the steering wheel in a motor vehicle crash. This typically gives rise to transverse sternal fractures. Because of the close proximity of the heart and great vessels, there is a high association of vascular and cardiac injuries with sternal fractures [17]. The sternum may also be fractured by axial compression, either of the entire chest, as in this case, or as a component of a flexion mechanism.

Case 6–27
Body of sternum fracture

(A)

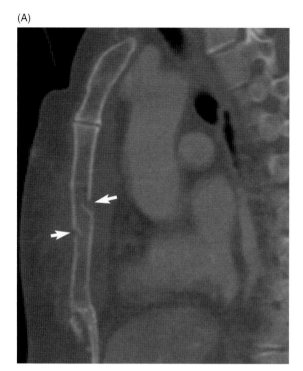

(B)

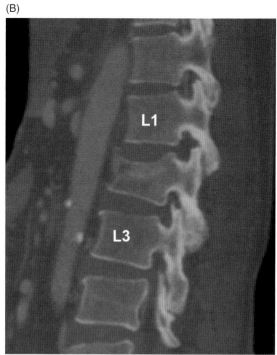

58-year-old woman who was a restrained passenger in a high-speed motor vehicle crash. Sagittal CT of the thorax in the midline, through the sternum (A) and upper lumbar spine (B). There are fractures of the body of the sternum where the superior and inferior fragments are impacted into each other (arrow). There is an associated anterior compression fracture of L2, confirming that the mechanism of injury was flexion of the body, compression the sternum into itself. Most sternal body fractures occur in motor vehicle crashes. In unrestrained drivers, direct impact into the steering wheel is another mechanism of injury. Airbags may reduce the incidence of sternal fractures from direct impact [18].

Case 6–28
Multiple left rib fractures

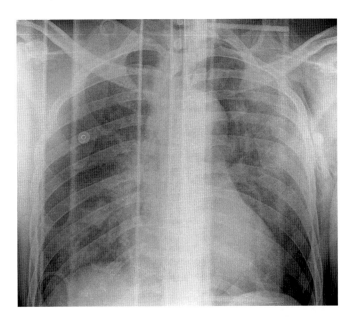

Man who was injured in a high speed motor vehicle crash. AP chest radiograph. There are multiple consecutive rib fractures on the left. Blunt chest trauma fractures the ribs more than any other bone. Consecutive fractures may cause a flail chest when two or more fractures (segmental fractures) occur in at least two ribs. This can produce paradoxical chest motion and interfere with breathing. Pneumothorax is a potential complication. The fourth through the ninth ribs are the ribs most frequently fractured. The posterior angle is the most susceptible to fracture. Fractures can occur at the site of direct impact.

Case 6–29
Segmental rib fractures with flail chest

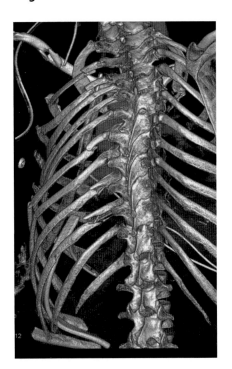

48-year-old involved in a high-speed T-bone motor vehicle collision requiring extrication from the wreckage. 3D surface-rendered CT of the left ribs, posterior view. The patient sustained multiple mildly displaced posterolateral rib fractures involving the first through eleventh left ribs with segmental fractures of the second through eighth, and tenth through eleventh ribs, raising a concern for flail chest. Comminuted fracture of the mid left clavicle and minimally displaced non-comminuted fracture through the proximal aspect of the same clavicle were also present. Flail chest is typically managed medically using ventilatory support, aggressive pulmonary toilet and pain management, with surgical stabilization often being reserved for those failing conservative measures [19]. Surgical stabilization of the thoracic cavity using either compression plates or intramedullary fixation being reserved in the immediate post-traumatic period for those unresponsive or unable to be weaned from ventilatory support [19]. Fixation may also occur in the post-traumatic setting to remedy painful rib malunion or nonunion [19–20].

References

1. Hill HA, Sachs MD. The grooved defect of the humeral head. A frequently unrecognized complication of dislocations of the shoulder joint. *Radiology.* 1940; 35:690–700.

2. George MS. Fractures of the greater tuberosity of the humerus. *J Am Acad Orthop Surg.* 2007 Oct;15(10):607–13. PMID: 17916784.

3. Gyftopoulos S, Albert M, Recht MP. Osseous injuries associated with anterior shoulder instability: what the radiologist should know. *AJR Am J Roentgenol.* 2014 Jun;202(6):W541–50. doi: 10.2214/AJR.13.11824. PMID: 24848847.

4. Aston JW Jr, Gregory CF. Dislocation of the shoulder with significant fracture of the glenoid. *J Bone Joint Surg Am.* 1973 Oct;55(7):1531–3. PMID: 4758724.

5. Hovelius L, Eriksson K, Fredin H, Hagberg G, Hussenius A, Lind B, Thorling J, Weckstrom J. Recurrences after initial dislocation of the shoulder. Results of a prospective study of treatment. *J Bone Joint Surg Am.* 1983 Mar;65(3):343–9. PMID: 6826597.

6. Larribe M, Laurent PE, Acid S, Aswad R, Champsaur P, Le Corroller T. Anterior shoulder instability: The role of advanced shoulder imaging in preoperative planning. *Semin Musculoskelet Radiol.* 2014 Sep;18(4):398–403. doi: 10.1055/s-0034-1384828. Epub 2014 Sep 3. PMID: 25184394.

7. Cisternino SJ, Rogers LF, Stufflebam BC, Kruglik GD. The trough line: A radiographic sign of posterior shoulder dislocation. *AJR Am J Roentgenol.* 1978 May;130(5):951–4. PMID: 417598.

8. Patel DN, Zuckerman JD, Egol KA. Luxatio erecta: Case series with review of diagnostic and management principles. *Am J Orthop (Belle Mead NJ).* 2011 Nov;40(11):566–70. PMID: 22263209.

9. Brogdon BG, Crotty JM, MacFeely L, McCann SB, Fitzgerald M. Intrathoracic fracture-dislocation of the humerus. *Skeletal Radiol.* 1995 Jul;24(5):383–5. PMID: 7570162.

10. Daffner SD, Cipolle MD, Phillips TG. Fracture of the humeral neck with intrathoracic dislocation of the humeral head. *J Emerg Med.* 2010 May;38(4):439–43. doi: 10.1016/j. jemermed.2007.09.064. Epub 2008 Jul 23. PMID: 18650050.

11. Mazzocca AD, Arciero RA, Bicos J. Evaluation and treatment of acromioclavicular joint injuries. *Am J Sports Med.* 2007;35:316–329. PMID: 17251175.

12. Simovitch R, Sanders B, Ozbaydar M, Lavery K, Warner JJ. Acromioclavicular joint injuries: Diagnosis and management. *J Am Acad Orthop Surg.* 2009 Apr;17(4):207–19. PMID: 19307670.

13. Davies EJ, Fagg JA, Stanley D. Subacromial, supracoracoid dislocation of the acromioclavicular joint with ipsilateral clavicle fracture: a case report with review of the literature and classification. *JRSM Open.* 2014 Jun 9;5(7):2054270414527281. doi: 10.1177/2054270414527281. eCollection 2014 Jul. PMID: 25057405; PMCID: PMC4100230.

14. Throckmorton T, Kuhn JE. Fractures of the medial end of the clavicle. *J Shoulder Elbow Surg.* 2007 Jan–Feb;16(1):49–54. Epub 2006 Dec 12. PMID: 17169583.

15. Veysi VT, Mittal R, Agarwal S, Dosani A, Giannoudis PV. Multiple trauma and scapula fractures: So what? *J Trauma.* 2003 Dec;55(6):1145–7. PMID: 14676662.

16. Herscovici D Jr, Fiennes AG, Allgower M, Ruedi TP. The floating shoulder: Ipsilateral clavicle and scapular neck fractures. *J Bone Joint Surg Br.* 1992 May;74(3):362–4. Comment in: J Bone Joint Surg Br. 1993 May;75(3):509. PMID: 1587877.

17. Johnson I, Branfoot T. Sternal fracture – A modern review. *Arch Emerg Med.* 1993 Mar;10(1):24–8. PMCID: PMC1285920; PMID: 8452609.

18. Knobloch K, Wagner S, Haasper C, Probst C, Krettek C, Otte D, Richter M. Sternal fractures occur most often in old cars to seat-belted drivers without any airbag often with concomitant spinal injuries: clinical findings and technical collision variables among 42,055 crash victims. *Ann Thorac Surg.* 2006 Aug;82(2):444–50. PMID: 16863741.

19. Pettiford BL, Luketich JD, Landreneau RJ. The management of flail chest. *Thorac Surg Clin.* 2007 Feb;17(1):25–33. PMID: 17650694.

20. Fowler TT, Taylor BC, Bellino MJ, Althausen PL. Surgical treatment of flail chest and rib fractures. *J Am Acad Orthop Surg.* 2014 Dec;22(12):751–760. PMID: 25425610.

Fractures and dislocations of the cervical spine

Refky Nicola, D.O., Felix S. Chew, M.D., and Catherine Maldjian, M.D.

Case 7–1
Atlanto-occipital dissociation

(A)

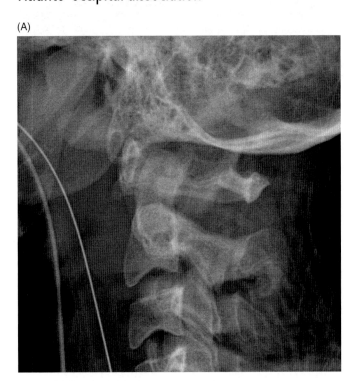

Young adult with complete high cervical cord injury from a high-speed motor vehicle crash. Lateral radiograph of the upper cervical spine. There is abnormal anterior position of the skull relative to the cervical spine. There is soft tissue swelling anterior to C1 and C2, but the relationship of C1 to C2 is normal.

(B)

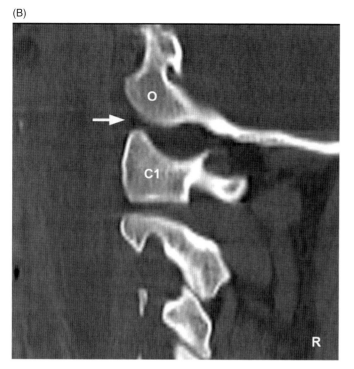

(C)

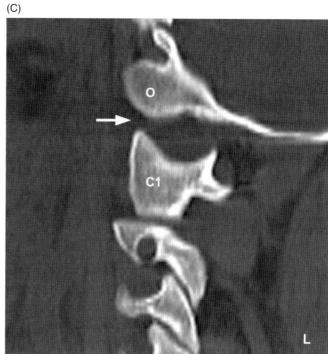

Sagittal CT of the upper cervical spine through the right (B) and left (C) atlanto-occipital joints. On both the right (R) and the left (L), there is marked anterior subluxation of the occipital condyles (O) over the superior articular facets of the atlas (C1).

(D)

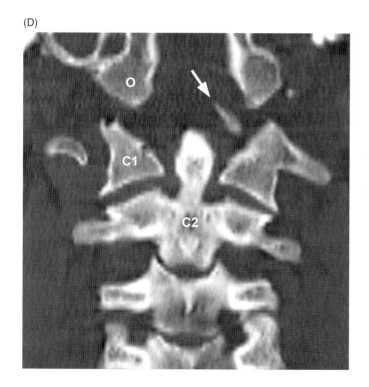

Coronal CT of the upper cervical spine. There is an avulsion fragment from the left occipital condyle (arrow). The occipital condyles are superiorly displaced relative to C1. Atlanto-occipital dissociation (AOD) is caused by hyperextension during high-energy deceleration trauma. The tectorial ligaments that normally tether the occipital condyles to the superior facets of C1 are disrupted. Dislocation and subluxation represent complete and incomplete dissociation, respectively. Atlanto-occipital dissociation is commonly fatal because stretching of the brainstem causes immediate respiratory arrest. (Source: Chew FS. Skeletal Radiology: The Bare Bones. 3rd Edition. Copyright © 2010 by Felix Chew.)

Case 7–2

Atlanto-occipital dissociation

(A)

(B)

(C)

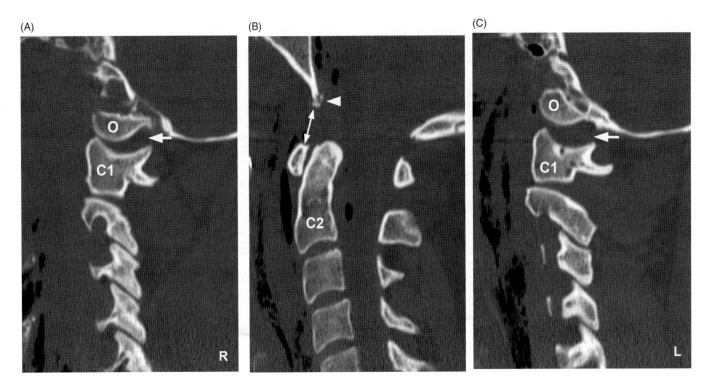

21-year-old man in high-speed motor vehicle crash with ASIA A spinal cord injury. Sagittal CT of the upper cervical spine, right (A) to left (C). There is widening of the distance (single-headed arrows) between the atlas (C1) and the occipital condyles (O) and the occiput is anteriorly displaced on both the right (R) and the left (L). There is retropharyngeal dissection of gas and soft tissue swelling. In the midline, there are small avulsion fragments at the tip of the clivus (arrowhead). The distance between the clivus and anterior arch of C1 (double-headed arrow) is abnormally increased. On CT, the increased distance between the occipital condyles and the lateral masses of C1 is diagnostic of atlanto-occipital dissociation (AOD). This type of trauma should be considered in patients with severe facial trauma. Subluxation of the atlanto-occipital articulation can be quantified by the distances between the occiput and axis, which are as follows: Basion-axial interval (BAI) is the distance from the basion (inferior tip of the clivus) to a line drawn along the posterior body of C2, which should normally measure less than 12 mm. Vertical Basion-dens distance should normally also measure less than 12 mm [1, 2]. Secondary radiologic signs of AOD include soft tissue swelling or subarachnoid/craniocervical junction/posterior cranial fossa hemorrhage [3].

Case 7–3

Atlanto-axial dissociation and odontoid fracture, Type I

(A)

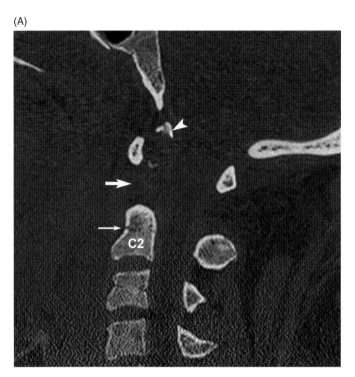

(B)

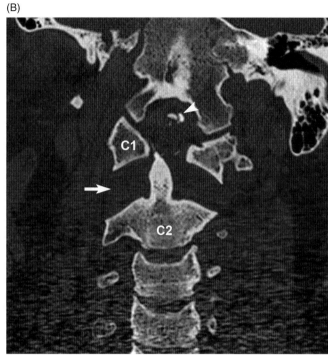

53-year-old man whose motor vehicle crashed into a tree. He was unresponsive at the scene. Sagittal (A) and coronal (B) CT of the upper cervical spine. There is an atlanto-axial distraction injury (arrows). In addition, there is an avulsion of the tip of the dens (odontoid fracture, type 1) (arrowheads), and a non-displaced fracture of the body of C2 (long arrow). The patient died shortly after hospital admission. In acute traumatic atlanto-axial dissociation (AAD), there is partial or complete derangement of the lateral atlanto-axial articulation. AAD is characterized by excessive motion between C1 and C2 caused by either a bony or a ligamentous injury. The three

mechanisms of AAD are flexion-extension, distraction, and rotation. Fielding and Hawkins provided a classification system for atlanto-axial dissociation. Type I AAD is rotatory fixation without anterior displacement of the atlas. Type II AAD is rotatory fixation with less than 5 mm of anterior displacement of the atlas. Type III AAD is rotatory fixation with greater than 5 mm of anterior displacement of the atlas. Type IV AAD is rotatory fixation with posterior displacement of the atlas. All of these injuries are typically associated with concurrent fractures, neurologic deficits, and/or vertebral artery injuries [4].

Case 7–4
Jefferson fracture

(A)

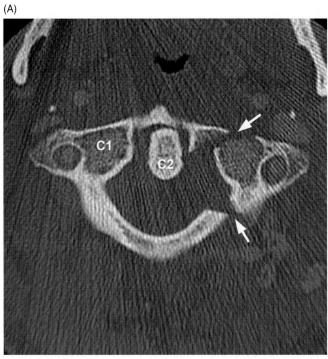

34-year-old man who fell on his head. Axial CT of C1. There are displaced fractures through the anterior and posterior portions of the ring of C1, on the left side (arrows). Because the spinal canal is wide at this level and the fracture fragments tend to displace peripherally, neurologic injury may be absent.

(B)

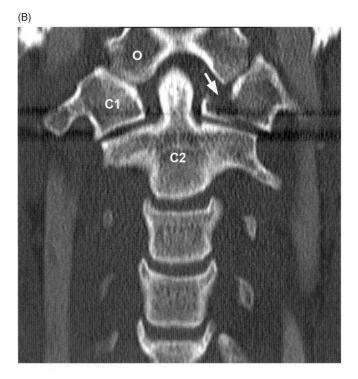

Coronal CT of the upper cervical spine. Image through the anterior C1 fracture shows displaced fracture (arrow) through the left lateral mass.

(C)

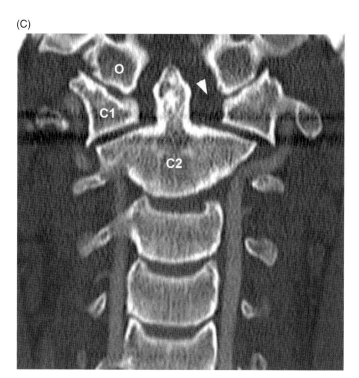

Coronal CT of the upper cervical spine. Image through the free left C1 fragment shows displacement of the left lateral mass, as indicated by the abnormally large gap (arrowhead) between the odontoid process and the left lateral mass. The injury is produced by axial loading, which causes compression of the lateral masses of C1 between the occipital condyles and C2 and gives rise to a burst fracture. The lateral masses are offset from the dens and the total amount of offset can be measured to determine the stability of the lesion. Less than 7mm total offset implies integrity of the transverse ligament and the injury would be deemed stable.

Case 7–5
Jefferson fracture

(A)

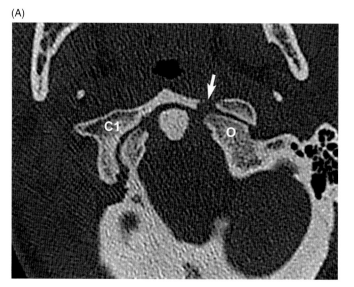

(B)

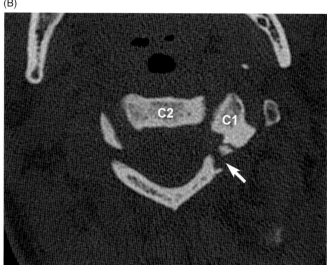

(C)

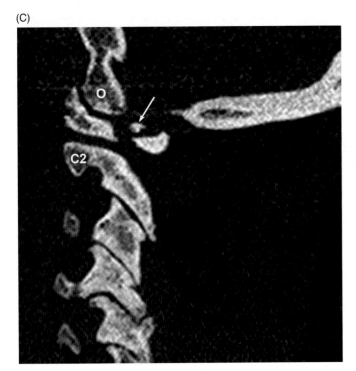

(D)

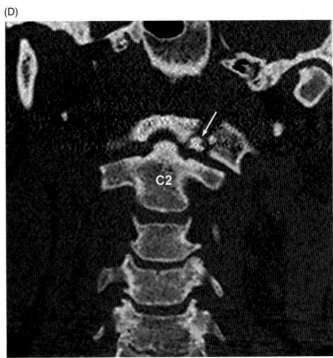

47-year-old woman who fell down a flight of stairs. Multiplanar CT of the upper cervical spine, axial (A-B), sagittal (C), and coronal (D). There are comminuted fractures of the ring of C1 involving both the anterior and posterior arches (arrows), characteristic of a Jefferson fracture. There is avulsion of the transverse ligament (long arrow). This injury results from axial loading and compression of the lateral masses of C1 between the occipital condyles and the articular facets of C2. The lateral masses are forced apart, resulting in fractures at the junctions of the anterior and posterior arch of lateral masses of C1 [5]. The classic Jefferson fracture is a four-part fracture of the anterior and posterior arches on both the right and the left. O=occipital condyle.

Case 7–6   Odontoid fracture, Type II-A

(A)   (B)   (C)

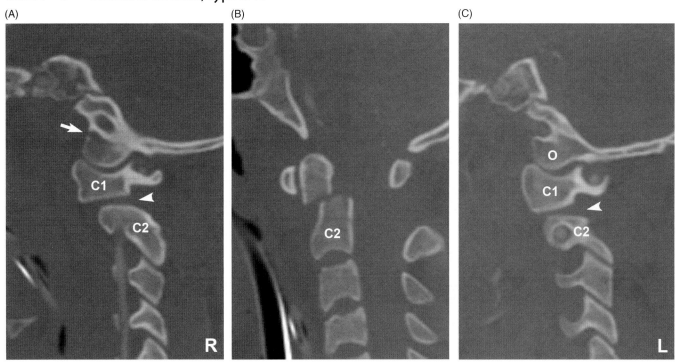

17-year-old male in severe motor vehicle crash. Traumatic brain injury with Glasgow coma score of 3 at presentation. Sagittal CT of the upper cervical spine, right (A) to left (C). Midline sagittal image shows a transverse fracture through the odontoid process of C2 (dens) with one-half width anterior displacement of the cranial fragment. Slice through the right facet joint (R) shows a non-displaced occipital condyle fracture (arrow) and anterior subluxation of C1 over C2 (arrowhead). Slice through the left facet joint (L) shows anterior subluxation of C1 over C2 (arrowhead).

(D)   (E)

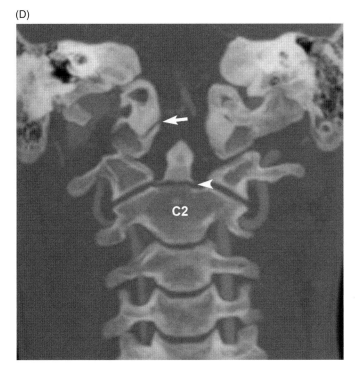 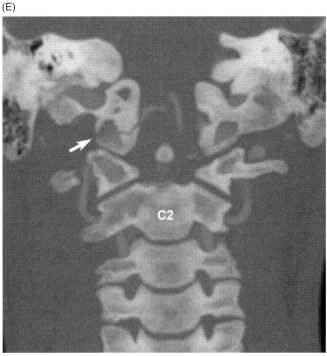

Coronal maximum intensity projection CT of the upper cervical spine, anterior (D) to posterior (E). There is a fracture transversely through the base of the odontoid process (arrowhead) and a right occipital condyle fracture (arrow).

(F)

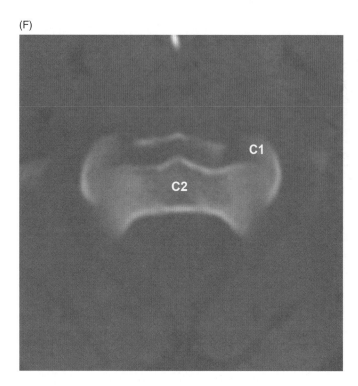

Axial CT at C1-C2 interspace. The fracture is not directly seen because it is in the axial plane, but there is anterior displacement of the cranial fragment and anterior subluxation of C1 over C2. Fractures of the odontoid are classified under the Anderson and D'Alonso system. Type I represents an avulsion fracture where the alar ligament attaches to the tip of the odontoid process. Type II, the most common type, is a transverse fracture through the base of the dens at the junction of the odontoid process with the body of C2. This fracture often fails to heal [6]. Type II fractures are further subdivided by Type II-A, II-B, and II-C. Type II-A fractures are defined as minimally displaced or non-displaced. Type II-B is displaced transverse fracture or fracture extending from anterior-superior to posterior-inferior. A Type II-C fracture is defined as a displaced fracture extending from anterior-inferior to posterior superior or with significant comminution. A Type III fracture is a fracture through the body of C2. Types II and III are considered unstable because they can result in atlanto-axial instability; the ligaments, dens fragment, C1, and occiput act as a single unit during movement [7]. In children, a synchondrosis at the base of the dens should not be confused for a Type II fracture.

Case 7–7   Odontoid fracture, Type II-A

(A)   (B)   (C)

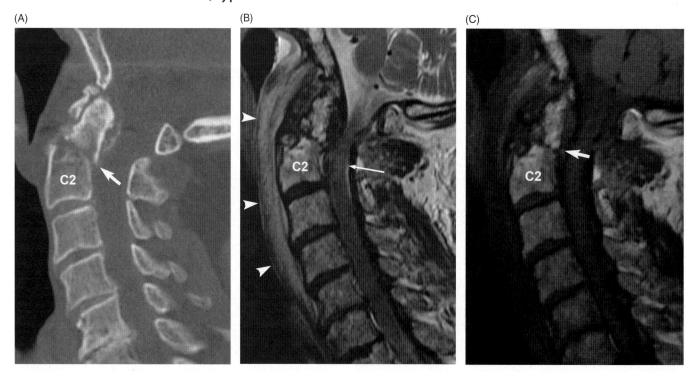

81-year-old man fell on the stairs, striking his head. Sagittal CT (A), T2 MRI (B), and T1 FLAIR MRI (C), of the upper cervical spine. There is minimally displaced fracture at the base of the odontoid (arrow). There is hyperintense signal with the prevertebral soft tissues (arrowheads). There is concerning for ligamentous injury as well as prevertebral hematoma. In addition, there is hyperintense signal within the cord consistent with cord edema at C2 (long arrow).

Case 7–8
Odontoid fracture, Type III

(A)

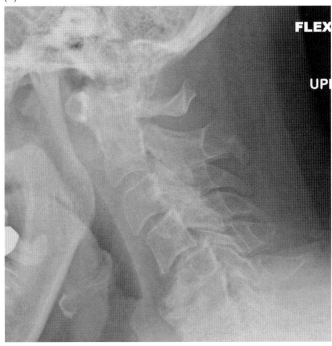

69-year-old woman who fell against a wall in her home, flexing her neck to the right. Lateral radiograph of the upper cervical spine in flexion. The odontoid process is displaced anteriorly, resulting in misalignment of the spinal canal at C1-C2. The posterior arch of C1 is anterior displaced relative to the posterior arch of C2.

(B)

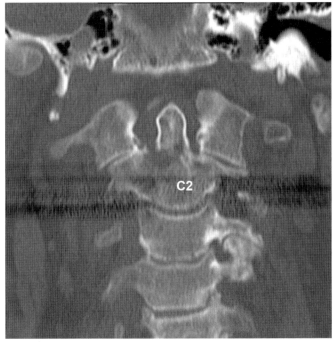

(C)

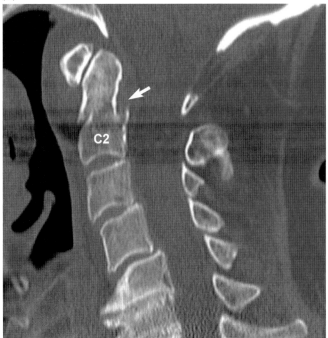

Coronal and sagittal CT of the upper cervical spine. (B) Coronal CT image shows the fracture extending through the base of the odontoid process, making this a type III odontoid fracture.

(C) Sagittal CT image shows impaction and anterior displacement of the odontoid. The posterior aspect of the spinal canal is misaligned at C1-C2.

(D)

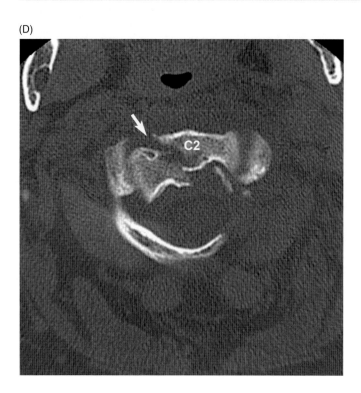

Axial CT at C2. Axial CT image through the upper body of C2 shows the displacement of the fracture. The most common mechanism of injury in the elderly is a ground-level fall. In this circumstance, as in this case, the upper cervical spine is the most common site of injury.

Case 7–9   Hangman fracture C2

(A)

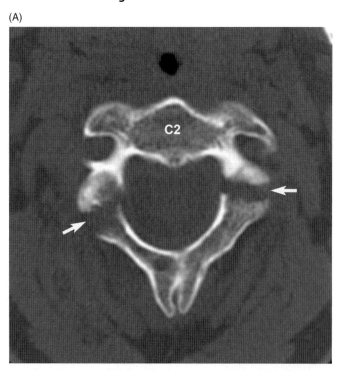

(B)

39-year-old man who fell when he was punched. Axial CT at C2 (A) and sagittal CT of the upper cervical spine (B). The axial CT shows bilateral fractures of the posterior elements of C2 (arrows). There is mild displacement of fracture fragments. Sagittal CT through the facet joints on one side shows the fracture passing between the articular facets of C2 (pars interarticularis); the contralateral side (not shown) was the same. The

hangman fracture draws its name from judicial hangings in which the knot was placed under the chin and the neck was forced into hyperextension [8]. In modern times, a similar mechanism occurs in car accidents when impact of the head against the windshield or of the chin on the steering wheel may force the neck into hyperextension, or in falls with a face-plant. This injury is most common in elderly adults.

Case 7–10
Hangman fracture C2

(A)

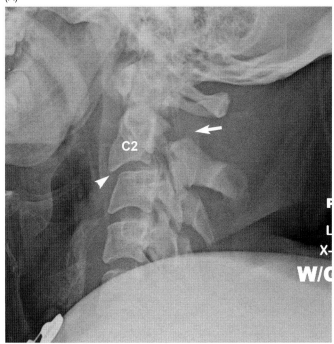

23-year-old man in high-speed motor vehicle crash into telephone pole. Lateral radiograph of the upper cervical spine. There are fractures of the neural arch of C2 at the pars interarticularis (arrow). The C2-C3 disc space is normal, but there is mild anterior displacement of C2 over C3 (arrowhead). A classification scheme exists for this fracture based on the severity of the associated soft tissue injuries and the degree of displacement of C2 over C3 [8].

(B) (C) (D)

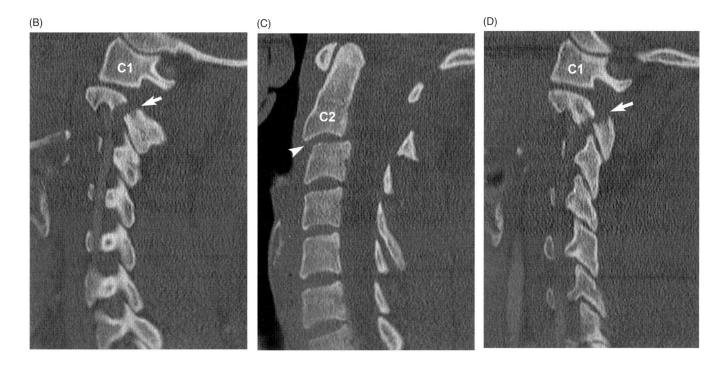

Sagittal CT of the upper cervical spine, right (B) to left (D). Sagittal CT through the right (B) and left (D) lateral masses of C2 show displaced fractures of the pars interarticularis (arrows). Sagittal CT through the midline (C) shows there is anterior displacement of C2 over C3 (arrowhead).

Case 7–11

Right lateral mass fracture C2

(A)

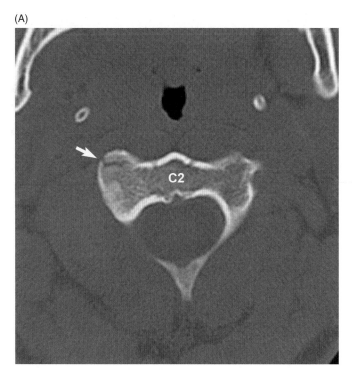

(B)

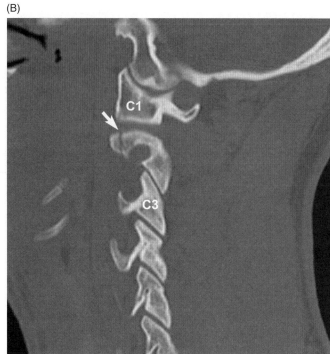

19-year-old man who was ejected during a motor vehicle crash. Axial CT at C2 (A) and sagittal CT of the upper cervical spine (B). There is a non-displaced fracture of the right lateral mass of C2 (arrow). Axial compression and lateral bending are the forces that lead to this fracture pattern, which is not common.

Case 7–12

Hyperextension teardrop fracture C2

(A)

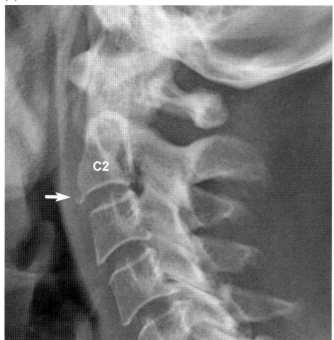

(B)

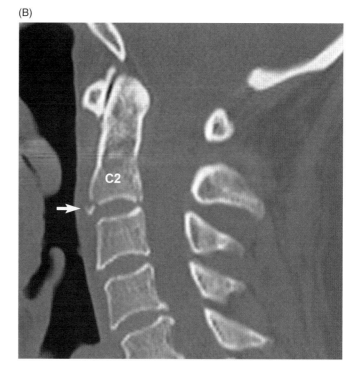

55-year-old woman who tripped and fell face-first into a parked vehicle, forcibly hyperextending her neck. Lateral radiograph (A) and sagittal CT (B) of the upper cervical spine. There is an avulsion of the anterior inferior endplate of C2 (arrow). In general, hyperextension strain causes a tear of the anterior longitudinal ligament and avulsion of the disc. In most of hyperextension strains, there is a bony avulsion where Sharpey's fibers insert on the annulus fibrosis [9]. A triangular fracture fragment results. In younger patients, there is usually high-energy trauma. Older patients may sustain the same injury with far less force, often in a ground-level fall [10].

Case 7–13
Hyperextension teardrop fracture C2

(A)

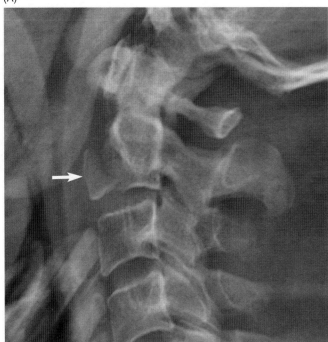

55-year-old female who was in a motor vehicle collision with a tractor trailer. The car was found buried under the dry cement load the truck was carrying. Lateral radiograph of the upper cervical spine. There is an avulsion fracture of the base of C2 (arrow). There is slight retrolisthesis of C2 over C3.

(B)

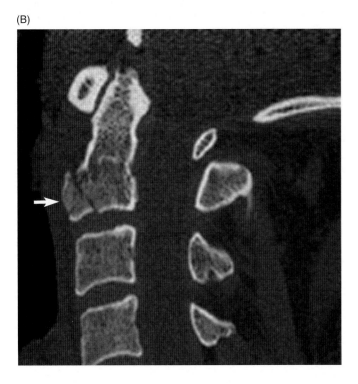

Sagittal CT of the upper cervical spine. There is an avulsion fracture of vertebral body of C2 (arrow). The vertical height of the avulsed fragment is greater than the horizontal width. Hyperextension teardrop fractures only involve the anterior column, and therefore are stable in flexion and unstable in extension. This type of injury is frequently associated with acute cervical central cord syndrome, thus MRI is often necessary to determine both the presence and the extent of spinal cord edema and contusion [10]. This type of fracture is most commonly seen in the elderly or in osteoporotic patients.

Case 7–14

Hyperextension injury C2

(A)

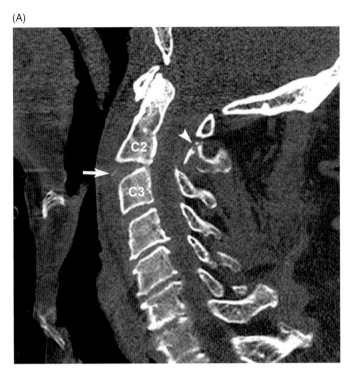

(B)

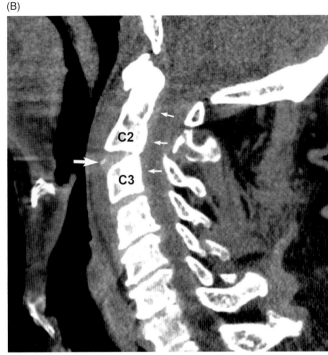

62-year-old male fell from 4 feet onto a concrete floor. Sagittal CT of the upper cervical spine (midline with bone (A) and soft tissue (B) settings). There is widening of the C2-C3 intervertebral disc space anteriorly and narrowing posteriorly, indicative of a hyperextension injury with tear of the anterior longitudinal ligament. There is extensive prevertebral swelling extending from C1 to C4. There is an avulsion fragment (arrow) from the anterior margin of the C2 endplate. There are also fractures of the posterior elements (arrowhead). There is an epidural hematoma extending along the posterior aspect of the vertebral bodies from C1 to C3 (small arrows). The patient had central cord syndrome. Hyperextension injuries are not uncommon and spinal cord injury may be present even with normal radiographs [11–12]. The neurologic impairment can vary from upper extremity paresthesias to complete quadriplegia [10]. The spectrum of hyperextension injuries ranges from minor muscle strains to more serious injuries. The anterior and posterior longitudinal ligaments may be disrupted, with the anterior more severely affected. The result may be hemorrhage beneath the prevertebral fascia and avulsion fragments anteriorly, and epidural hemorrhage posteriorly. Davis et al. noted incomplete avulsion of the annulus fibrosus with hyperextension and whiplash injuries [12]. Frequently, the radiographs may show normally aligned vertebrae owing to the immediate realignment following the impacting force. Therefore, the presence of diffuse paravertebral soft tissue swelling with normally aligned vertebrae may indicate injury [9–11].

Case 7–15

Hyperflexion injury C5-C7

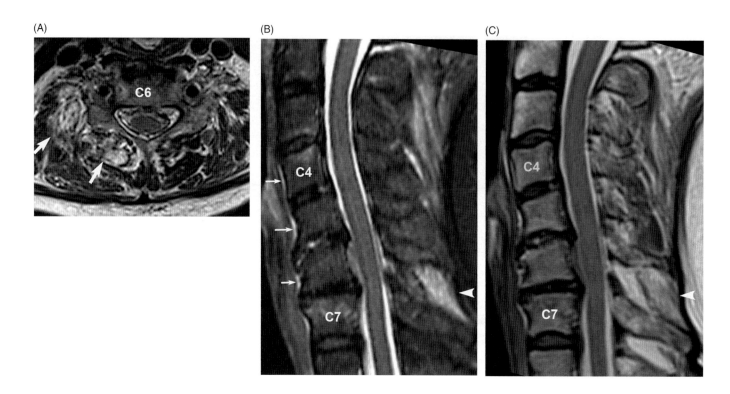

51-year-old woman who has neck pain following a motor vehicle crash a few days ago. Axial T2 MRI at C6 (A), sagittal STIR (B), and sagittal T2 (C) of the middle cervical spine. Hyperintense signal is present within the right paraspinal muscles (arrows). There is abnormal signal within the interspinous ligaments at C6-C7 (arrowhead), with widening of the interspinous distance. Abnormal marrow signal at C7 suggests fracture. The anterior longitudinal ligament from the C4-C7 is also abnormal (long arrows). Hyperflexion injuries of the cervical spine may cause partial or complete disruption of the posterior cervical complex, which is comprised of the posterior articulations stabilized by the joint capsule, interspinous ligaments, supraspinous ligaments, and ligamenta flava [13, 14]. Harris et al. proposed that, with a hyperflexion injury, there is compression in the anterior column and distraction of the posterior column [15]. Anterior subluxation of the cervical spine is an unstable injury, thus a prompt diagnosis is essential. The soft tissue damage in the anterior cervical spine may be severe. MRI may be appropriate in the evaluation of neck injuries because it is capable of direct visualization of the relevant structures [14].

Case 7–16

Hyperextension teardrop injury

(A)

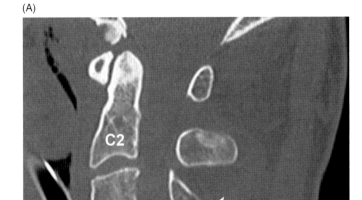

40-year-old man injured in a diving accident. Sagittal CT of the upper cervical spine. There is an avulsion fracture of the anterior inferior corner of the C3 vertebral body. The fragment is mildly displaced, and the C3-C4 disc space is slightly widened. Soft tissue swelling anterior to the C3 body suggests rupture of the anterior longitudinal ligament. There is a fracture of the C3 spinous process (arrowhead) with the fragment outside of the imaging volume.

(B)

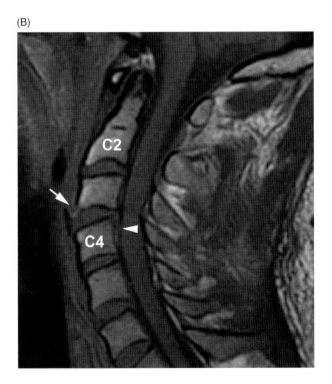

Sagittal T1 FLAIR MRI of the upper cervical spine. There is a tear (arrow) of the anterior longitudinal ligament just superior to the teardrop fragment. There is also a tear (arrowhead) of the posterior longitudinal ligament at the C4 level. The C3-C4 disc space is widened anteriorly, and there is mild retrolisthesis of C3 over C4.

(C)

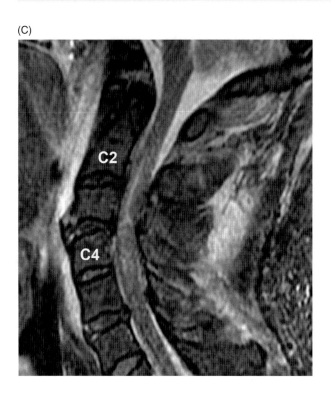

Sagittal T2 MRI of the upper cervical spine. There is prevertebral hematoma. There is hematoma in the posterior soft tissues that corresponded to fractures of the spinous process of C3 and C4, interspinous ligament injury, and nuchal ligament injury. There is contusion of the spinal cord centered at C3 and C4.

Case 7–17

Hyperflexion injury C5-C6

(A)

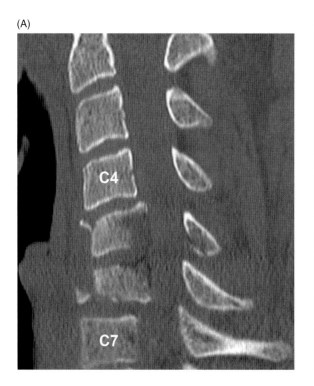

(B)

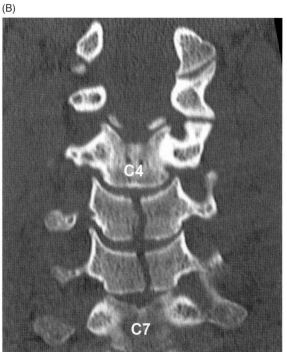

30-year-old man injured in a diving accident. Sagittal (A) and coronal (B) CT of the middle cervical spine. There is an avulsion fracture of the anterior superior margin of C5 and an avulsion fracture of the anterior inferior margin of C6, with retrolisthesis of C5 on C6. There are fractures in the sagittal plane through the bodies of C5 and C6.

(C)

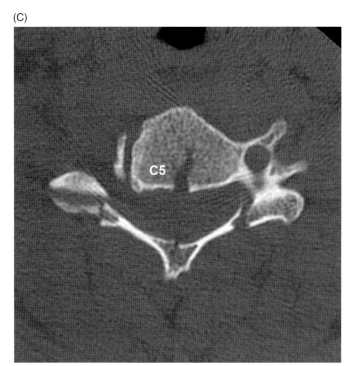

(D)

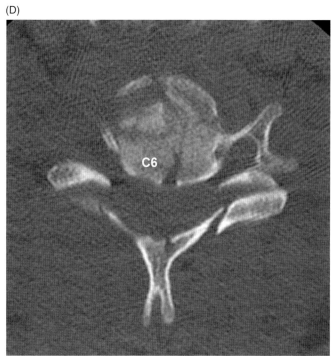

Axial CT at C5 (C) and C6 (D). Axial CT through C5 shows fracture of the vertebral body in the sagittal plane and segmental fractures of the posterior neural arch. Axial CT through C6 shows comminuted fractures of the body with retropulsion and segmental fractures of the posterior neural arch. The spinal canal is narrowed by the retropulsed C6 fragments. Patients with cervical spine fractures should be screened for blunt cerebrovascular injury (BCVI) [16]. CT angiography is commonly used for this purpose.

Case 7–18

Unilateral jumped facet C3-C4

(A)

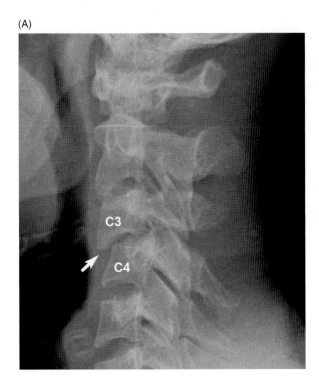

(B)

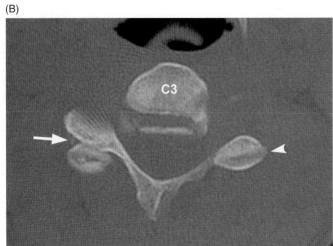

35-year-old woman in motor vehicle crash. Lateral radiograph of the cervical spine (A) and axial CT of C3-C4 (B). There is anterolisthesis of C3 on C4 (arrow), with the facet joints at the C3 level and above projecting at a different rotation than the facet joints at the levels below. The mechanism of injury involves flexion, distraction, and rotation. The inferior articular process displaces anteriorly and superiorly to the superior articular process of the subjacent level. On the axial CT, the right C3 inferior articular facet is anterior to the C4 superior articular facet (arrow), whereas the left facet joint is normally located (arrowhead). These injuries comprise 12–16% of all cervical spine injuries. This is considered a stable injury. 75% of unilateral facet dislocation are associated with fractures of the involved articular processes [17]. (Source: Chew FS. Skeletal Radiology: The Bare Bones. 3rd Edition. Copyright © 2010 by Felix Chew.)

Perched facet C6-C7

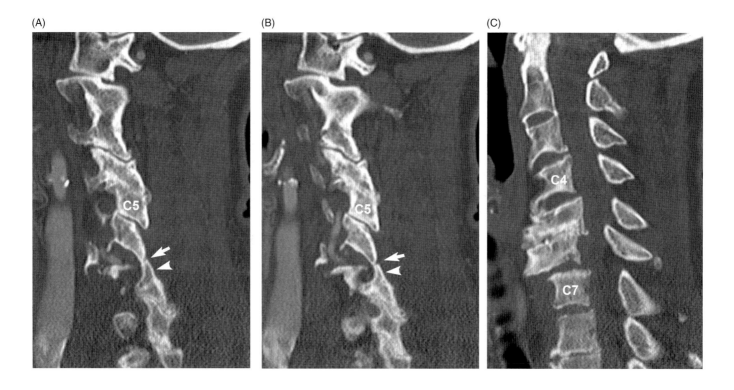

(A)   (B)   (C)

88-year-old woman in motor vehicle crash. Sagittal CT angiogram through the left facet joints, lateral (A) to medial (C). The inferior corner of the C6 inferior facet is perched on top of the superior corner of the C7 superior facet (arrows). The articular surface of the C7 superior facet is uncovered (arrowheads) because of the abnormal position of the C6 inferior facet. The near-midline image (C) shows anterolisthesis of C6 over C7, including the vertebral body and posterior neural arch. This patient has advanced multilevel degenerative changes with bony proliferation throughout the cervical spine. Hyperflexion force may disrupt the facet joint and other posterior ligaments. The superior vertebra rotates and subluxates forward, uncovering of the inferior articulating facet surface. Uncovering may be partial or complete. With further flexion, perched facets may become locked facets [18].

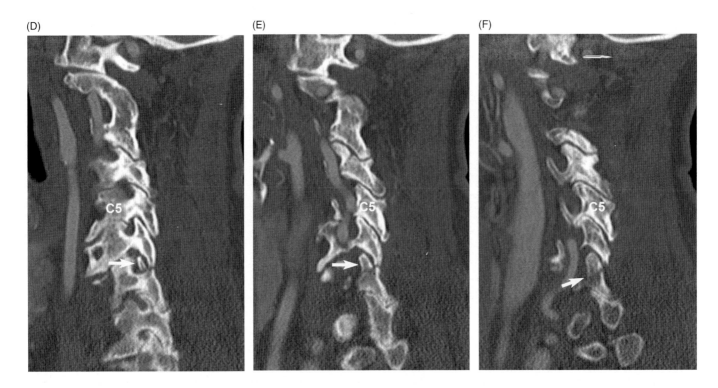

(D) (E) (F)

Sagittal CT angiogram through the right facet joints, medial (D) to lateral (F). There is a fracture of the superior articular process of the C7 superior facet (arrow), with anterior displacement of the fragment into the neural foramen. Thus, this patient had a perched facet on one side and a fractured facet on the other, both at the same level. The CT angiogram was performed to screen for blunt cerebrovascular injury.

Case 7–20
Bilateral jumped facets C5-C6

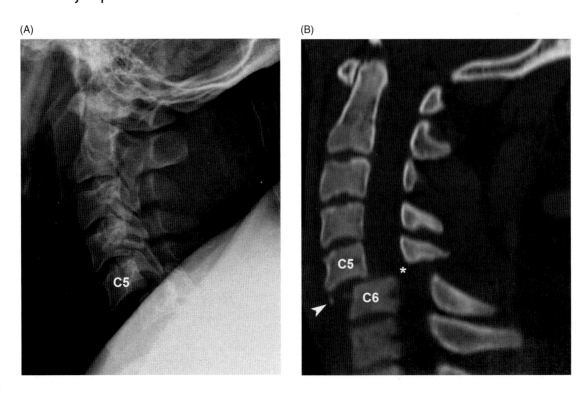

(A) (B)

29-year-old man who was an unrestrained driver in a three-car pileup. His car was struck twice. Lateral radiograph (A) and midline sagittal CT (B) of the upper cervical spine. There is forward translation of C5 over C6, greater than half of the vertebral body. There are bilateral jumped facets of C5 on C6. There is also prominence of the prevertebral soft tissues. The sagittal

CT shows the forward translation of C5 over C6 with severe bony compromise of the spinal canal (*) between the body of C6 and the posterior arch of C5. There is also a small anterior superior avulsion fracture fragment (arrowhead) of C6 that remains attached to C5. The patient had an ASIA A spinal injury and was subsequently treated with fusion.

(C)

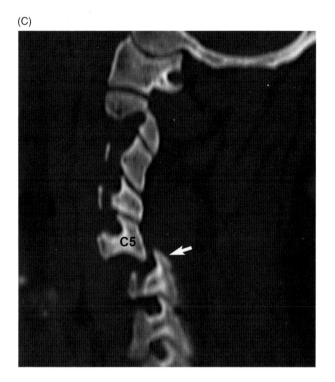

(D)

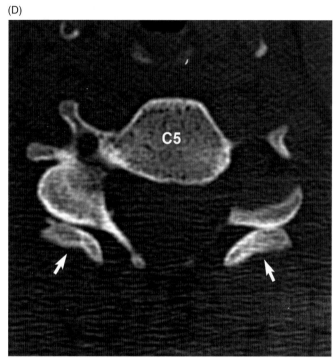

Sagittal CT (C) through the articular facets of the cervical spine; axial CT (D) at C5-C6. Sagittal CT through one set of facet joints shows that the inferior articular process of C5 has jumped over the superior articular process of C6 (arrow) and is resting anterior to it. The superior facet of C6 is consequently uncovered (naked facet). On the axial CT images, there is reversal of the relation between the facet joints where the inferior facets of the C5 are displaced anterior to the superior facet of the C6 (arrows). This is described as the reverse hamburger bun sign, where the convex surfaces of the articular processes face each other rather than the flat surfaces. Bilateral interfacetal dislocation results from severe flexion force to the head and neck causing anterior displacement of the spine and ligamentous disruption at the level of the injury. The dislocated facet joints are either perched on or jumped over one another

to become locked. There is subluxation of the vertebral body by more than 50%, and both the anterior and posterior ligamentous structures are disrupted at the site of the injury with fracture of the superior and inferior articular facets and disc extrusion. Bilateral interfacetal dislocation is associated with compression fractures of the subjacent vertebrae and/or disc herniation at the level of the injury. In addition, there is a high degree of neurologic injury with this type of spinal injury. These are highly unstable injuries. A study by Carrino et al. of patients with bilateral facet dislocation demonstrated the following associated injuries: anterior longitudinal ligament abnormality (26.7%), disc herniation or disruption (90%), posterior longitudinal ligament disruption (40%), facet fracture (63.3%), and disruption of the posterior column ligament complex (97%) [19].

Case 7–21
Clay shoveler fracture C7

(A)

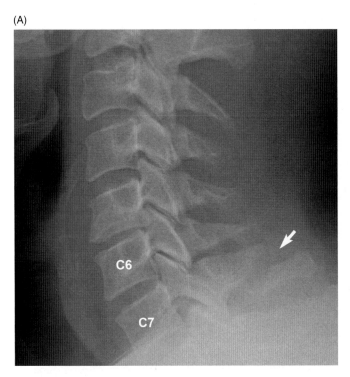

(B)

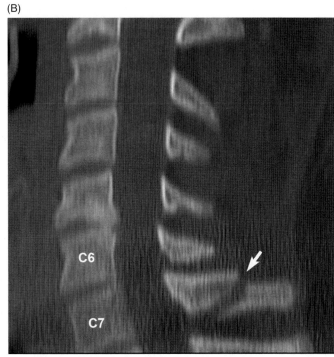

(C)

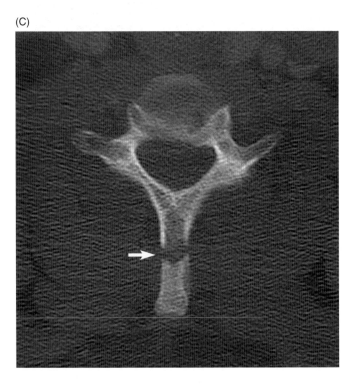

44-year-old man with neck pain after motor vehicle crash. Lateral radiograph (A) and sagittal CT (B) of the cervical spine; axial CT (C) through C7. The lateral radiograph and sagittal CT show an avulsion fracture (arrow) of the spinous process of C7. Axial CT confirms only the fracture of the spinous process (arrow). The clay shoveler fracture is an oblique avulsion fracture of a lower spinous process, typically from C6 to T1. This fracture originated from laborers who sustained this pattern of injury when shoveling clay out of ditches. The sudden strenuous exertion of the paraspinal muscles – mainly the trapezius, rhomboid, and supraspinous ligament – results in an avulsion of the spinous process. The clay shoveler fracture is considered a stable fracture.

Case 7–22
Ankylosing spondylitis with fracture C5

(A)

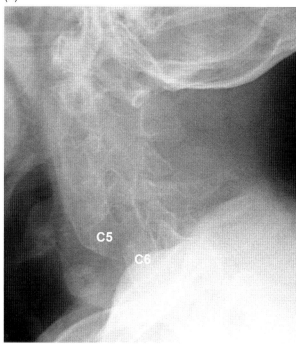

50-year-old man with ankylosing spondylitis who was injured in a fall. Lateral radiograph of the cervical spine. There is fusion of the entire cervical spine with ossification of the anterior longitudinal ligament along its entire length, and posterior element and interbody fusion of the upper segments. There is profound osteopenia. There is fracture through the C5 vertebra with anterior displacement of nearly 100%.

(B)

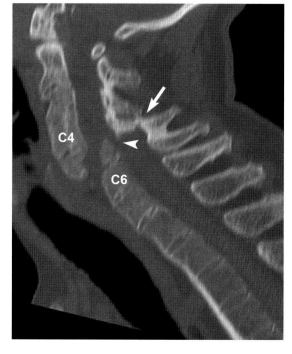

Sagittal CT of the cervical spine. There are features of longstanding ankylosing spondylitis, with complete fusion of the vertebral bodies and fusion of the upper cervical posterior elements. The fracture extends through the C5 body and exits posterior between C4 and C5 (arrow). The upper cervical spine is translated anteriorly by nearly one vertebral body, resulting in severe bony compromise of the spinal canal at C4-C5 (arrowhead).

(C)

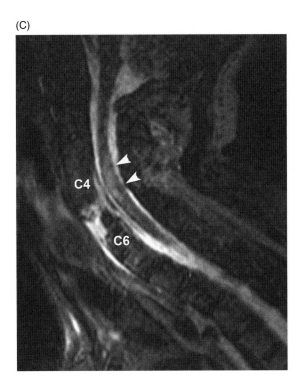

Sagittal STIR MRI of the cervical spine following reduction and external stabilization. There is severe compromise of the vertebral canal and there is extensive cord contusion. Anklyosis of the spine results in a rigid, fragile vertebral column that is vulnerable to low-energy trauma and may even fail under physiologic loads [20–21]. The appearance of fractures may be subtle on radiographs because of osteopenia.

Case 7–23

Diffuse idiopathic skeletal hyperostosis with fracture C5-C6

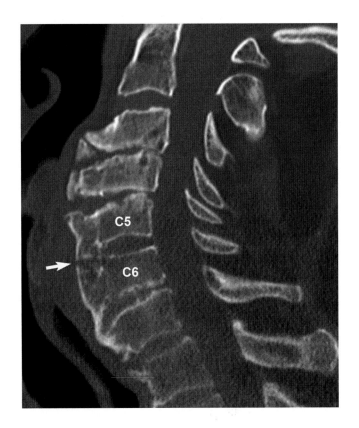

67-year-old man with diffuse idiopathic skeletal hyperostosis (DISH) who was injured in ground-level fall. Sagittal CT of the cervical spine. There is diffuse hyperostosis along the anterior cervical spine with a thick layer of bone. A minimally displaced fracture (arrow) is present through the anterior phyte bridging C5 and C6, with posterior extension below the superior endplate. There has been no translation of the vertebral column, nor compromise of the spinal canal. Patients who have spine fusion from DISH are vulnerable to low-energy trauma such as ground-level falls [22].

References

1. Roche C, Carty H. Spinal trauma in children. *Pediatr Radiol*. 2001 Oct;31(10):677–700. PMID: 11685436.

2. Maves CK, Souza A, Prenger EC, Kirks DR. Traumatic atlanto-occipital disruption in children. *Pediatr Radiol*. 1991;21(7):504–7. PMID: 1771115.

3. Astur N, Sawyer JR, Klimo P Jr, Kelly DM, Muhlbauer M, Warner WC Jr. Traumatic atlanto-occipital dislocation in children. *J Am Acad Orthop Surg*. 2014 May;22(5):274–82. doi: 10.5435/JAAOS-22-05-274. PMID: 24788443.

4. Looby S, Flanders A. Spine trauma. *Radiol Clin North Am*. 2011 Jan;49(1):129–63. doi: 10.1016/j.rcl.2010.07.019. PMID: 21111133.

5. Pratt H, Davies E, King L. Traumatic injuries of the C1/C2 complex: Computed tomographic imaging appearances. *Curr Probl Diagn Radiol*. 2008 Jan–Feb;37(1):26–38. PMID: 18054664.

6. Clark CR, White AA III. Fractures of the dens. A multicenter study. *J Bone Joint Surg Am*. 1985 Dec;67(9):1340–8. PMID: 4077905.

7. Roberts A, Wickstrom J. Prognosis of odontoid fractures. *Acta Orthop Scand*. 1973;44(1):21–30. PMID: 4702606.

8. Effendi B, Roy D, Cornish B, Dussault RG, Laurin CA. Fractures of the ring of the axis. A classification based on the analysis of 131 cases. *J Bone Joint Surg Br*. 1981;63-B(3):319–27. PMID: 7263741.

9. Edeiken-Monroe B, Wagner LK, Harris JH Jr. Hyperextension dislocation of the cervical spine. *AJR Am J Roentgenol*. 1986 Apr;146(4):803–8. PMID: 3485356.

10. Rao SK, Wasyliw C, Nunez DB Jr. Spectrum of imaging findings in hyperextension injuries of the neck. *Radiographics*. 2005 Sep–Oct;25(5):1239–54. PMID: 16160109.

11. Cintron E, Gilula LA, Murphy WA, Gehweiler JA. The widened disk space: A sign of cervical hyperextension injury. *Radiology*. 1981 Dec;141(3):639–44. PMID: 7302217.

12. Davis SJ, Teresi LM, Bradley WG Jr, Ziemba MA, Bloze AE. Cervical spine hyperextension injuries: MR findings. *Radiology*. 1991 Jul;180(1):245–51. PMID: 2052703.

13. Webb JK, Broughton RB, McSweeney T, Park WM. Hidden flexion injury of the cervical spine. *J Bone Joint Surg Br*. 1976 Aug;58(3):322–7. PMID: 956249.

14. Stäbler A, Eck J, Penning R, Milz SP, Bartl R, Resnick D, Reiser M. Cervical spine: Postmortem assessment of accident injuries – Comparison of radiographic, MR imaging, anatomic, and pathologic findings. *Radiology*. 2001 Nov;221(2):340–6. PMID: 11687673.

15. Harris JH Jr, Edeiken-Monroe B, Kopaniky DR. A practical classification of acute cervical spine injuries. *Orthop Clin North Am*. 1986 Jan;17(1):15–30. PMID: 3511428.

16. Liang T, Tso DK, Chiu RY, Nicolaou S. Imaging of blunt vascular neck injuries: A review of screening and imaging modalities. *AJR Am J Roentgenol*. 2013 Oct;201(4):884–92. doi: 10.2214/AJR.12.9664. PMID: 24059380.

17. Shanmuganathan K, Mirvis SE, Levine AM. Rotational injury of cervical facets: CT analysis of fracture patterns with implications for management and neurologic outcome. *AJR Am J Roentgenol*. 1994 Nov;163(5):1165–9. PMID: 7976894.

18. Lingawi SS. The naked facet sign. *Radiology*. 2001 May;219(2):366–7. PMID: 11323458.

19. Carrino JA, Manton GL, Morrison WB, Vaccaro AR, Schweitzer ME, Flanders AE. Posterior longitudinal ligament status in cervical spine bilateral facet dislocations. *Skeletal Radiol*. 2006 Jul;35(7):510–4. Epub 2006 Mar 25. PMID: 16565835.

20. Caron T, Bransford R, Nguyen Q, Agel J, Chapman J, Bellabarba C. Spine fractures in patients with ankylosing spinal disorders. *Spine (Phila Pa 1976)*. 2010 May 15;35(11):E458–64. doi: 10.1097/BRS.0b013e3181cc764f. PMID: 20421858.

21. Wang YF, Teng MM, Chang CY, Wu HT, Wang ST. Imaging manifestations of spinal fractures in ankylosing spondylitis. *AJNR Am J Neuroradiol*. 2005 Sep;26(8):2067–76. PMID: 16155161.

22. Taljanovic MS, Hunter TB, Wisneski RJ, Seeger JF, Friend CJ, Schwartz SA, Rogers LF. Imaging characteristics of diffuse idiopathic skeletal hyperostosis with an emphasis on acute spinal fractures: Review. *AJR Am J Roentgenol*. 2009 Sep;193(3 Suppl):S10–9, Quiz S20–4. doi: 10.2214/AJR.07.7102. PMID: 19696239.

Fractures and dislocations of the thoracolumbosacral spine

Refky Nicola, D.O., Felix S. Chew, M.D., and Catherine Maldjian, M.D.

Case 8–1

Hyperextension fracture-dislocation T4-T5

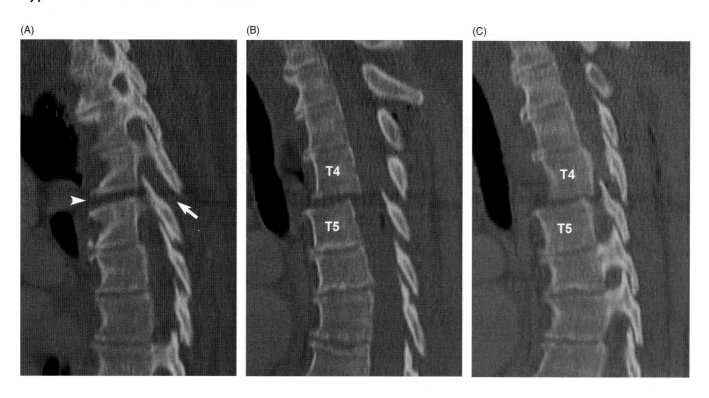

(A) (B) (C)

73-year-old woman in high-speed motor vehicle crash. Sagittal CT of the upper thoracic spine (left to right). There is retrolisthesis of T4 on T5 with widening of the facet joints (arrow) and widening of the anterior intervertebral disc space (arrowhead). There are multilevel underlying degenerative changes. This is a hyperextension fracture-dislocation injury. This injury is rare and usually grossly unstable. T4-T5 and T5-T6 constitute the most common locations for thoracic spine fracture-dislocations [1]. (Source: Chew FS. Skeletal Radiology: The Bare Bones. 3rd Edition. Copyright © 2010 by Felix Chew.)

Case 8–2

Thoracic spine fracture-dislocation T10-T11

(A)

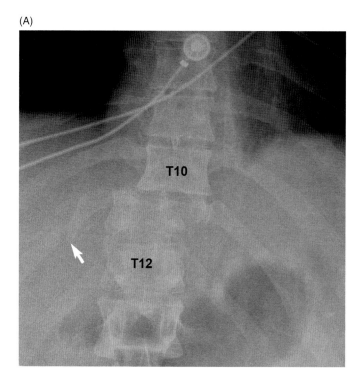

(B)

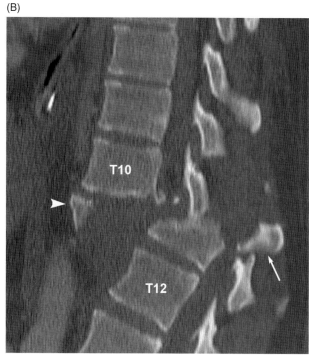

35-year-old man in high-speed motor vehicle crash. AP radiograph (A) and sagittal CT (B) of the lower thoracic spine. The AP radiograph shows gross lateral misalignment of the spine at T10-T11. The left eleventh rib has stayed with T10, while the right eleventh rib is fractured (arrow) but has stayed with T11, indicating the severity of the T11 fractures. The sagittal CT shows gross anterior dislocation of T10 over T11 and complete obliteration of the spinal canal. An anterior superior avulsion fragment of T11 has remained with T10 (arrowhead). The T10 spinous process (long arrow) has been avulsed. This is a flexion distraction injury. All three columns are disrupted, the anterior column on the compression side and the middle and posterior column on the tensile side. The ligamentum flavum, interspinous ligaments, and supraspinous ligaments are disrupted. When all three columns are disrupted from shear forces, dislocation can occur. The extent of translational injury or dislocation determines the degree of instability. In fracture-dislocations of the thoracic spine caused by flexion injury, the three main forces are axial compression, axial distraction, and translation. Compression and distraction may occur simultaneously at the opposite sides of the same level. Displacement of the spinal column, as seen in this case, indicates a translational component.

Case 8–3 Hyperflexion injury T3-T4

(A)

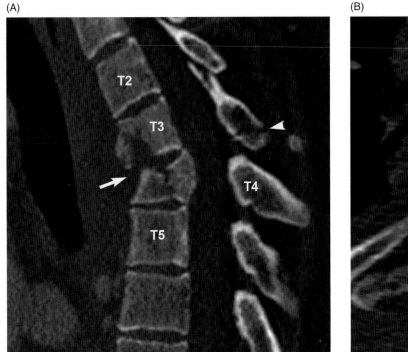

(B)

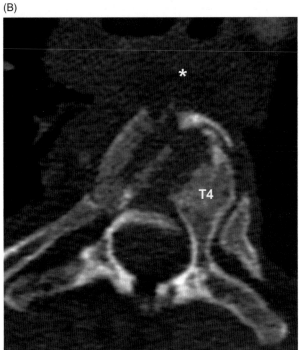

45-year-old woman who crashed her motorcycle into a guardrail at 50 mph. Sagittal CT (A) of the upper thoracic spine and axial CT (B) of T4. There are fractures of T3 and T4. The T3 fracture involves the body and extends into the posterior elements, including the spinous process (arrowhead). The T4 fracture is a burst fracture that has resulted in loss of approximately 30% height and mild retropulsion. The T4 body is split into multiple fragments and the posterior elements are involved. There is a prevertebral hematoma (*) at T3-T4 displacing the esophagus.

(C)　　　　　　　　　　　(D)

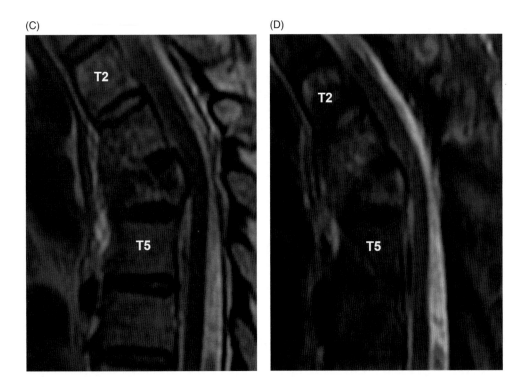

Sagittal T2 (C) and STIR (D) MRI of the upper thoracic spine. There is diffuse bone marrow edema within the vertebral bodies T3 and T4 with mild retropulsion. There is disruption of the anterior longitudinal ligament, posterior longitudinal ligament, and disc space of T3-T4, However, there is no cord edema. Robertson [2] compared spine injuries in motorcycles and cars and found thoracic spine injuries were more common in motorcyclists, whereas cervical spine injuries were more common in car occupants. The most common site of injury in motorcyclists was mid-thoracic, whereas the most common site in car occupants was upper cervical [2]. Thoracic spine injuries in motorcyclists occur with hyperflexion [3]. Axial loading is concentrated at the point of maximal flexion and results in injuries predominantly in the mid-thoracic spine (T4-T7), with T6 being the most common location [4].

Case 8–4
Fracture-dislocation T5-T6

(A)

(B)

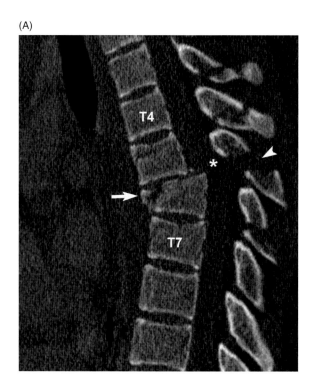
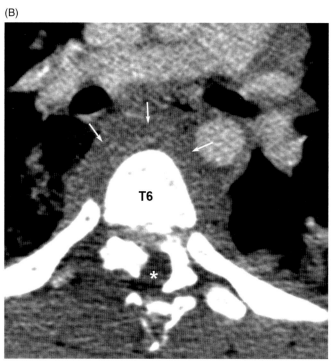

17-year-old woman who was ejected during a motor vehicle crash. Sagittal CT (A) of mid-thoracic spine and axial CT (B) at T6. There is anterior subluxation of T5 on T6 with compression fracture involving the superior endplate of T5 and compression fracture of T6 (arrow). There is a widely displaced spinous process fracture of T5 (arrowhead) that indicates a flexion-distraction mechanism of injury. There are also fractures of the spinous process of T3, T4, and T6. The spinal canal narrowing (*) caused by the anterior subluxation of T5 on T6 is concerning for transection of the cord, with spinal canal narrowing confirmed on the axial CT. There is prevertebral hematoma (long arrows). The patient had an ASIA A spinal cord injury at T5.

(C)

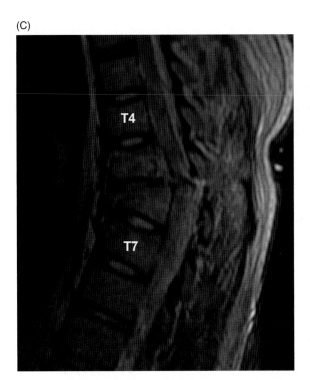

(D)

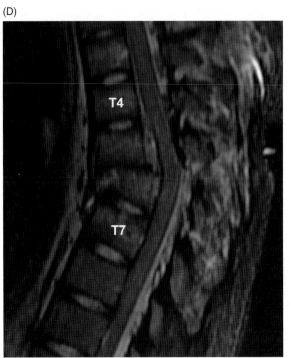

Sagittal T2 (C) and STIR (D) MRI of the mid-thoracic spine. There is anterior subluxation of T5 on T6 with disruption of the anterior longitudinal, posterior longitudinal, intraspinous, and interspinous ligaments. There is spinal cord edema. There is also hyper-intense signal within the paraspinal muscles from T4 to T7. Fracture-dislocation injuries result from compression and/or distraction forces combined with some degree of shear or rotation [5]. These injuries are unstable and have the highest incidence of complete neurologic injury of any of the thoracolumbar injury patterns [5]. The most common location is the thoracolumbar junction. Pickett et al. [6] looked at spinal cord injuries in Canada between 1997 and 2001 and found the most common cause of spinal cord injuries was motor vehicle collisions, whereas the second most common cause was falls. Car crashes were more frequently seen in younger patients, whereas ground-level falls were more frequently seen in elderly patients. Complete spinal cord injuries were most closely associated with burst fractures and bilateral facet fracture-dislocations [7]. A recent study of patients with thoracic and lumbar spine injuries from motor vehicle collisions from the Crash Injury Research and Engineering Network (CIREN) database identified 57.5% of the injuries with compression fractures, 24.9% with burst fractures, 8.8% with flexion-distraction injuries, 2.4% with flexion-dislocation injuries, and 6.4% with extension injuries [8].

Case 8–5

Compression fracture T12

(A)

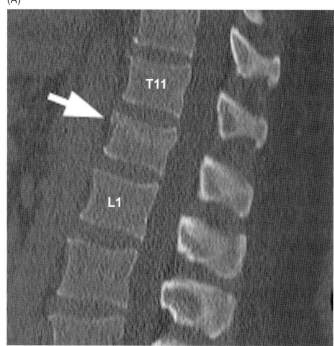

44-year-old man whose motorcycle collided at high speed with a deer. Sagittal CT of the thoracolumbar junction. There is a wedge compression fracture at the superior endplate body of T12 (arrow). The posterior elements are not distracted, and there is no translation of T12 over L1.

(B)

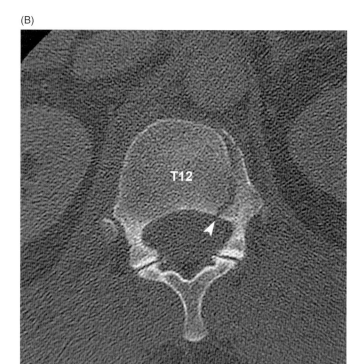

(C)

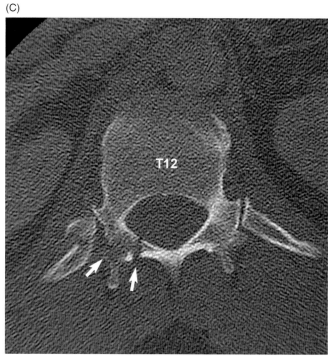

Axial CT at T12, superior (B) and inferior (C). A wedge compression fracture can be seen along the left lateral aspect of the superior endplate of T12 (arrowheads). There are comminuted fractures involving the right costovertebral junction, right twelfth rib, right pedicle, and right lamina. No translational component is present and the spinal canal is patient and unobstructed. This is likely an axial compression injury in which the vertebral body failed on the left and the posterior elements failed on the right.

Case 8–6
Hyperflexion fracture-dislocation T9-T10

(A)   (B)   (C)

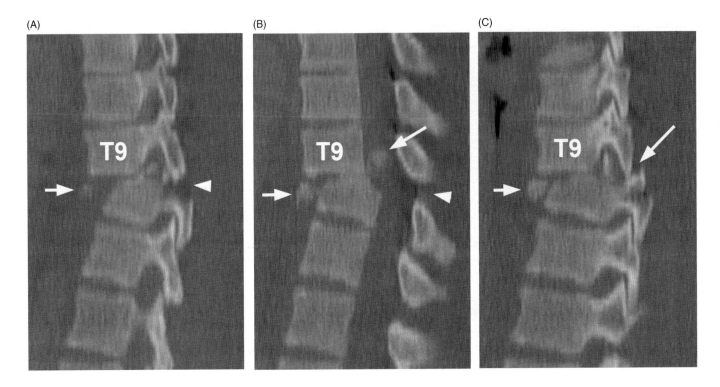

17-year-old man who was ejected from his vehicle during a motor vehicle collision. He was unrestrained. Sagittal CT of the lower thoracic spine, right (A) to left (C). There is a comminuted burst fracture of the T10 vertebral body (short arrows) with retropulsion of fragments. The fracture extends through the posterior elements (arrowheads). There is anterolisthesis of T9 over T10, and focal kyphosis. The retropulsed fragment (long arrow) occupies the spinal canal and the patient has a complete spinal cord transection. These injuries are consistent with a hyperflexion fracture-dislocation pattern. The posterior column fails under tension while the anterior and middle columns fail under compression. (Source: Chew FS. Skeletal Radiology: The Bare Bones. 3rd Edition. Copyright © 2010 by Felix Chew.)

Case 8–7
Distraction/shearing injury T11-T12

(A)

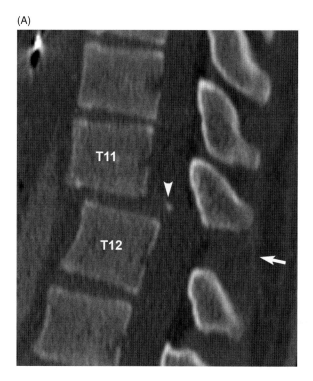

(B)

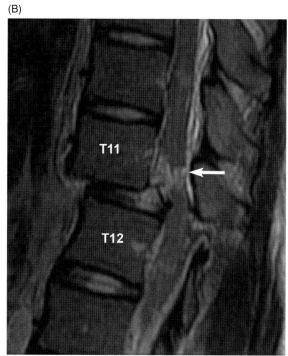

19-year-old man who crashed his car into a telephone pole that then fell onto his vehicle. Sagittal CT (A) and T2 MRI (B) of the lower thoracic spine. There is anterior translation of T11 over T12. The anterior disc space of T11-T12 is narrowed, while their spinous processes are splayed apart (short arrow). There is a small avulsion fracture of the posterior inferior margin of the T11 body (arrowhead). There is extensive edema and hemorrhage in the spinal cord (long arrow).

(C)

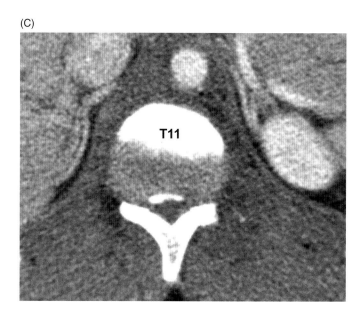

(D)

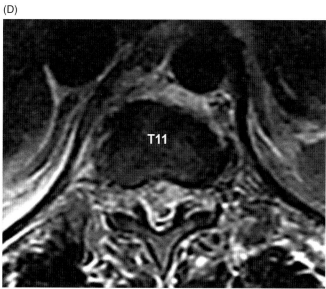

Axial CT (C) and T2 MRI (D) at T11. There is disruption of the anterior and posterior longitudinal ligaments as well as hyper-intense signal within the spinal cord at the level of T11. There was also hemorrhage at the level of the transection, which is not well visualized on these images. In a study of 100 patients with thoracolumbar spine fractures, Hsu et al. demonstrated that imaging was required in patients with high-energy injuries who met any of the following criteria: back pain/midline tenderness, local signs of thoracolumbar spine injuries, abnormal neurologic signs, cervical spine fractures, GCS less than 15, major distracting injury, and ETOH/drug intoxication [9]. In a study of 407 trauma patients in Korea, of which 123 were intoxicated and 284 were not, there was no significant correlation between alcohol consumption and spine injury severity although head and face injuries appeared worse [10]. Cord transection is evident on T2 MRI as interruption of the normal low-signal intensity of the cord. Frequently, a post-traumatic syrinx will develop months or years after the injury to the spinal cord. This begins as myelomalacia, which represents a softening of the cord as a result of the injury, eventually coalescing to form larger cyst or syrinx. However, it is important to distinguish myelomalacia from syrinx, as the syrinx can be shunted to restore neurologic function, but the myelomalacia cannot be shunted and does not respond to surgery. Spinal cord atrophy may also occur [11].

Case 8–8

Diffuse idiopathic skeletal hyperostosis with fracture T7

(A) (B) (C)

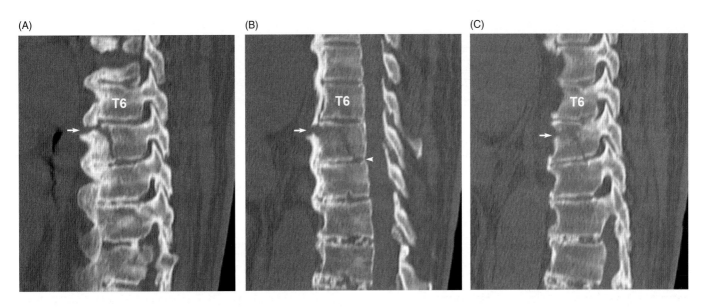

82-year-old man injured in ground-level fall. Sagittal CT of the mid-thoracic spine, right (A) to left (C). There is diffuse idiopathic skeletal hyperostosis (DISH) with flowing ossification of the anterior longitudinal ligament bridging the vertebral bodies at multiple contiguous levels. The intervertebral disc spaces are not narrowed, although several are calcified. At T6-T7, there is a horizontal fracture through bridging phytes (arrows) that extends in the axial plane through the T7 vertebral body, just inferior to the superior endplate, and then passes in the coronal plane to the posterior portion of T7-T8 disc space (arrowhead).

There is mild lordotic angulation at the fracture site, in keeping with an extension mechanism of injury. The posterior elements are intact, and the facet joints are not ankylosed. This patient also sustained a C7 fracture (not shown). Spine fractures through DISH were first described in the cervical region [12] and later described in the thoracic region [13]. Rigidity of the spine predisposes it to fracture with minimal trauma, usually by hyperextension mechanism. Associated neurologic injuries are common.

Case 8–9
Ankylosing spondylitis with fracture T7

(A)

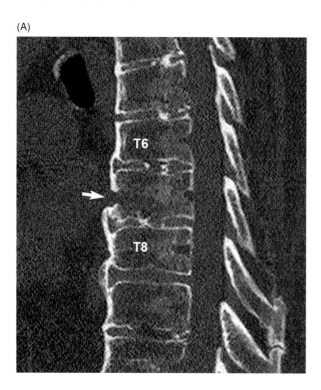

86-year-old man fell backward down the stairs. Sagittal CT of the mid-thoracic spine. There is a non-displaced fracture line through the vertebral body of T7 (arrow). There is diffuse osteopenia throughout the thoracic spine. There is ossification of the spinal ligaments, joints, and discs at multiple levels. There is no evidence of retropulsion or narrowing of the spinal canal.

(B)

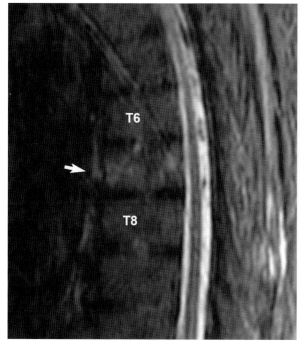

Sagittal T2 MRI of the mid-thoracic spine. There is diffuse bone marrow edema and fracture through the vertebral body of T7 (arrow). There is no spinal cord edema. Fractures of the ankylosed spine can occur with minor trauma owing to rigidity and osteoporosis [14–15]. One study found the prevalence of vertebral fractures among patients with ankylosing spondylitis to be approximately 19% [16]. The incidence of spinal cord injury in spine trauma patients with underlying ankylosing spondylitis is 2% [17]. Caron et al. [18] found a 32% mortality rate following a traumatic fracture through an ankylosed spine (including both ankylosing spondylitis and DISH).

Case 8–10
Chance fracture L1

(A)

(B)

(C)

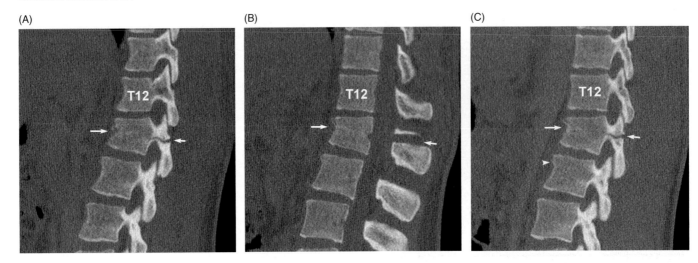

17-year-old man who fell from a 30-foot height and landed upright on his buttocks. Sagittal CT of the thoracolumbar junction, right (A) to left (C). There is a fracture in the axial plane extending through the L1 vertebral body (long arrows) and pedicles and into the spinous process (short arrows). There is mild focal kyphosis with minimal anterior wedging of the vertebral body. There is a mild compression fracture of the anterior superior corner of the L2 vertebral body (arrowhead). The Chance fracture pattern is caused by flexion-distraction without compression [19]. It is a horizontal fracture through the vertebral body and posterior elements, typically sustained in motor vehicle crash with a lap belt (but neither shoulder belt, nor airbag). It has been described as a fulcrum fracture because the seat belt acts as a fulcrum and absorbs the flexion or compression force and the spine, being posterior to the fulcrum, sustains the tensile forces through all its columns, thereby making it a distraction injury [20–21]. In a conventional flexion distraction type injury, the anterior column of the spine acts as the fulcrum and absorbs the compressive forces that leads to significant anterior wedging, a finding that is not typically seen with Chance fractures.

(D)

(E)

(F)

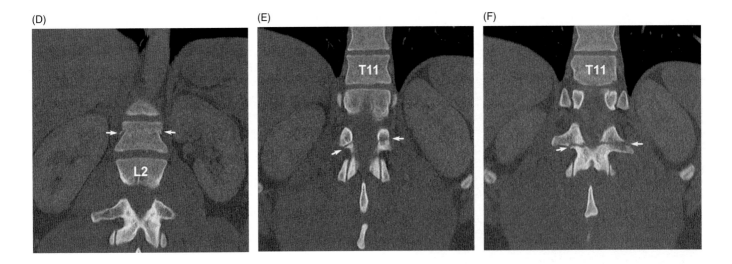

Coronal CT of the thoracolumbar junction, anterior (D) to posterior (F). Three patterns are seen with Chance fractures and variants. One involves disruption of the posterior ligaments and facet joints and posterior disc. Another involves a horizontal fracture through the posterior elements. The third is a horizontal fracture that dissects through the posterior elements and vertebral body. When a compression deformity occurs it is confined to the anterior superior part of the vertebral body. Associated bowel, pancreas, and mesenteric injury can be seen 15–20% of the time [21].

(G)

(H)

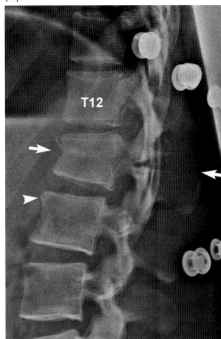

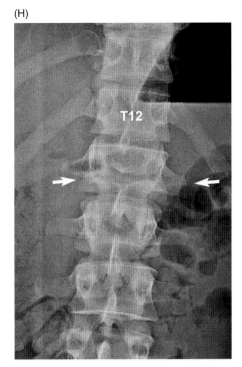

Lateral (G) and AP (H) radiographs of the thoracolumbar junction. The patient has been mobilized and is wearing a brace. The fracture plane (arrows) extends through the body and posterior elements of L1, with minimal impaction anteriorly and persistent distraction posteriorly. The fracture at the anterior superior corner of the L2 body is visible (arrowhead).

Case 8–11
Chance fracture L1

(A)

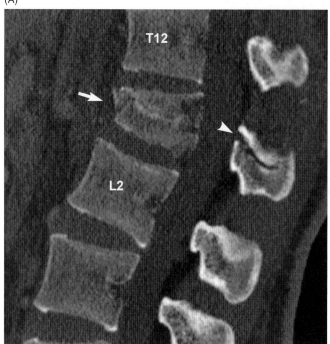

(B)

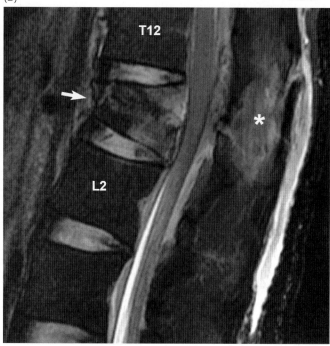

23-year-old man who rolled his car into a ditch. Sagittal CT (A) and T2 MRI (B) of the thoracolumbar junction. There is a horizontally oriented fracture through the vertebral body of L1 with loss of approximately 50% height (arrow) with fractures extending into the right pedicle, lamina, and spinous process

(arrowhead). MRI shows the L1 vertebral body fracture (arrow) and marrow edema within the vertebral body. There is extensive edema in the posterior elements and posterior paraspinal soft tissue, including the interspinous ligaments (*).

(C)

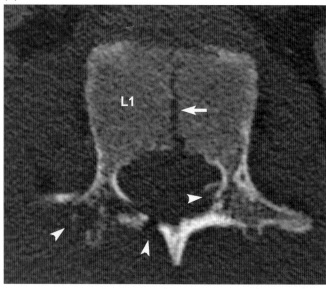

Axial CT at L1. There is a fracture of the vertebral body, right pedicle, lamina, and spinous process of L1. No retropulsion is identified. The Chance fracture was first described by Q. Chance in 1948 [19], but it was not until 1965 that Howland et al. related these fractures to use of lap belts during motor vehicle accidents [22]. The most common locations are between T11 and L2. However, with the advent of the three-point safety belts in the late 1960s, seat belt injuries became less common [23]. The indications for surgery include ligamentous involvement of the posterior column or initial kyphotic angulation more than 15 degrees [24–26].

Case 8–12

Thoracolumbar flexion-distraction injury

(A) (B) (C)

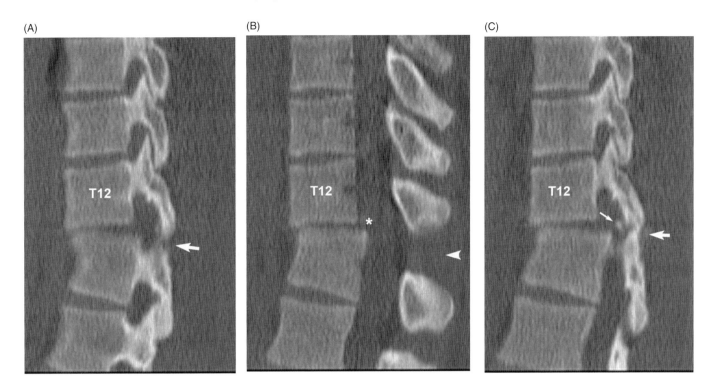

35-year-old man injured on a construction site when he fell 12 feet while inspecting a pipe. Sagittal CT of the thoracolumbar junction, right (A) to left (C). On both the right and the left, the facet joints at T12-L1 are perched (short arrows), with distraction evident between the spinous processes in the midline (arrowheads). There is a small posterior element fracture fragment visible on the right side within the neural foramen. There is mild compression of the superior endplate of L1 (long arrows) with narrowing of the intervertebral disc space anteriorly. There is anterolisthesis of T11 over L1 (*), mildly compromising the spinal canal. There is a mild kyphosis at the T12-L1 level.

Case 8–13

Superior endplate compression fracture T12

(A)

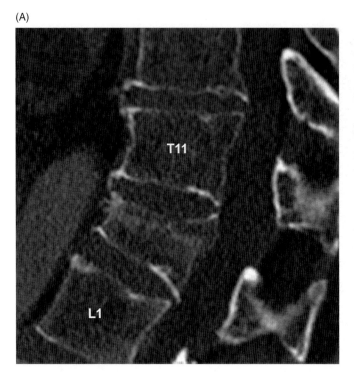

(B)

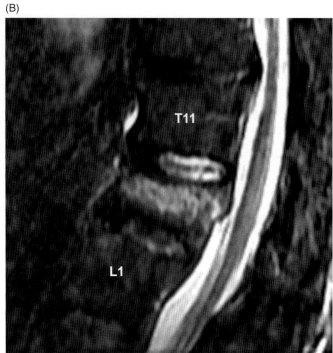

(C)

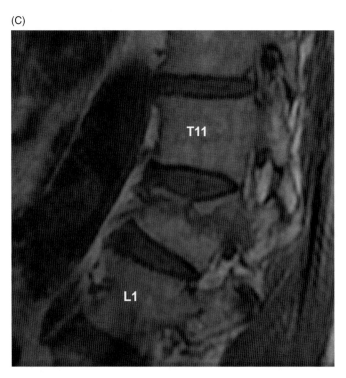

68-year-old man injured when an all-terrain vehicle fell on top of him. Sagittal CT (A) and STIR (B) and T1 (C) MRI of the thoracolumbar junction. There is a compression fracture of the superior endplate of T12 with approximately 30–40% loss of height. No retropulsion is identified. MRI demonstrates compression fracture of the superior endplate of T12 with high bone marrow signal, consistent with bone marrow edema in an acute fracture. There is no associated posterior distraction injury. This patient had no neurologic deficit. Anterior wedge compression fractures account for almost 50% of all thoracolumbar fractures [7]. The mechanism of injury typically involves axial loading with or without an element of flexion. The two populations that are commonly associated with compression fractures are trauma patients and osteoporosis patients. Compression fractures primarily involve the anterior cortex and retropulsion is infrequent. The fracture is often not well visualized on axial CT images because the axial plane is parallel to the fracture line. However, the fracture should be clearly seen on the sagittal and coronal reformatted CT images. On MRI, vertebral body bone marrow edema should suggest an acute fracture.

Case 8–14
Compression fractures of multiple vertebral bodies

(A)

(B)

(C)

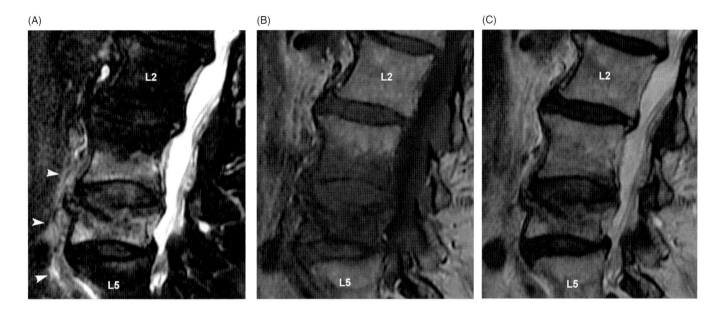

91-year-old woman with progressive weakness in the hips. Sagittal STIR (A), T1 (B), and T2 (C) MRI of the mid-lumbar spine. There is a compression fracture of the inferior endplate of L3 with 50% height loss. There is bone marrow edema at the inferior endplates of the L3 and L4 vertebral bodies. No retropulsion is identified. There were no neurologic deficits. Vertebral compression fractures are often multiple and are common and painful features associated with osteoporosis, a condition affecting 25% of women aged 70 or older and 40% of women aged 80 or older. Osteoporosis affects 33% of men aged 75 or older [27]. The typical appearance of osteoporotic compression fractures is anterior wedging of the vertebral bodies in the mid-thoracic, lower thoracic, and upper lumbar regions. This is considered significant when the anterior height is less than 80% of the posterior height [28]. Osteoporotic vertebral fractures typically have no cortical break when acute and lack significant fracture callus when healing. Involvement of multiple levels can lead to kyphosis, reducing pulmonary capacity and impairing physical activity. Osteoporotic fractures typically result from minimal trauma. The most frequent management is conservative treatment. However, persistent neurologic symptoms from cord compression may require surgical decompression [28].

Case 8–15

Osteoporotic compression fractures

(A) (B) (C)

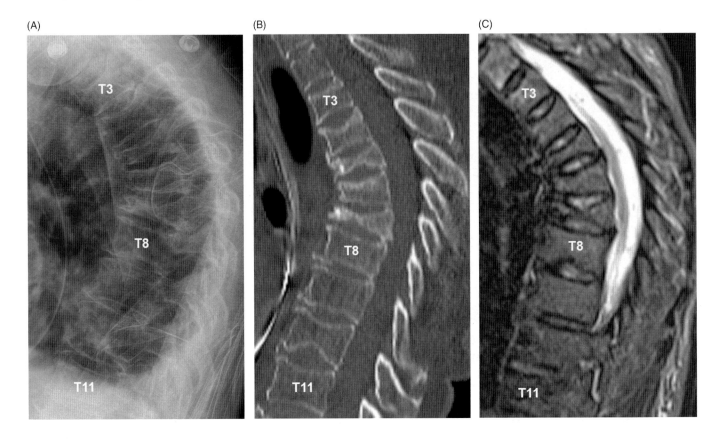

68-year-old woman with back pain and increasing kyphosis. Lateral radiograph (A), sagittal CT (B), sagittal T2 MRI (C) of the thoracic spine. Lateral thoracic spine radiograph shows multiple osteoporotic compression fractures. The CT scan shows involvement of T4-T7 and T10. The T2 MRI shows no bone marrow edema at any of these levels, indicating that these fractures are not acute. The treatment of osteoporotic vertebral compression fractures by percutaneous vertebroplasty, while commonly done, does not appear to have better outcomes for patients than placebo [29].

Case 8–16
Burst fracture L1

(A)

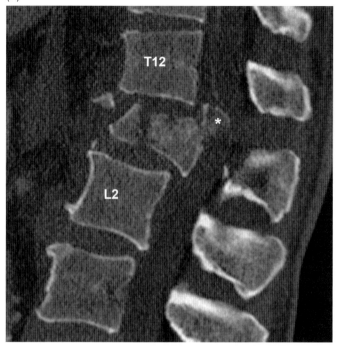

(B)

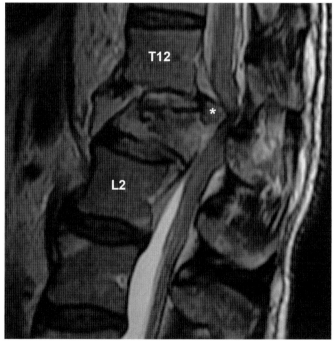

(C)

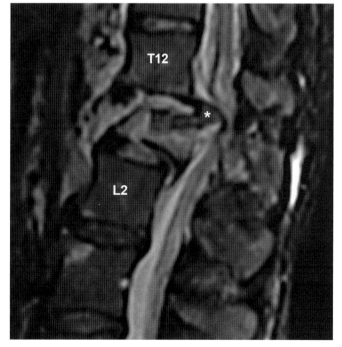

54-year-old man who was hit by a car and ejected 30 feet from his motorcycle. Sagittal CT of the thoracolumbar junction. There is a comminuted fracture of the vertebral body of L1 with greater than 50% loss of height and retropulsion of a posterior fragment that compromises the spinal canal. There is a prevertebral hematoma.

Sagittal T2 (B) and STIR (C) MRI of the thoracolumbar junction. There is disruption of the anterior longitudinal, posterior longitudinal, and interspinous ligaments at L1. There is also edema within the cord. Burst fractures result from severe axial loading [30] and consequent failure of the anterior and middle columns under compression. However, the unstable burst fracture also involves the posterior column [30]. There is a greater degree of neurologic impairment in patients with disruption of the posterior elements than in patients with intact posterior elements [31]. Meves et al. demonstrated a positive correlation between the degree of spinal canal narrowing and the presence and severity of neurologic deficits [32].

Case 8–17

Burst fracture L2 and multiple transverse process fractures

(A)

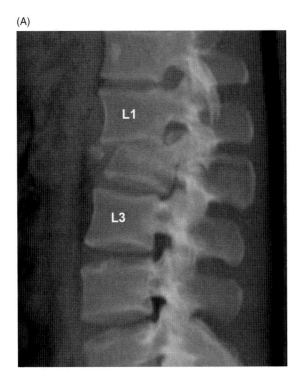

(B)

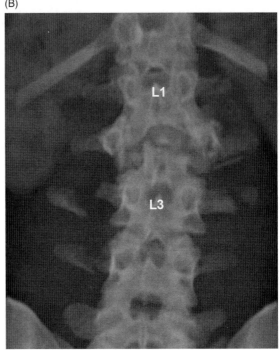

29-year-old man who was injured at a construction site when a wall collapsed onto his back. 3D volume-rendered sagittal (A) and coronal CT (B) of the lumbar spine. There is a comminuted fracture of the superior endplate and body of L2, with anterolisthesis of L1.

(C)

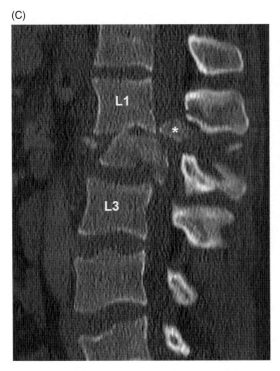

(D)

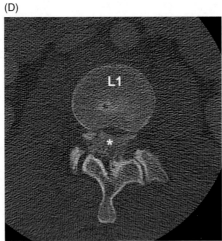

Sagittal CT (C) of the upper lumbar spine and axial CT (D) at L1. The fracture involves the entire L2 body as well as the posterior elements. There is a large fragment (*) of L2 that has been retropulsed into the spinal canal at the L1-L2 level, completely obliterating the spinal canal.

(E)

(F)

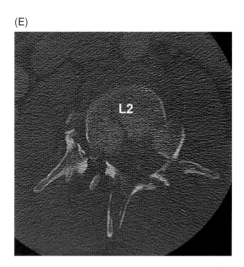

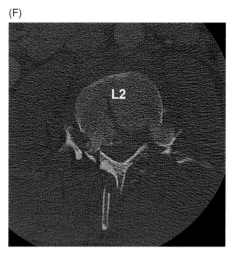

Axial CT of L2, superior (E) and inferior (F). There are fractures of the body and posterior elements of L2 with retropulsion of bone into the spinal canal. There is widening of the interpedicular distance. The spinal canal has been completely obliterated by the retropulsed fracture fragment. About 90% of burst fractures demonstrate a sagittal component [33]; 85% demonstrate sagittal fractures of the posterior elements, commonly at the spinolaminar junction. Sagittal fractures of the anterior and posterior columns lead to the interpedicular widening of more than 4 mm that is seen in 80% of these fractures and denotes an unstable injury [34]. Other signs of instability include greater than 50% compression of the vertebral body, translational component, and posterior element fractures.

Case 8–18

Transverse process fracture L2

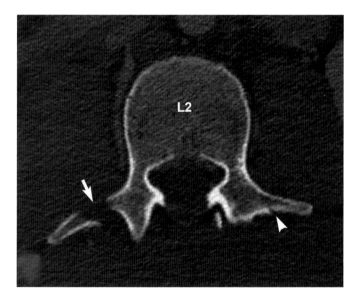

28-year-old man who was ejected during a motor vehicle crash. Axial CT of L2. There are fractures of the right (arrow) and left (arrowhead) transverse processes of L2. There were also other spine fractures (not shown). Fractures of the transverse processes occur secondary to a direct blow to the lumbar area, or can also be attributed to avulsion injuries caused by excessive muscular forces acting on the transverse processes. The two major muscles acting on the lumbar transverse processes are the quadratus lumborum, which originates from the twelfth rib and the tips of the transverse processes of L1-L5 and the psoas, which originates from the anterior surfaces of the lumbar transverse processes. These fractures are typically associated with rotary fracture-dislocations and seat belt injuries of the spine. Abdominal organ injuries have also been associated with transverse process fractures when associated with very large impacts or when deceleration/acceleration forces have been involved, but are infrequent when the transverse process fractures are the result of moderate energy blunt force. Miller et al. found that 48% of trauma patients with lumbar spine fractures that included transverse process fractures also had abdominal organ injuries while only 6% of those whose lumbar spine fractures did not include transverse process fractures also had abdominal organ injuries [35–37].

Case 8–19
Comminuted sacral fractures

(A)

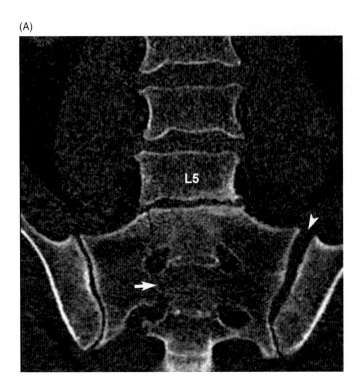

(B)

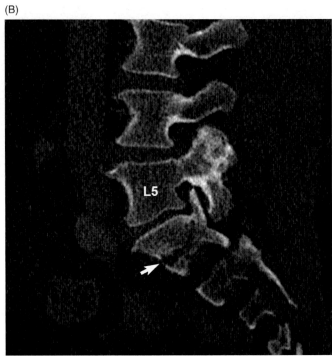

(C)

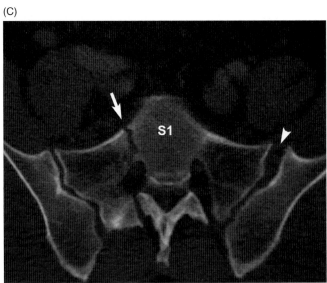

54-year-old male fell 15 feet from a tree and landed on his back. Coronal (A) and sagittal (B) CT of the lumbosacral junction and axial CT (C) of S1. There is a comminuted fracture (arrows) through the right sacral ala extending into the S1 and S2 neural foramina (Zone II), and widening of the left sacroiliac joint (arrowhead). There was also disruption of the pubic symphysis (not shown). Because of the location of lumbosacral plexus in regards to the sacrum, 25% of sacral fractures are associated with neurologic injury [38]. In the setting of pelvic ring trauma, sacral fractures may be classified using the Denis classification. Zone 1 fractures involve the sacral ala lateral to the sacral foramina and are rarely associated with neurologic deficit. Zone II fractures involve the sacral foramina and are often associated with neurologic deficit, which may present as unilateral lumbar or sacral radiculopathies. Zone III fractures involve the sacral canal and often present with significant bilateral neurologic damage [39].

Case 8–20

Spinopelvic dissociation

(A)

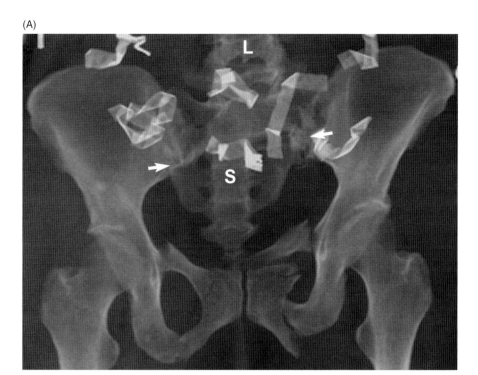

41-year-old woman injured in a high-speed automobile crash. 3D volume-rendered CT of the pelvis. Volume-rendered anterior projection from CT shows misalignment of the lumbar spine (L) and S1 with the lower sacrum (S). There are transverse fractures (arrows) separating S1 from the lower sacrum. There is fracture-dislocation of the left hemi-pelvis and bilateral fractures of the superior and inferior pubic rami, more displaced on the left. The radiopaque ribbons overlying the upper pelvis indicate surgical packing material placed following the emergent laparotomy that preceded the CT scan.

(B)

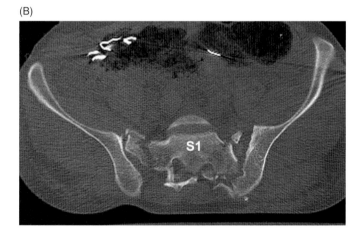

Axial CT at the S1 level. There are highly comminuted fractures of the sacrum involving bilateral ala, bilateral neural foramina, and the posterior neural arch. There is an axial component of the fracture that traverses the entire sacrum (not shown). The left SI joint is dislocated with posterior iliac avulsion fractures, and the right SI joint is subluxated.

(C)

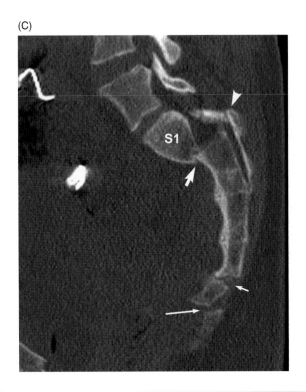

Sagittal CT of the lumbosacral junction near the midline. There is a transverse fracture at S1 extending from the body (arrow) to the posterior elements (arrowhead) with nearly 100% posterior displacement of the inferior fragment. The inferior fragment is impacted into the superior fragment. This fracture forms the horizontal limb of an H-shaped sacral fracture that separates the spine from the pelvis. There has been anterior angulation at S4-S5 (small arrow), and there is also injury of the coccyx with posterior subluxation (long arrow). U-shaped sacral fractures may also result in spinopelvic dissociation. Typical treatment would be internal fixation of the lumbar spine, sacrum, and iliac wings [40–41].

Case 8–21
Bilateral sacral wing fractures

(A)

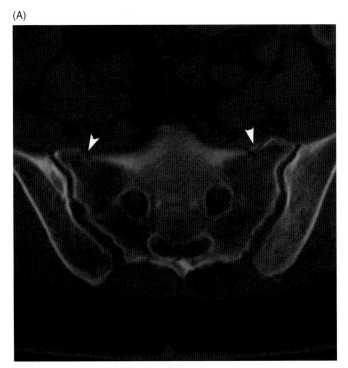

(B)

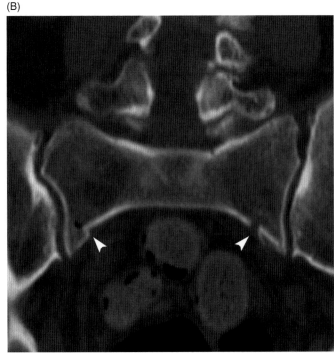

63-year-old woman with a ground-level fall. Axial (A) and coronal (B) CT of the sacrum. There are fractures (arrowheads) of the right and left sacral ala that are slightly medial to the sacroiliac joints and minimally displaced. Because the bones are diffusely demineralized and the trauma was low energy, these may be considered fragility fractures. Vertical sacral wing fractures (such as in this patient) may occur from vertical shear, when the patient sits too hard or falls into a sitting position. In older adults, fragility fractures of the pelvis are more common than high-energy fractures [42].

Case 8–22
Comminuted coccyx fracture

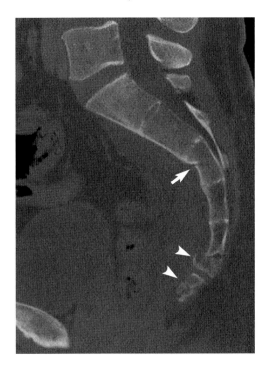

38-year-old-man in a BASE (building, antenna, span, or earth) jumping accident. Midline sagittal CT of the sacrum and coccyx. There is a comminuted fracture of the coccyx involving two levels (arrowheads). There is also an anteriorly impacted fracture of S3 (arrow). BASE jumping with a parachute, wingsuit, or other device is a recreational activity that has a five- to eightfold risk of injury or death compared with skydiving [43], estimated at one severe injury (or death) per 500 jumps [44].

Case 8–23
Coccyx fracture

(A)

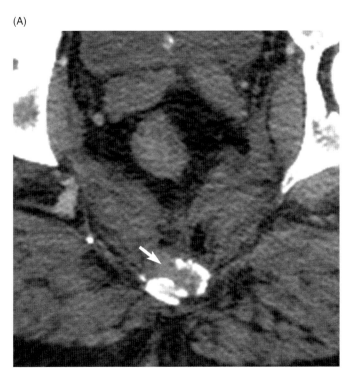

(B)

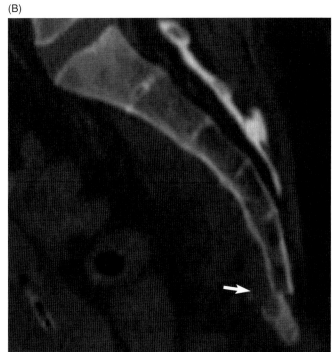

34-year-old man with polytrauma following an all-terrain vehicle crash into a tree. Axial CT (A) of the coccyx and midline sagittal CT (B) of the sacrum and coccyx. There is a fracture of the distal coccyx with anterior displacement of the distal fracture fragment and surrounding hematoma (arrows). Isolated fractures of the coccyx may occur as a result of a fall into the seated position or during a difficult vaginal childbirth. The muscles of the levator ani and several pelvic floor ligaments attach to the coccyx, making immobilization for healing difficult. Treatment is generally limited to analgesics, air cushions, stool softeners, local steroid injections, and time [45–46].

References

1. Hanley EN Jr, Eskay ML. Thoracic spine fractures. *Orthopedics*. 1989 May;12(5):689–96. PMID: 2657681.

2. Robertson A, Branfoot T, Barlow IF, Giannoudis PV. Spinal injury patterns resulting from car and motorcycle accidents. *Spine (Phila Pa 1976)*. 2002 Dec 15;27(24):2825–30. PMID: 12486355.

3. Drysdale WF, Kraus JF, Franti CE, Riggins RS. Injury patterns in motorcycle collisions. *J Trauma*. 1975 Feb;15(2):99–115. PMID: 1113363.

4. Kupferschmid JP, Weaver ML, Raves JJ, Diamond DL. Thoracic spine injuries in victims of motorcycle accidents. *J Trauma*. 1989 May;29(5):593–6. PMID: 2724376.

5. Nagel DA, Koogle TA, Piziali RL, Perkash I. Stability of the upper lumbar spine following progressive disruptions and the application of individual internal and external fixation devices. *J Bone Joint Surg Am*. 1981 Jan;63(1):62–70. PMID: 7451527.

6. Pickett GE, Campos-Benitez M, Keller JL, Duggal N. Epidemiology of traumatic spinal cord injury in Canada. *Spine (Phila Pa 1976)*. 2006 Apr 1;31(7):799–805. PMID: 16582854.

7. Looby S, Flanders A. Spine trauma. *Radiol Clin North Am*. 2011 Jan;49(1):129–63. doi: 10.1016/j.rcl.2010.07.019. PMID: 21111133.

8. Rao RD, Berry CA, Yoganandan N, Agarwal A. Occupant and crash characteristics in thoracic and lumbar spine injuries resulting from motor vehicle collisions. *Spine J*. 2014 Oct 1;14(10):2355–65. doi: 10.1016/j.spinee.2014.01.038. Epub 2014 Jan 31. PMID: 24486471.

9. Hsu JM, Joseph T, Ellis AM. Thoracolumbar fracture in blunt trauma patients: Guidelines for diagnosis and imaging. *Injury*. 2003 Jun;34(6):426–33. PMID: 12767788.

10. Yoonhee C, Jung K, Eo E, Lee D, Kim J, Shin D, Kim S, Lee M. The relationship between alcohol consumption and injury in ED trauma patients. *Am J Emerg Med*. 2009 Oct;27(8):956–60. doi: 10.1016/j.ajem.2008.07.035. PMID: 19857414.

11. Gray L, Vandemark R, Hays M. Thoracic and lumbar spine trauma. *Semin Ultrasound CT MR*. 2001 Apr;22(2):125–34. PMID: 11327527.

12. Fardon DF. Odontoid fracture complicating ankylosing hyperostosis of the spine. *Spine (Phila Pa 1976)*. 1978 Jun;3(2):108–12. PMID: 663759.

13. Bernini PM, Floman Y, Marvel JP Jr, Rothman RH. Multiple thoracic spine fractures complicating ankylosing hyperostosis of the spine. *J Trauma*. 1981 Sep;21(9):811–4. PMID: 7277549.

14. Hitchon PW, From AM, Brenton MD, Glaser JA, Torner JC. Fractures of the thoracolumbar spine complicating ankylosing spondylitis. *J Neurosurg*. 2002 Sep;97(2 Suppl):218–22. PMID: 12296682.

15. Wade W, Saltzstein R, Maiman D. Spinal fractures complicating ankylosing spondylitis. *Arch Phys Med Rehabil*. 1989 May;70(5):398–401. PMID: 2719544.

16. Ghozlani I, Ghazi M, Nouijai A, Mounach A, Rezqi A, Achemlal L, Bezza A, El Maghraoui A. Prevalence and risk factors of osteoporosis and vertebral fractures in patients with ankylosing spondylitis. *Bone*. 2009 May;44(5):772–6. doi: 10.1016/j.bone.2008.12.028. Epub 2009 Jan 14. PMID: 19442629.

17. Ticó N, Ramon S, Garcia-Ortun F, Ramirez L, Castelló T, Garcia-Fernández L, Lience E. Traumatic spinal cord injury complicating ankylosing spondylitis. *Spinal Cord*. 1998 May;36(5):349–52. PMID: 9601116.

18. Caron T, Bransford R, Nguyen Q, Agel J, Chapman J, Bellabarba C. Spine fractures in patients with ankylosing spinal disorders. *Spine (Phila Pa 1976)*. 2010 May 15;35(11):E458-64. doi: 10.1097/BRS.0b013e3181cc764f. PMID: 20421858.

19. Chance GQ. Note on type of flexion fracture of the spine. *Br J Radiol*. 1948 Sep;21(249):452. PMID:19078456.

20. Smith WS, Kaufer H. Patterns and mechanisms of lumbar injuries associated with lap seat belts. *J Bone Joint Surg Am*. 1969 Mar;51(2):239–54. PMID: 5767317.

21. Gertzbein SD, Court-Brown CM. Flexion-distraction injuries of the lumbar spine. Mechanisms of injury and classification. *Clin Orthop Relat Res*. 1988 Feb;227:52–60. PMID: 3338223.

22. Howland WJ, Curry JL, Buffington CB. Fulcrum fractures of the lumbar spine. Transverse fracture induced by an improperly placed seat belt. *JAMA*. 1965 Jul 19;193:240–1. PMID: 14310340.

23. Triantafyllou SJ, Gertzbein SD. Flexion distraction injuries of the thoracolumbar spine: A review. *Orthopedics*. 1992 Mar;15(3):357–64. PMID: 1553330.

24. Rennie W, Mitchell N. Flexion distraction fractures of the thoracolumbar spine. *J Bone Joint Surg Am*.

1973 Mar;55(2):386–90. PMID: 4696170.

25. Anderson PA, Henley MB, Rivara FP, Maier RV. Flexion distraction and chance injuries to the thoracolumbar spine. *J Orthop Trauma*. 1991;5(2):153–60. PMID: 1861190.

26. Neumann P, Nordwall A, Osvalder AL. Traumatic instability of the lumbar spine. A dynamic in vitro study of flexion-distraction injury. *Spine (Phila Pa 1976)*. 1995 May 15;20(10):1111–21. PMID: 7638653.

27. Kim DH, Vaccaro AR. Osteoporotic compression fractures of the spine; current options and considerations for treatment. *Spine J*. 2006 Sep–Oct;6(5):479–87. PMID: 16934715.

28. Cheong HW, Peh WC, Guglielmi G. Imaging of diseases of the axial and peripheral skeleton. *Radiol Clin North Am*. 2008 Jul;46(4):703–33, vi. doi: 10.1016/j. rcl.2008.04.007. PMID: 18922289.

29. Kroon F, Staples M, Ebeling PR, Wark JD, Osborne RH, Mitchell PJ, Wriedt CH, Buchbinder R. Two-year results of a randomized placebo-controlled trial of vertebroplasty for acute osteoporotic vertebral fractures. *J Bone Miner Res*. 2014 Jun;29(6):1346–55. PMID: 24967454.

30. Denis F. The three column spine and its significance in the classification of acute thoracolumbar spinal injuries. *Spine (Phila Pa 1976)*. 1983 Nov–Dec;8(8):817–31. PMID: 6670016.

31. Kim NH, Lee HM, Chun IM. Neurologic injury and recovery in patients with burst fracture of the thoracolumbar spine. *Spine (Phila Pa 1976)*. 1999 Feb 1;24(3):290–3; discussion 294. PMID: 10025025.

32. Meves R, Avanzi O. Correlation between neurological deficit and spinal canal compromise in 198 patients with thoracolumbar and lumbar fractures. *Spine (Phila Pa 1976)*. 2005 Apr 1;30(7):787–91. PMID: 15803082.

33. Kilcoyne RF, Mack LA, King HA, Ratcliffe SS, Loop JW. Thoracolumbar spine injuries associated with vertical plunges: reappraisal with computed tomography. *Radiology*. 1983 Jan;146(1):137–40. PMID: 6849034.

34. Atlas SW, Regenbogen V, Rogers LF, Kim KS. The radiographic characterization of burst fractures of the spine. *AJR Am J Roentgenol*. 1986 Sep;147(3):575–82. PMID: 3488659.

35. Miller CD, Blyth P, Civil ID. Lumbar transverse process fractures–a sentinel marker of abdominal organ injuries. *Injury*.

2000 Dec;31(10):773–6. PMID: 11154746.

36. Sturm JT, Perry JF Jr. Injuries associated with fractures of the transverse processes of the thoracic and lumbar vertebrae. *J Trauma*. 1984 Jul;24(7):597–9. PMID: 6748119.

37. Tewes DP, Fischer DA, Quick DC, Zamberletti F, Powell J. Lumbar transverse process fractures in professional football players. *Am J Sports Med*. 1995 Jul–Aug;23(4):507–9. PMID: 7573665.

38. Mehta S, Auerbach JD, Born CT, Chin KR. Sacral fractures. *J Am Acad Orthop Surg*. 2006 Nov;14(12):656–65. PMID: 17077338.

39. Denis F, Davis S, Comfort T. Sacral fractures: An important problem. Retrospective analysis of 236 cases. *Clin Orthop Relat Res*. 1988 Feb;227:67–81. PMID: 3338224.

40. Sullivan MP, Smith HE, Schuster JM, Donegan D, Mehta S, Ahn J. Spondylopelvic dissociation. *Orthop Clin North Am*. 2014 Jan;45(1):65–75. doi: 10.1016/j. ocl.2013.08.002. Epub 2013 Oct 12. PMID: 24267208.

41. Vaccaro AR, Kim DH, Brodke DS, Harris M, Chapman JR, Schildhauer T, Routt ML, Sasso RC. Diagnosis and management of sacral spine fractures. *Instr Course Lect*. 2004;53:375–85. PMID: 15116628.

42. Soles GL, Ferguson TA. Fragility fractures of the pelvis. *Curr Rev Musculoskelet Med*. 2012 Sep;5(3):222–8. doi: 10.1007/ s12178-012-9128-9. PMID: 22589010; PMCID: PMC3535080.

43. Soreide K, Ellingsen CL, Knutson V. How dangerous is BASE jumping? An analysis of adverse events in 20,850 jumps from the Kjerag Massif, *Norway. J Trauma*. 2007 May;62(5):1113–7. PMID: 17495709.

44. Mei-Dan O, Carmont MR, Monasterio E. The epidemiology of severe and catastrophic injuries in BASE jumping. *Clin J Sport Med*. 2012 May;22(3):262–7. doi: 10.1097/ JSM.0b013e31824bd53a. PMID: 22450590.

45. Coppola PT, Coppola M. Emergency department evaluation and treatment of pelvic fractures. *Emerg Med Clin North Am*. 2000 Feb;18(1):1–27, v. PMID: 10678158.

46. Hodges SD, Eck JC, Humphreys SC. A treatment and outcomes analysis of patients with coccydynia. *Spine J*. 2004 Mar–Apr;4(2):138–40. PMID: 15016390.

Fractures and dislocations of the pelvis

Felix S. Chew, M.D., and Hyojeong Mulcahy, M.D.

Case 9–1

Pelvis anterior compression injury

(A)

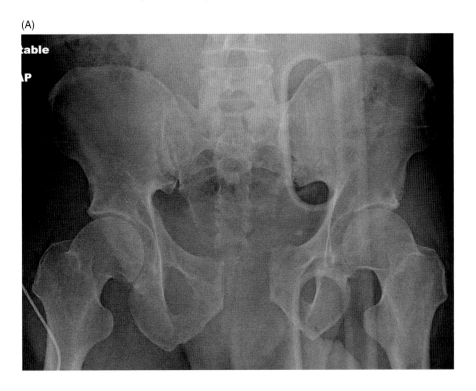

45-year-old man who was the passenger on a motorcycle that crashed into the back of a parked truck. AP radiograph of the pelvis. There is mild widening of the right sacroiliac joint and gross diastasis of the symphysis pubis.

(B)

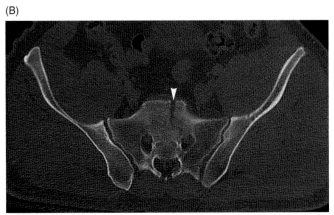

(C)

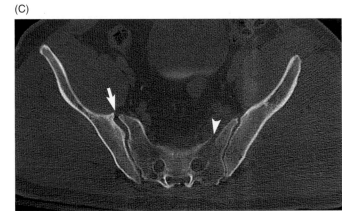

Axial CT of the pelvis, superior (B) to inferior (C). There is mild widening of the anterior aspect of the right SI joint (arrow), and a fracture of the sacrum that begins near the midline and extends through the left neural foramina (arrowheads). With severe anterior compression, the pelvis is flattened. The iliac wings rotate externally, resulting in disruption of the anterior and posterior arches of the pelvis under tension [1–2].

The anterior arch injury is typically diastasis of the symphysis pubis, vertical fractures of one or both obturator rings, or some combination; the posterior arch injury may be diastasis of one or both SI joints, fractures of the sacral wing, or some combination. Anterior compression injury is commonly sustained in automobile vehicle crashes in which the victim's car hits head-on.

Case 9–2

Pelvis anterior compression injury

(A)

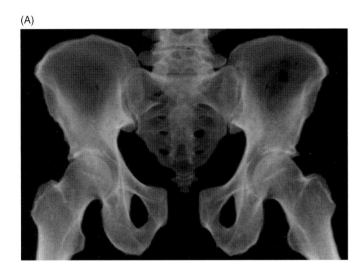

59-year-old man who was injured in a horseback riding accident. 3D volume-rendered CT of the pelvis. There is subtle bilateral sacroiliac joint diastasis and marked symphysis pubis diastasis. There are no fractures.

(B)

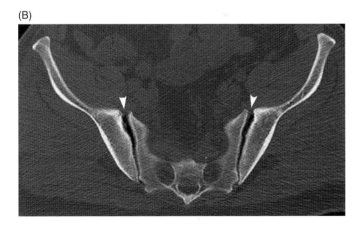

Axial CT of the pelvis. There is mild, symmetric widening of the anterior sacroiliac joints bilaterally (arrowheads). This pattern of injury is that of AP compression, sometimes called open-book injury.

Case 9–3
Pelvis straddle fractures

(A)

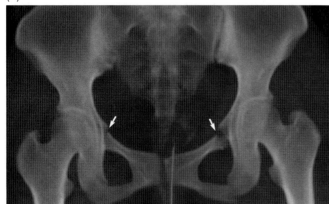

25-year-old woman in high-speed motor vehicle crash. 3D volume-rendered CT of the pelvis. There are fractures of the right and left superior (arrows) and right and left inferior pubic rami. This combination of fractures is descriptive of the appearance, but not of the mechanism. The straddle fracture is generally caused by tensile loading of the anterior pelvic arch, as occurs in anterior compression of the pelvis.

(B)

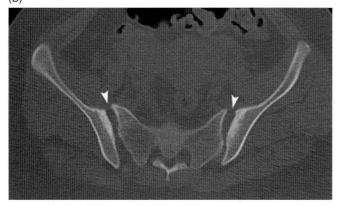

Axial CT of the pelvis. There is posterior dislocation of both SI joints. The bilateral SI joints are widened (arrowheads) and the iliac wings are posteriorly translated relative to the sacrum.

Case 9–4

Pelvis lateral compression injury

(A)

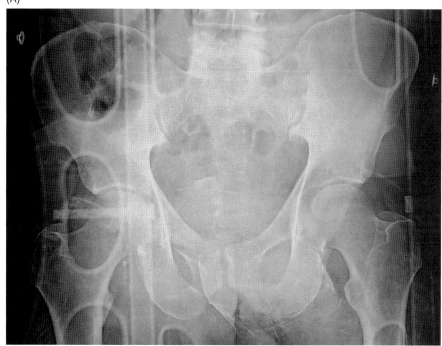

60-year-old man who fell 20 feet off a ladder, landing on his right side. AP radiograph of the pelvis. There are fractures of the right sacral wing and right obturator ring.

(B)

(C)

(D)

(E)

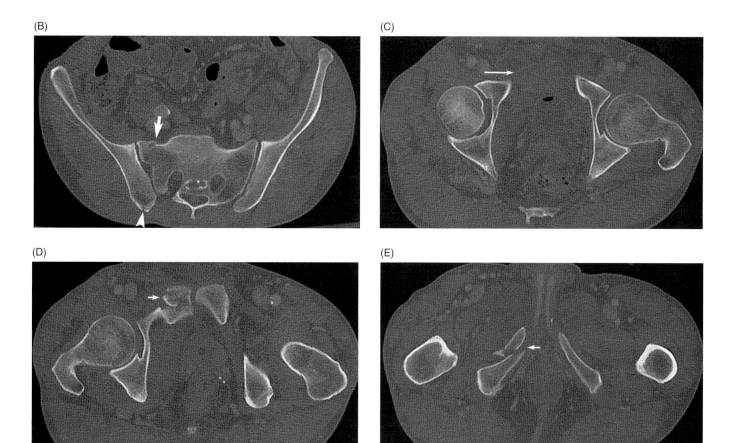

Axial CT of the pelvis, superior (B) to inferior (E). (B) There is a compression fracture of the right sacral wing (arrow), and a posterior distraction fracture of the right ilium (arrowhead). (C) At the level of the hip joints, the right acetabulum is intact but there is slight internal rotation of the right hemi-pelvis (long arrow shows direction of rotation). (D-E) There are fractures of the right pubis and right interior pubic ramus (small arrows). With lateral compression of the pelvis, the outboard iliac wing is rotated inward, typically resulting in some combination of an ipsilateral iliac wing fracture, impacted ipsilateral sacral wing fracture, or ipsilateral posterior sacroiliac joint distraction. The posterior sacroiliac may have sprains or avulsion fractures that are caused by the iliac wing rotating on the fulcrum of the sacrum. Fractures from a shearing mechanism will typically involve the anterior pelvic arch as it is compressed together [1–2].

Case 9–5

Windswept pelvis from lateral compression injury

(A)

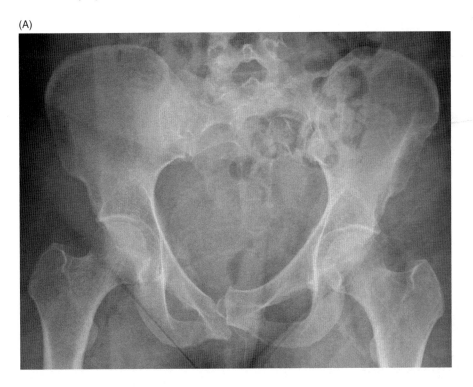

Woman injured in a motor vehicle crash. AP radiograph of the pelvis. The symphysis pubis has been disrupted, with overlap of the right and left pubic bones in the axial plane. There are fractures of the left sacral wing and subtle diastasis of the right sacroiliac joint. There is inward rotation of the left iliac wing and outward rotation of the right iliac wing.

(B)

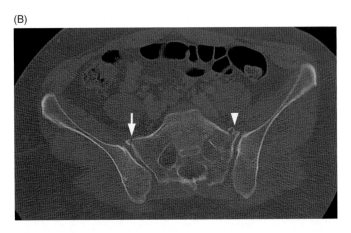

Axial CT of the pelvis. At the upper sacrum (B), there is an impaction fracture (arrowhead) of the left sacral wing that involves the neural foramen. There is an avulsion fracture of the right sacral wing (short arrow).

(C)

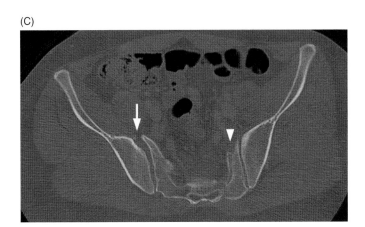

At the lower sacrum (C), the right sacroiliac joint is widened anteriorly (long arrow), but not posteriorly. The impaction fracture of the left sacrum (arrowhead) is seen. There is inward rotation of the left iliac wing, and outward rotation of the right iliac wing.

(D)

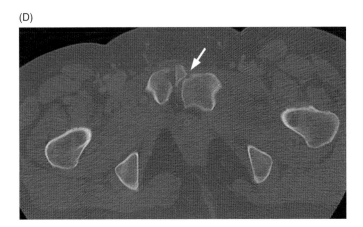

At the symphysis pubis (D), there is diastasis with the left pubis posterior to the right pubis, and a fragment sheared off the right pubis anteriorly (angled arrow).

(E)

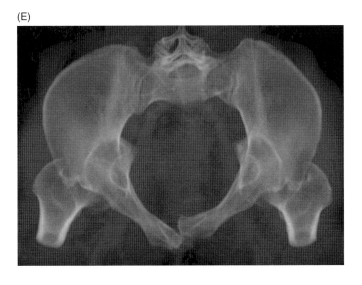

3D volume-rendered CT of the pelvis. 3D volume-rendered CT inlet view shows inward rotation of the left hemi-pelvis and outward rotation of the right hemi-pelvis. The windswept pelvis is the result of severe lateral compression [1–2].

Case 9–6

Pelvis vertical shear injury

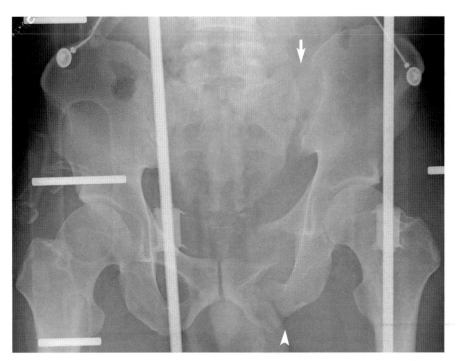

36-year-old man who fell 40 feet and landed on his buttocks. AP radiograph of the pelvis. There are fractures through the left superior and inferior pubic rami (arrowhead), and superior dislocation of the left hemi-pelvis through the left sacroiliac joint (arrow). In vertical shear injuries, one hemi-pelvis is typically displaced superiorly relative to the other, with disruptions involving both the anterior and posterior arches. The anterior disruption may be through the symphysis pubis or either obturator ring, and the posterior disruption may be through either sacroiliac joint, either sacral wing, either iliac wing, or some combination [1–2].

Case 9–7

Left hemi-pelvis dislocation

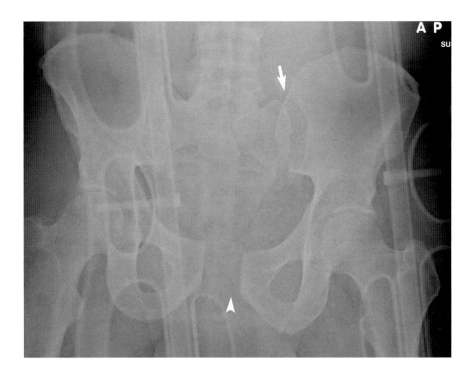

38-year-old man bucked from a horse. AP radiograph of the pelvis. The left sacroiliac joint (arrow) and symphysis pubis (arrowhead) are widely diastatic with lateral displacement of the otherwise intact left hemi-pelvis. There is a vertical fracture through the left L5 transverse process. In general, the outcome of pelvic ring injuries is less dependent on the morphology of the injury and more dependent on the associated visceral injuries that the patient has sustained [3].

Case 9–8
Anterior column acetabular fracture

(A)

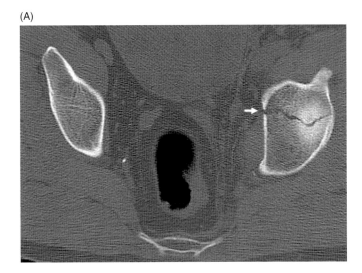

(B)

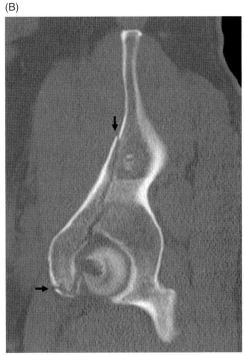

(C)

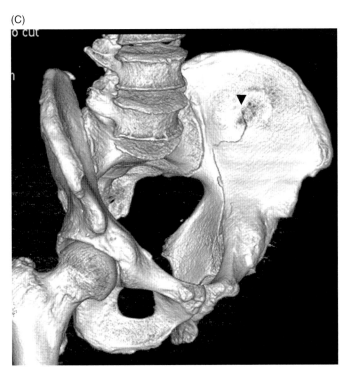

54-year-old man who fell from a ladder. Axial (A), sagittal (B), and 3D surface-rendered (C) CT of the left hip. Axial CT image shows a transversely oriented fracture line involving the anterior column (white arrow). Sagittal CT image shows a vertically oriented fracture line involving the anterior column (black arrows). 3D surface-rendered CT shows anterior column fracture extending to the left ilium (black arrowhead). Anatomically, the acetabulum consists of anterior and posterior columns, configured like an inverted Y. The anterior column extends from the upper sacrum to the anterior pubic ramus, forming two limbs of the Y, and the posterior column extends from the posterosuperior iliac spine to the ischial tuberosity, forming the third limb of the Y. Each column has an articular surface or wall. Acetabular fractures may be described according to involvement of columns and walls and direction of fracture [4–5].

Case 9–9

Anterior column acetabular fracture

(A)

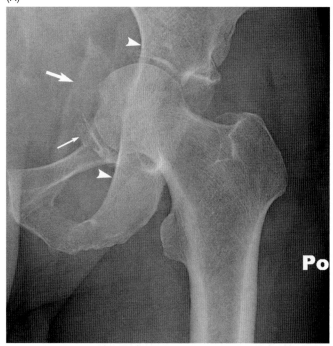

54-year-old man in motor vehicle crash. AP radiograph of the left hip. The femoral head appears as if it had been punched through the acetabulum into the pelvic cavity. The iliopubic line is interrupted where there are displaced fractures of the anterior column (long arrow) and anteromedial displacement of the femoral head. A large fragment of the medial wall (arrow) has been displaced medially with the femoral head. The ilioischial line (arrowheads) has not been interrupted indicating that the posterior column is intact. In all likelihood, this patient was the driver of a car that was struck by another vehicle from the left side.

(B)

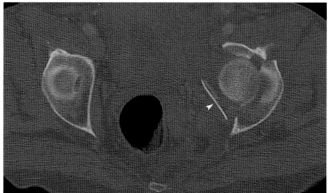

(C)

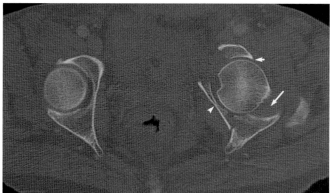

(D)

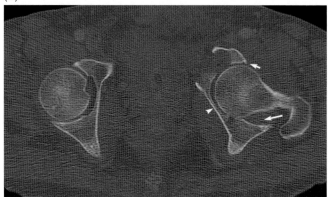

Axial CT of the pelvis, superior (B) to inferior (D). The medial wall of the acetabulum is fractured and displaced medially (arrowhead). The femoral head is dislocated medially from the posterior acetabulum (long arrow), which is still attached to the pelvis, but the articular surfaces of the displaced medial and anterior acetabular fragments remain in contact with the femoral head (short arrow).

Case 9–10

T-type acetabular fracture

(A)

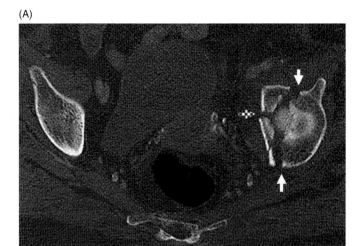

(B)

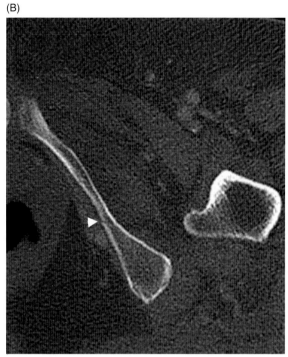

(C)

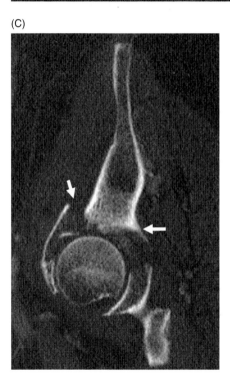

(D)

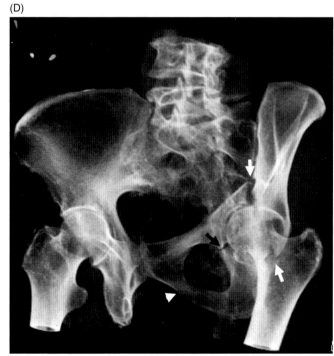

76-year-old woman who fell on her left hip while golfing. Multiplanar (A, B, C) and 3D volume-rendered (D) CT of the left hip. (A) Axial CT shows a sagittally oriented fracture line at the level of acetabular roof (white arrows). There is a coronally oriented second fracture line (dotted white arrow). (B) Axial CT at the level of ischium shows a non-displaced fracture at left ischium (white arrowhead). (C) Sagittal CT at the columnar junction shows that the fracture involves anterior and posterior columns as well as the quadrilateral plate (white arrows). (D) 3D volume-rendered CT shows that the fracture has a transverse fracture (white arrows) and a second fracture (black arrow) with a component extending into the obturator ring (white arrowhead).

Case 9–11

Both column acetabular fracture

(A)

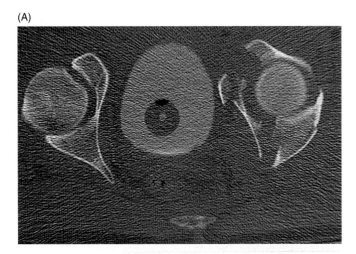

(B)

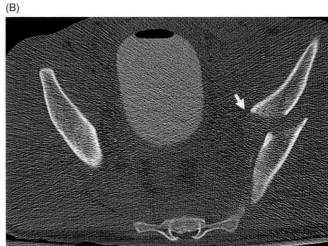

(C)

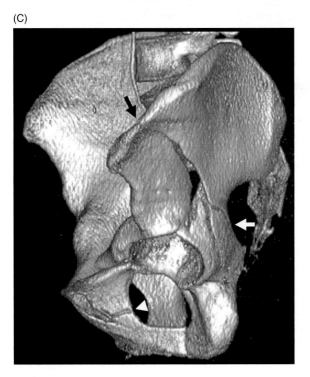

20-year-old man with motor vehicle crash injuries. Axial (A, B) and 3D surface-rendered (C) CT of the left hip. (A) Axial CT at the level of the quadrilateral plate shows comminuted fracture involving anterior and posterior columns of left acetabulum. (B) Axial CT at the level of the ilium shows a spur sign. A spur sign is only seen in both column fractures, and it is a differential point from T-type fracture (white arrow). The spur sign is shown only on the ipsilateral obturator oblique view and is created by medial translation of the distal fragment. The visualized spur fragment is simply the inferior end of the weight-bearing strut of bone in communication with the axial skeleton. On CT, this fragment is easier to see because one can trace down the weight-bearing strut of bone in continuity with the axial skeleton from the sacroiliac joint across the sciatic buttress. The fragment of bone never descends down to the acetabular surface in the setting of a both-column fracture, thus creating the "CT spur" sign. (C) 3D surface-rendered CT shows fracture involving anterior column (white arrow), posterior column (black arrow), and the obturator ring (white arrowhead).

Case 9–12

Posterior column acetabular fracture

(A)

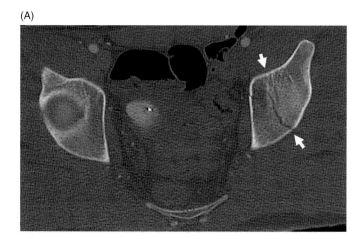

(B)

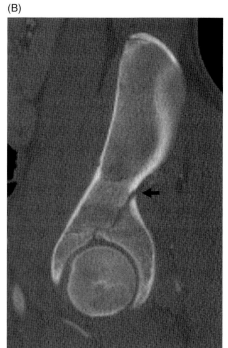

(C)

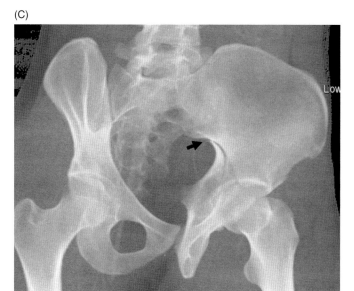

21-year-old man with injuries from a high-speed motor vehicle crash. Multiplanar (A, B) and 3D volume-rendered (C) CT of the pelvis and left hip. (A) Axial CT at the level of the sciatic notch shows sagittally oriented fracture line involving the posterior column (white arrows). (B) Sagittal CT at the level of columnar junction shows the fracture extending to the sciatic notch (black arrow). (C) 3D volume-rendered CT shows fracture extending to the sciatic notch (black arrow). The fracture extends inferiorly to involve the obturator ring (not shown).

Case 9–13   Transverse and posterior wall acetabular fracture

(A)

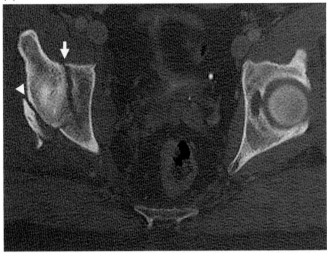

(B)

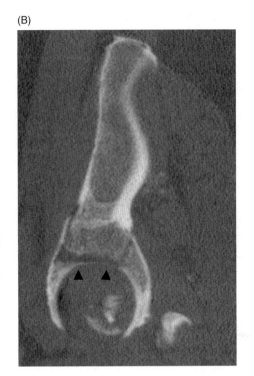

44-year-old man injured in a motor vehicle crash. Multiplanar CT of the right hip. (A) Axial CT just proximal to the level of quadrilateral plate shows sagittally oriented fracture (white arrow) with a displaced posterior wall fragment (white arrowhead). (B) Sagittal CT at the level of columnar junction shows transverse fracture. The quadrilateral plate is not involved (black arrowheads), distinguishing this from a T-type fracture.

Case 9–14   Posterior column posterior wall acetabular fracture

(A)

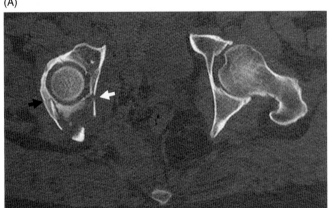

(B)

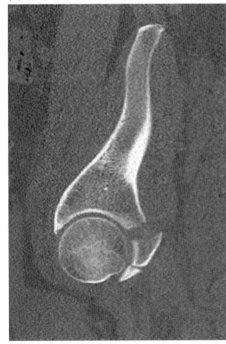

49-year-old man injured in a motorcycle-versus-car accident. Multiplanar CT of the right hip. (A) Axial CT at the level of quadrilateral plate shows posterior column fracture (white arrow) with minimally displaced posterior wall (black arrow) fracture. (B) Sagittal CT at the level of columnar junction shows fractures involving the posterior column and posterior wall.

Case 9–15

Anterior column posterior hemi-transverse acetabular fracture

(A)

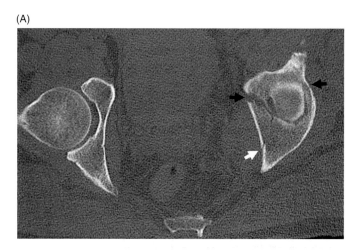

(B)

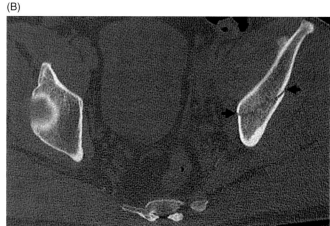

(C)

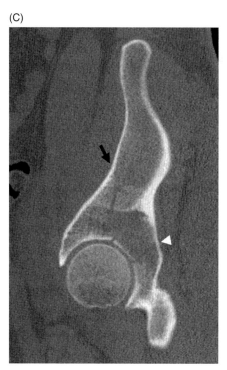

54-year-old man injured in a 7-foot fall from a ladder, landing on to his left hip. Multiplanar CT of the left hip. (A) Axial CT at the level of quadrilateral plate shows a coronally oriented fracture involving the anterior column (black arrows). The second fracture line is sagittally oriented and involves the posterior column (white arrow). (B) Axial CT at the level of sciatic notch shows coronally oriented fracture without a spur sign. This is a differential point from both column fractures (black arrows). (C) Sagittal CT at columnar junction shows vertically oriented fracture line extending to the ilium (black arrow). A transverse fracture involves the posterior column without extending to the sciatic notch (white arrowhead).

Case 9–16
Anterior column posterior hemi-transverse acetabular fracture

(A)

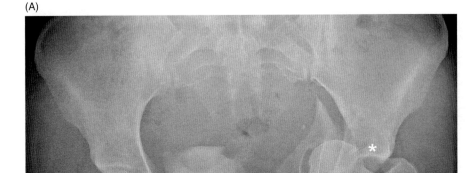

22-year-old woman whose car was struck from the side. AP radiograph of the pelvis. Loading of the left hip from the impact of the crash has pushed the femoral head into the acetabulum and resulted in these fractures. The posterior column of the acetabulum has been fractured from the pelvis, displaced medially, and rotated internally. The ischium is seen in a nearly lateral orientation (arrowhead). The anterior column is also fractured; the fractures extend to the pubis (arrow). One portion of the acetabular dome remains intact (asterisk). Both the iliopubic and the ilioischial lines have been disrupted on the left, indicative of anterior column and posterior column fractures, respectively. The bladder has a balloon catheter and is filled with contrast; there has been no rupture, but it is severely displaced to the right by hematoma originating from the fracture site.

(B)

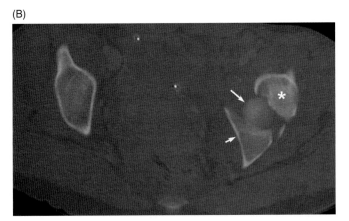

(C)

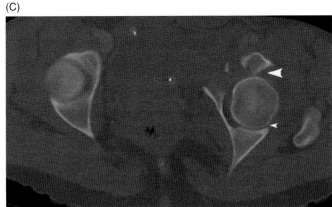

Axial CT of the left hip. (B) Axial CT at the level of the acetabular dome shows a displaced fracture with inward rotation of the posterior column (short arrow). The femoral head is centered in the middle of the fracture (long arrow). A small portion of the dome remains intact (asterisk). (C) Axial CT at the level of the middle of the femoral head shows the femoral head has maintained its articulation with the posterior wall of the acetabulum (small arrowhead), but it is dislocated from the anterior wall fragment (large arrowhead).

(D)

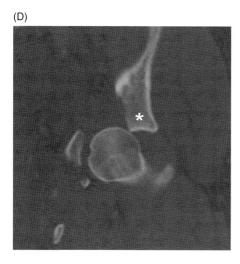

(E)

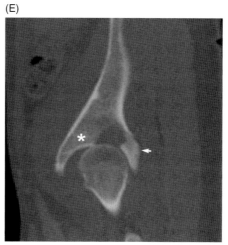

Coronal (D) and sagittal (E) CT of the left hip. (D) Coronal CT through the left femoral head shows it is medially dislocated from the remaining portion of the intact acetabular dome (asterisk). This intact portion of articular surface is important because it becomes the key to the operative reduction of the fracture. (E) Sagittal CT through the femoral head shows the intact portion of anterior acetabular dome (asterisk) and the widely displaced hemi-transverse fracture fragment of the posterior column (arrow).

Case 9–17
Anterior acetabular wall fracture

(A)

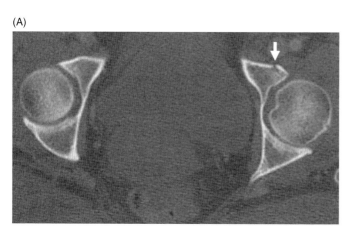

(B)

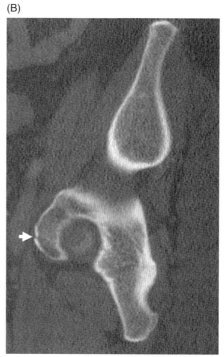

32-year-old woman injured in motor vehicle crash. Multiplanar CT of the left hip. Axial CT (A) at the level of quadrilateral plate shows a minimally displaced anterior acetabular wall fracture (white arrow). Sagittal CT (B) at columnar junction shows anterior acetabular wall fracture (white arrow).

Case 9–18
Posterior hip dislocation

(A)

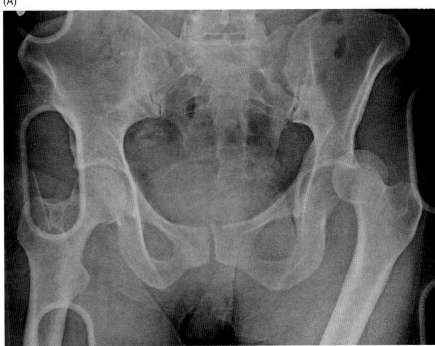

30-year-old woman injured in a rollover motor vehicle crash. AP radiograph of the pelvis. The patient is on a trauma board. The left femoral head is dislocated from the hip and has moved to a position that is superior and lateral to its normal location. The thigh is adducted. Because the lesser trochanter is obscured by the shaft, it is evident that the femur is internally rotated. The bony pelvis is intact.

(B)

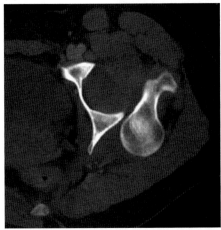

Axial CT of the left hip. The acetabulum is empty. The femoral head is dislocated posteriorly and internally rotated, so that the anterior aspect of the femoral head is resting against the posterior aspect of the posterior acetabular rim. There are no fractures of either the acetabulum or the femoral head.

(C)

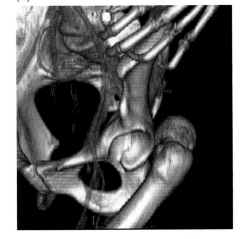

3D surface-rendered CT of the left hip, anterior view. The posterior dislocation of the hip and the internal rotation of the femur are evident. The Thompson-Epstein classification of posterior hip dislocations has five types [6]. Type I is a posterior dislocation without fracture. Type II is a posterior dislocation with a single large posterior acetabular wall fracture fragment. Type III has a comminuted posterior acetabular wall fracture. Type IV has a fracture of the acetabular floor (roof). Type V has a fracture of the femoral head. This case represents Type I, because there is no associated fracture.

Case 9–19
Posterior hip dislocation with comminuted posterior wall acetabular fractures

(A)

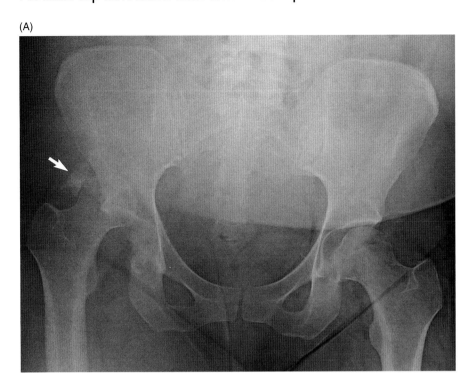

33-year-old woman who crashed her motor scooter into a car when it veered into her path. AP radiograph of the pelvis. The right hip is posteriorly dislocated and has displaced fragments (arrow) of the posterior acetabular wall.

(B) (C)

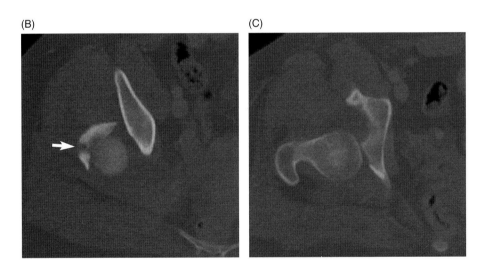

Axial CT of the right hip, superior (B) to inferior (C). The right femoral head is posteriorly dislocated from the acetabulum. The posterior wall of the acetabulum has been fractured and fragments have been displaced posteriorly and superiorly by the dislocated femoral head. The major posterior wall fragment is comminuted (arrow). The acetabular roof remains intact.

(D)

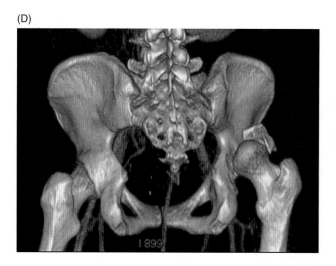

(E)

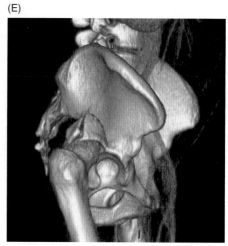

3D surface-rendered CT of the right hip, posterior (D) and lateral (E) views. The right hip is posteriorly dislocated and has displaced fragments of the posterior acetabular wall. Traumatic hip dislocations are commonly caused by motorcycle and automobile crashes [7–8]. Prompt recognition and reduction improves the long-term prognosis [8–9]. Posterior dislocation is the most common type of hip dislocation (approximately 90%) [7–10]. Hip dislocations may be classified by the direction of dislocation (anterior or posterior) and the associated fractures (acetabulum or femoral head) [10].

Case 9–20

Posterior hip dislocation with acetabular roof fracture

(A)

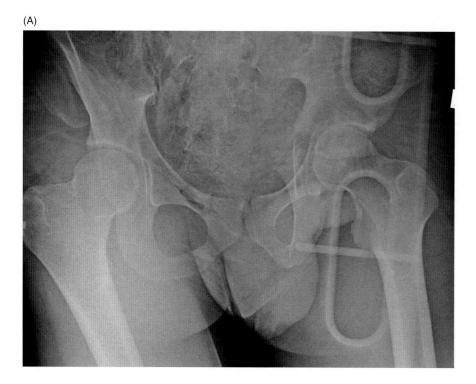

19-year-old man who was crushed beneath a motor vehicle that he was repairing. AP radiograph of the pelvis. The patient is on a trauma board. There is a fracture of the left obturator ring and left acetabulum, which is difficult to characterize because of the nonstandard position of the patient. The left femoral head projects over the acetabulum, but the incongruity of the femoral head with the acetabular roof indicates that there is misalignment and suggests dislocation.

(B) (C) (D)

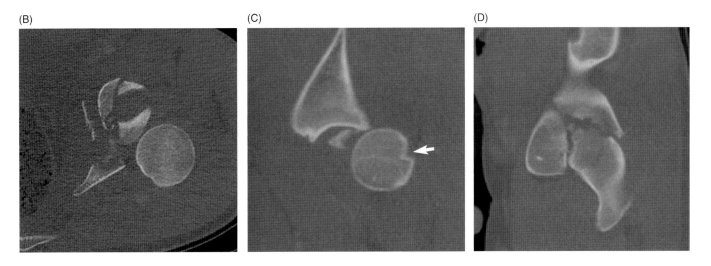

Multiplanar CT of the left hip. Axial CT (B) shows a comminuted fracture of the acetabular roof with posterior dislocation of the hip. Sagittal CT (C) through the femoral head shows posterior dislocation of the hip and a displaced fragment within the acetabulum. There is also an impaction fracture of the posterior aspect of the femoral head (arrow). Sagittal CT (D) through the medial wall of the acetabulum shows that the fracture has T-shaped morphology.

(E) (F) (G)

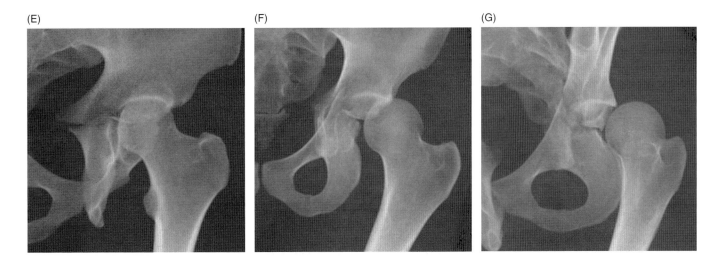

3D volume-rendered CT of the pelvis and left hip. Bilateral oblique (E and G) and anterior (F) volume-rendered views of the pelvis show the left acetabular fracture and the left posterior hip dislocation. On the left oblique view (E), corresponding to the positioning of the initial trauma radiograph, the femoral head is superimposed over the acetabulum, spuriously simulating normal location.

Case 9–21

Posterior hip dislocation with femoral head fracture

(A)

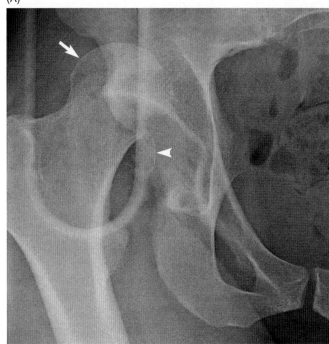

27-year-old man involved in a motor vehicle crash. AP radiograph of the right hip. Initial trauma radiograph shows posterior dislocation of the right hip. A curvilinear fragment (arrow) of the femoral head adjacent to the medial cortex of the femoral neck is partially obscured by the trauma board. There is no acetabular fracture. During posterior dislocation, a femoral head fragment may be sheared off by the sharp posterior rim of the acetabulum. The posterior dislocation in this case may be classified as Thompson-Epstein Type V.

(B)　　　　　(C)　　　　　(D)

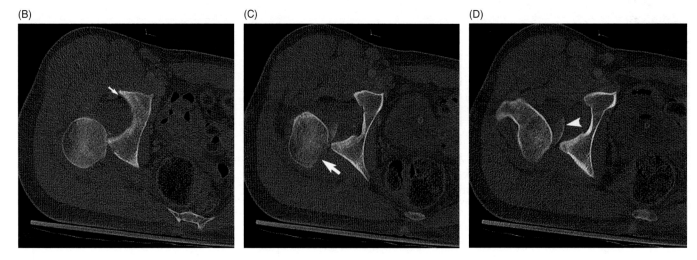

Axial CT of the right hip, superior (B) to inferior (D). There is posterior dislocation of the right hip, with the femoral head engaged with the posterior acetabular rim. There is a defect in the posterior femoral head (arrow) where a fragment of bone has been sheared off below the fovea. The fragment itself is anterior to the posterior acetabular rim, still within the acetabulum

(arrowhead). The small bubble of nitrogen gas (small arrow) is a characteristic CT feature of acute traumatic hip dislocation [11]. Femoral head fractures are high energy injuries typically associated with posterior hip dislocation [12]. Femoral head fractures may be classified by the Pipkin system. The femoral head fracture in this case could be classified as Pipkin Type 1.

Case 9–22

Posterior hip dislocation with femoral head fracture

(A)

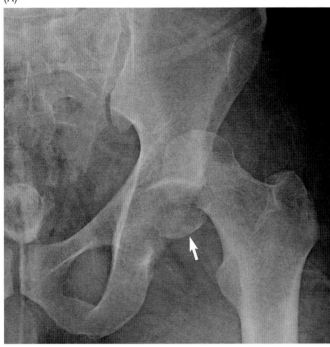

30-year-old man injured in a motorcycle crash. AP radiograph of the left hip. There is posterior dislocation of the hip. A curvilinear fracture fragment (arrow) of the femoral head projects over the posterior wall of the acetabulum. The posterior dislocation in this case may be classified as Thompson-Epstein Type V. The patient had multiple pelvic injuries including disruption of the left sacroiliac joint.

(B)

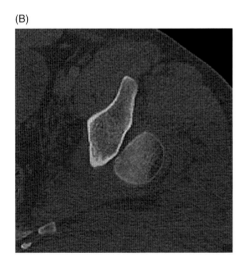

(C)

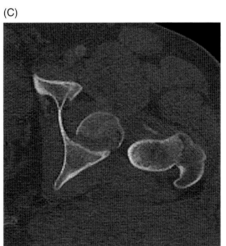

Axial CT of the left hip. (B) Above the level of the acetabulum, the dislocated femoral head is posterior to the ilium. The anteromedial aspect of the head is flattened. (C) At the level of the acetabulum, there is a large femoral head fragment within, and markedly displaced from, the dislocated head. Some femoral head fractures associated with dislocations may be classified by the Pipkin system. Type I does not involve the weight-bearing portion of the head (below the fovea); Type II involves the weight-bearing portion (above the fovea). Type III has an associated femoral neck fracture, and Type IV has an associated acetabular fracture.

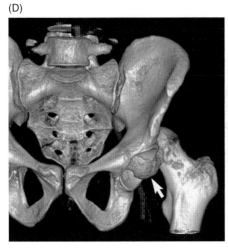

(D)

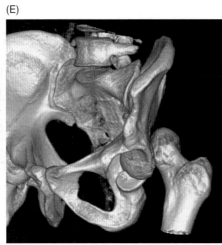

(E)

3D surface-rendered CT of the left hip. There is posterior dislocation of the left hip with a large femoral head fragment within the acetabulum. On the frontal view (D), the fovea of the femoral head (arrow) is part of the displaced fragment. On the oblique view (E), the flattened anteromedial aspect of the femoral head represents the donor site. The femoral head fracture in this case could be classified as Pipkin Type II.

Case 9–23

Partially reduced hip dislocation with incarcerated fragment

(A)

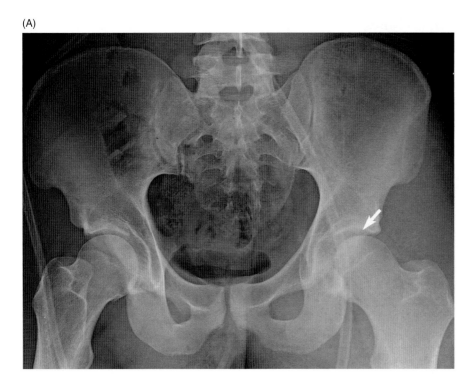

19-year-old man who accidentally stepped off the path while hiking, falling approximately 100 feet. AP radiograph of the pelvis. There has been partial relocation of the left hip following posterior dislocation. The articular surfaces of the acetabulum and the femoral head are not congruent (arrow), indicating that there may be incarcerated tissues preventing complete reduction.

(B)

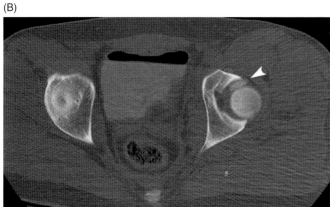

(C)

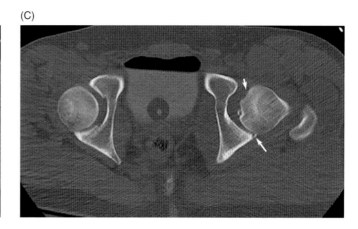

Axial CT of the pelvis, superior (B) to inferior (C). The hip has been dislocated and partially reduced. There is at least one large fracture fragment trapped anteriorly between the articular surfaces; the shape of the fragment (arrowhead) indicates that it is

a piece of the femoral head, and the donor site is anterior and inferior (short arrow), making this a Pipkin Type I fracture. There is a small posterior acetabular rim fracture (long arrow).

Case 9–24

Anterior hip dislocation, inferior

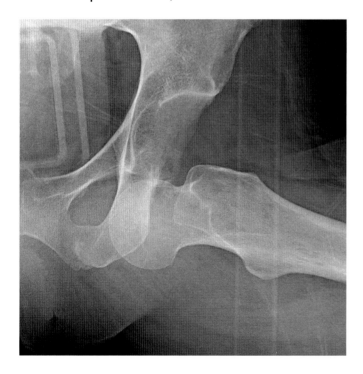

43-year-old female pedestrian who was struck by a car. AP radiograph of the left hip. The hip is dislocated anteriorly, with the femoral head resting on the anterior aspect of the ischium. The thigh is abducted, unlike a posterior dislocation, in which the femur typically would be adducted. Anterior hip dislocations represent approximately 10% of traumatic hip dislocations in adults, and may be inferior or superior. The Epstein classification [9–12] of anterior hip dislocation has Type I (superior) and Type II (inferior), each modified by the absence of fractures (subtype A), presence of femoral head fractures (subtype B), or presence of acetabular fractures (subtype C). This case would be Epstein Type II-A, anterior-inferior hip dislocation without fracture.

Case 9–25

Anterior hip dislocation, inferior

(A)

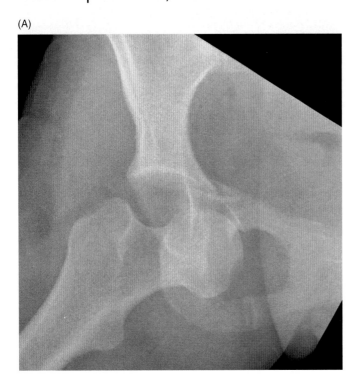

22-year-old woman who fell next to a moving car and was run over at low speed. AP radiograph of the right hip. There is an anterior fracture-dislocation of the right hip. There are fractures of the anterior acetabulum and inferior pubic ramus, and the femoral head is dislocated inferomedially. The thigh is abducted.

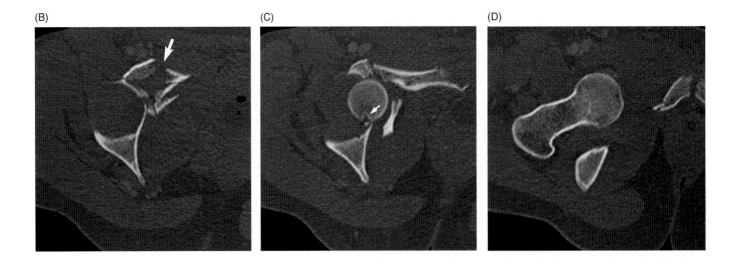

(B)　　　　　　　(C)　　　　　　　(D)

Axial CT of the left hip. Axial CT (B) through the acetabulum shows absence of the femoral head and fractures of the anterior wall and superior pubic ramus (arrow). Axial CT (C) through the top of the femoral head shows the anterior dislocation. The acetabular fractures include the medial wall, and there is an impaction fracture (small arrow) of the femoral head. Axial CT (D) through the femoral head and neck shows its location anterior to the obturator ring. This case would be Epstein Type II-C, anterior-inferior hip dislocation with acetabular fracture.

Case 9–26

Anterior hip dislocation, superior

(A)

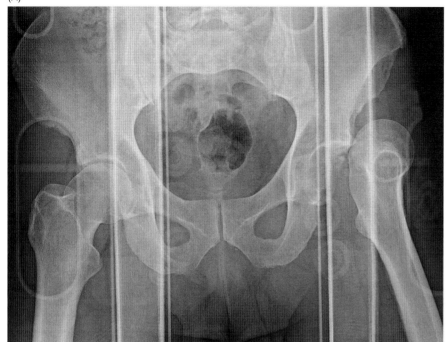

68-year-old man who was injured when the tree he was cutting down landed on him. AP radiograph of the pelvis. The left hip is dislocated, and the femoral head is lateral and superior to the empty acetabulum. The femur is externally rotated such that the head, neck, and greater trochanter are overlapping, while the lesser trochanter projects medially. There is abduction of the thigh. No fracture is evident. This case could be classified as Epstein Type 1-A, anterior-superior without fracture [6, 13].

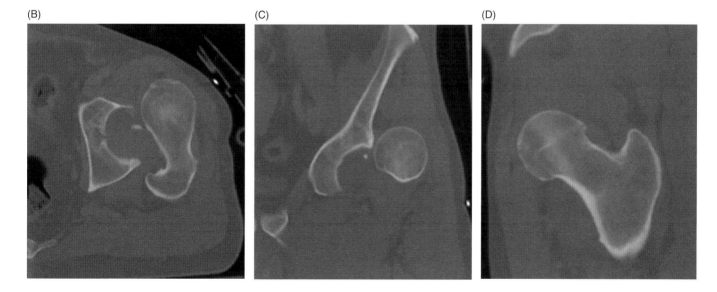

(B) (C) (D)

Multiplanar CT of the left hip. (B) Axial CT shows the lateral and anterior dislocation of the femoral head. The femur is externally rotated such that the head is pointing anteriorly.

(C) The coronal CT shows the empty acetabulum and the dislocated femoral head. (D) The sagittal CT shows the rotated proximal femur without contact with the acetabulum.

(E)

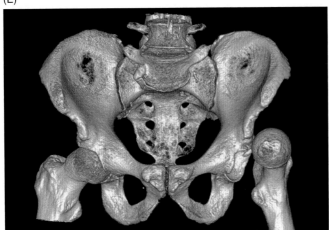

3D surface-rendered CT of the left hip. The femur always rotates externally when the head is dislocated anteriorly. The posterolateral position of the lesser trochanter is an anatomic marker for rotation of the femur. When visible in profile, there is external rotation; when obscured by the shaft, there is internal rotation.

References

1. Olson SA, Burgess A. Classification and initial management of patients with unstable pelvic ring injuries. *Instr Course Lect.* 2005;54:383–93. PMID: 15948467.

2. Young JW, Burgess AR, Brumback RJ, Poka A. Pelvic fractures: Value of plain radiography in early assessment and management. *Radiology.* 1986 Aug;160(2):445–51. PMID: 3726125.

3. Poole GV, Ward EF, Muakkassa FF, Hsu HS, Griswold JA, Rhodes RS. Pelvic fracture from major blunt trauma. Outcome is determined by associated injuries. *Ann Surg.* 1991 Jun;213(6):532–8; discussion 538–9. PMID: 2039283; PMCID: PMC1358569.

4. Lawrence DA, Menn K, Baumgaertner M, Haims AH. Acetabular fractures: Anatomic and clinical considerations. *AJR Am J Roentgenol.* 2013 Sep;201(3):W425–36. doi: 10.2214/AJR.12.10470. Review. PubMed PMID: 23971473.

5. Potok PS, Hopper KD, Umlauf MJ. Fractures of the acetabulum: Imaging, classification, and understanding. *Radiographics.* 1995 Jan;15(1):7–23; discussion 23–4. Review. PubMed PMID: 7899615.

6. Sanders S, Tejwani N, Egol KA. Traumatic hip dislocation – A review. *Bull NYU Hosp Jt Dis.* 2010;68(2):91–6. Review. PubMed PMID: 20632983.

7. Yang RS, Tsuang YH, Hang YS, Liu TK. Traumatic dislocation of the hip. *Clin Orthop Relat Res.* 1991 Apr;(265):218–27. PMID: 2009661.

8. Clegg TE, Roberts CS, Greene JW, Prather BA. Hip dislocations – Epidemiology, treatment, and outcomes. *Injury.* 2010 Apr;41(4):329–34. doi: 10.1016/j.injury.2009.08.007. Epub 2009 Sep 30. Review. PubMed PMID: 19796765.

9. Sahin V, Karakas ES, Aksu S, Atlihan D, Turk CY, Halici M. Traumatic dislocation and fracture-dislocation of the hip: A long-term follow-up study. *J Trauma.* 2003 Mar;54(3):520–9. PMID: 12634533.

10. Stephenson JW, Davis KW. Imaging of traumatic injuries to the hip. *Semin Musculoskelet Radiol.* 2013 Jul;17(3):306–15. doi: 10.1055/s-0033-1348097. Epub 2013 Jun 20. Review. PMID: 23787985.

11. Fairbairn KJ, Mulligan ME, Murphey MD, Resnik CS. Gas bubbles in the hip joint on CT: An indication of recent dislocation. *AJR Am J Roentgenol.* 1995 Apr;164(4):931–4. PMID: 7726051.

12. Droll KP, Broekhuyse H, O'Brien P. Fracture of the femoral head. *J Am Acad Orthop Surg.* 2007 Dec;15(12):716–27. Review. PMID: 18063712.

13. Erb RE, Steele JR, Nance EP, Edwards JR. Traumatic anterior dislocation of the hip: Spectrum of plain film and CT findings. *American Journal of Roentgenology.* 1995 Nov;165(5):1215–9. PMID: 7572506

Fractures and dislocations of the femur

Felix S. Chew, M.D.

Case 10–1

Impacted subcapital femoral neck fracture

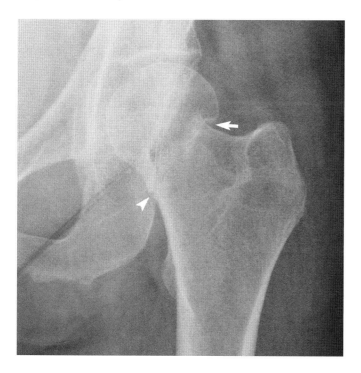

Elderly woman injured in ground-level fall. AP radiograph of the left hip. There is a subcapital fracture of the femoral neck with impaction of the superior cortex (arrow) and minimal displacement at the inferior cortex (arrowhead). A major goal of surgical therapy for fractures such as this is to restore mobility to the patient. Approximately 80% of hip fractures in elderly patients occur in women [1]. The Garden classification for femoral neck fractures is related to the degree of valgus displacement: Type I is impacted (sometimes incomplete) and valgus; Type II is non-displaced (but complete); Type III is varus angulation but only minimal displacement; Type IV is displaced. This case is an example of Garden Type I.

Case 10–2
Displaced subcapital femoral neck fracture

(A)

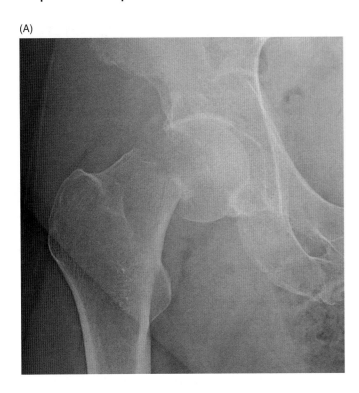

54-year-old man with severe left hip pain, unable to walk. AP radiograph of the right hip. There is a complete subcapital fracture of the femoral neck with varus angulation of the shaft relative to the head, and proximal translation of the neck relative to the head. The risk of osteonecrosis of the femoral head fragment is high when the fracture is displaced. Therefore, fractures such as these are usually treated with hip replacement. This case is an example of Garden type IV.

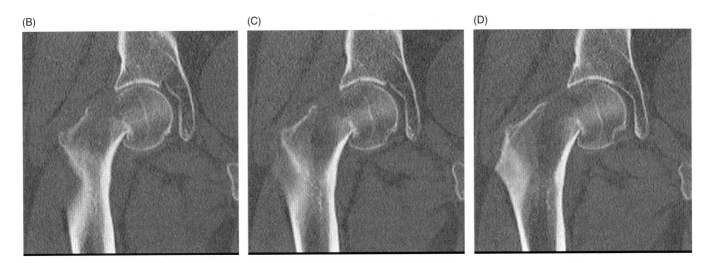

(B) (C) (D)

Coronal CT of the right hip, anterior (B) to posterior (D). The inferior portion of the neck is proximally translated and impacted into the middle of the head fragment. The separation of the superior margins of the head and neck fragments reflects the varus angulation of the shaft fragment relative to the head fragment.

Case 10–3
Transcervical femoral neck fracture

(A)

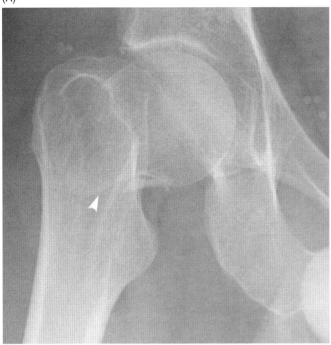

(B)

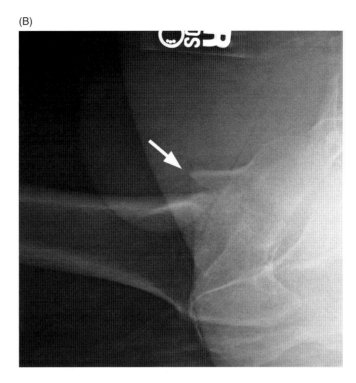

Elderly man injured in ground-level fall. AP (A) and lateral (B) radiographs of the right hip. There is apparent external rotation of the right proximal femur that makes the fracture easy to overlook because the greater trochanter is overlapping the femoral neck. In the appropriate clinical setting, asymmetry of

hip rotation when compared with the contralateral side (not shown) should prompt further investigation. The fracture itself is difficult to see (arrowhead). Cross-table lateral radiograph of the right hip shows the fracture (arrow) extending through the middle of the femoral neck.

(C)

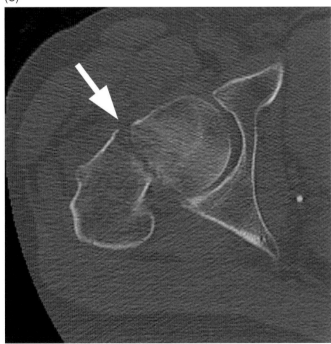

Axial CT of the right hip at the level of the femoral neck. There is a fracture traversing the femoral neck. The fracture is more displaced anteriorly (arrow) than posteriorly because of the greater external rotation of the distal fragment (including the shaft and trochanters) relative to the proximal fragment (including the neck and head).

Case 10–4
Basicervical femoral neck fracture

(A)

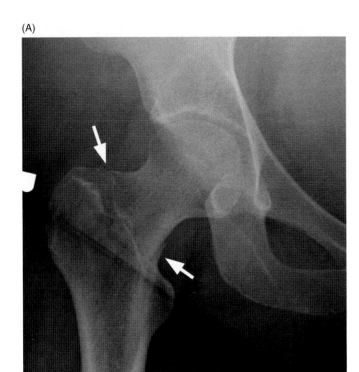

Middle-aged woman injured in a fall while in the bathroom. AP radiograph of the right hip. There is a fracture (arrow) extending along the base of the femoral neck.

(B)

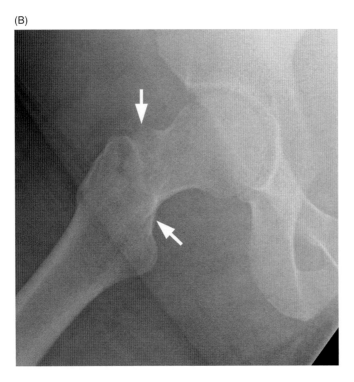

Frog lateral radiograph of the right hip. The fracture (arrows) extends through the base of the femoral neck, but does not involve the trochanters.

(C)

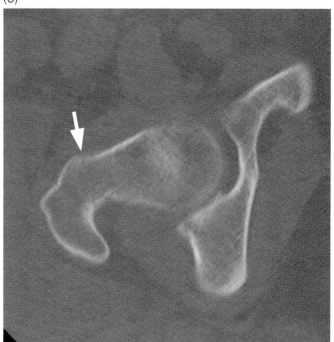

Axial CT of the right hip at the level of the femoral neck. The fracture (arrows) traverses the base of the femoral neck, medial to the greater trochanter.

Case 10–5
Greater trochanteric fracture

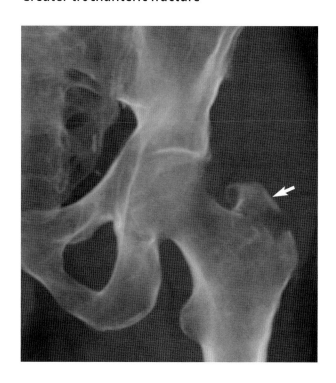

55-year-old man injured in ground-level fall. 3D volume-rendered CT of the left hip. There is an isolated fracture of the greater trochanter with superior displacement (arrow). The gluteus medius and gluteus minimus muscles insert on the greater trochanter.

Case 10–6
Intertrochanteric fracture

(A)

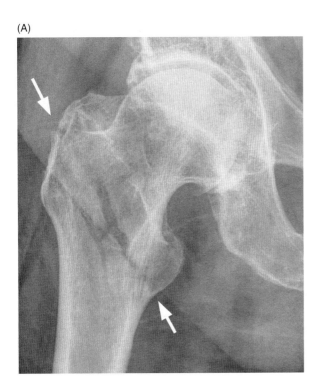

Elderly woman injured in a fall from standing. AP radiograph of the right hip. There is a fracture (arrows) extending obliquely from the greater trochanter to the lesser trochanter. The fracture is lateral to the base of the femoral neck. The right hip is externally rotated.

(B)

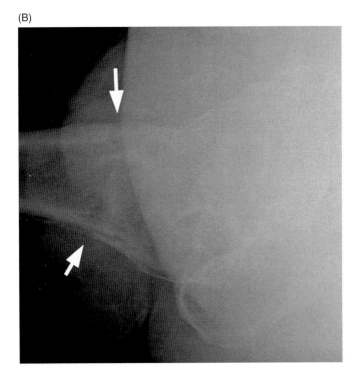

Cross-table lateral radiograph of the right hip. This view does not show the fracture (arrows) very well. The risk of osteonecrosis of the femoral head as a complication of an intertrochanteric fracture is low because the fracture is outside of the hip capsule and extends through cancellous bone with a good blood supply [2].

Case 10–7

Intertrochanteric femur fracture, comminuted

(A)

(B)

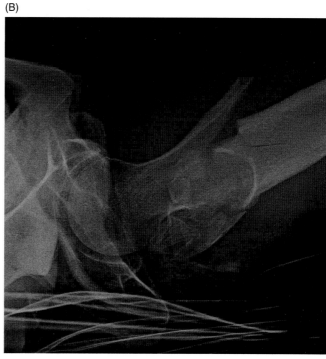

50-year-old woman injured in bicycle accident. AP (A) and true lateral (B) of the left hip. There is a comminuted intertrochanteric fracture of the proximal femur with comminution of the greater trochanter and subtrochanteric extension. There is varus angulation and medial displacement of the shaft.

(C)   (D)   (E)

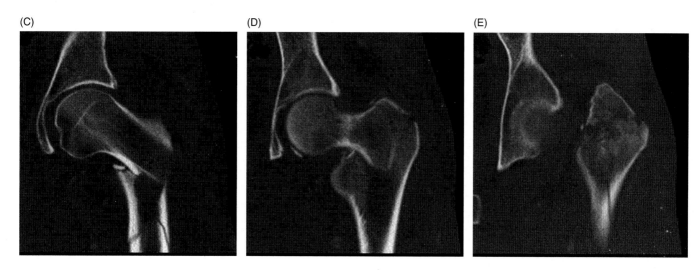

Coronal CT of the left hip, anterior (C) to posterior (E). The major head-neck fragment is impacted into the major shaft fragment. There is comminution of the greater trochanter, but the lesser trochanter is part of the shaft fragment. There are minimally displaced fractures extending into the proximal shaft.

Case 10–8   Intertrochanteric femur fracture, comminuted

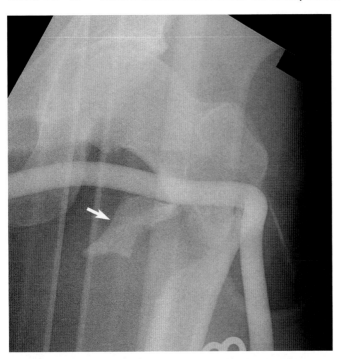

27-year-old man in a motorcycle crash. AP radiograph of the left hip. There is a three-part intertrochanteric fracture with displaced lesser trochanter fragment (arrow). Most hip fractures in adults aged 40 years or younger are the result of high-energy trauma such as motor vehicle crashes.

Case 10–9   Intertrochanteric femur fracture, comminuted

(A)

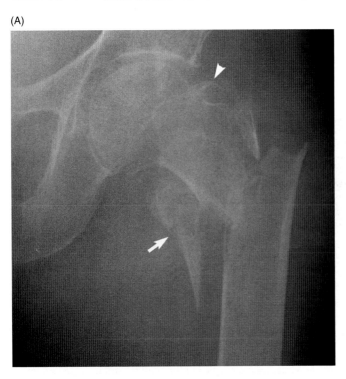

(B)

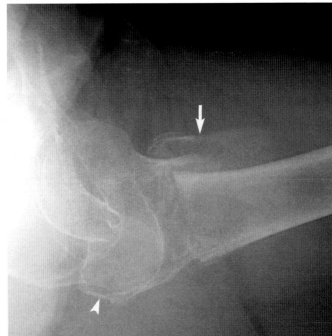

Elderly woman injured in ground-level fall. AP (A) and cross-table lateral (B) radiographs of the left hip. There is a four-part intertrochanteric fracture of the left proximal femur. The lesser (arrows) and greater (arrowheads) trochanters are separate fragments; the head and neck comprise another fragment; the shaft is the fourth fragment. Intertrochanteric fractures tend to occur in young adults with high-energy trauma and in very elderly adults with low-energy trauma. Unlike subcapital fractures, for which there is a strong preponderance of women, intertrochanteric fractures in very elderly patients have equal incidence between men and women.

Case 10–10

Intertrochanteric-subtrochanteric (peritrochanteric) femur fracture

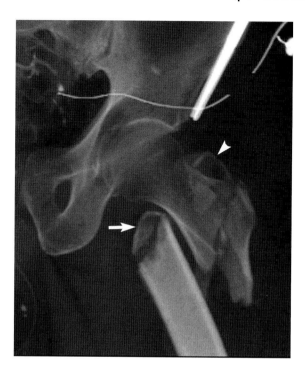

72-year-old man in rollover tractor accident. 3D volume-rendered CT of the left hip. There is a four-part intertrochanteric fracture that extends to the subtrochanteric portion of the femoral shaft, with wide displacement.

Case 10–11

Bilateral subtrochanteric femur fractures

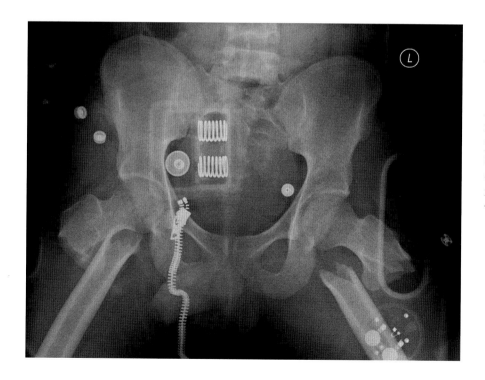

Young man in high-speed motor vehicle crash. AP radiograph of the pelvis. There are bilateral subtrochanteric femoral shaft fractures with proximal and medial displacement. The proximal femurs are abducted by the gluteus medius and gluteus minimus; the shaft is pulled proximally by the thigh adductors. Subtrochanteric fractures have a bimodal distribution – that is, typically young men from severe trauma and elderly women from ground-level falls.

Case 10–12   Segmental femur fracture

(A)

(B)

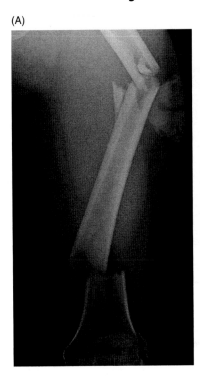
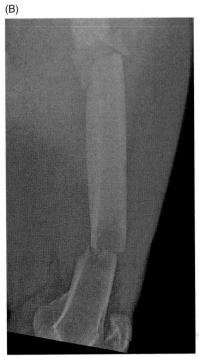

34-year-old man with polytrauma from high-speed motor vehicle crash. AP (A) and lateral (B) radiographs of the left femur. There is a segmental fracture of the femur with comminution at the proximal fracture. There is also a patella fracture.

Case 10–13   Spiral shaft of femur fracture

(A)

(B)

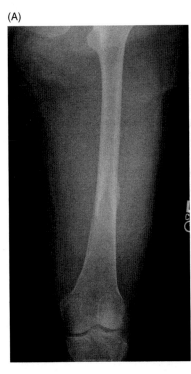
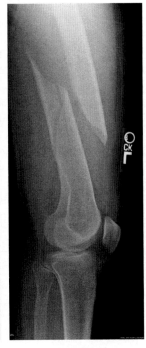

46-year-old woman who fell while skiing. AP (A) and lateral (B) radiographs of the left femur. There is a comminuted, displaced spiral fracture of the femoral shaft in bayonet apposition. The fracture line extends circumferentially around the femoral cortex, and is joined by a vertical component. The alignment and overlap of fragments on the AP view may delay visual recognition of the fracture.

Case 10–14
Shaft of femur fracture

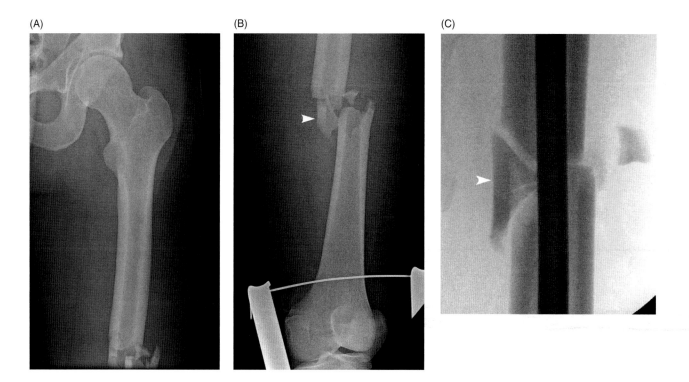

23-year-old man injured when his motorcycle collided with an automobile. AP radiographs (A-B) of the right femur; intraoperative radiograph (C). Initial AP radiographs show a comminuted femoral shaft fracture with a butterfly fragment (arrowhead) along the medial cortex. The limb has already been placed in traction, pending operative reduction and fixation.

On the intraoperative radiograph following placement of an intramedullary nail, the butterfly morphology (arrowhead) of the fragment is more apparent. The biomechanics of this fracture imply that the femur was loaded in bending until it broke, with the butterfly fragment on the medial concave side of the bend.

Case 10–15

Bisphosphonate-related insufficiency femur fracture

(A)

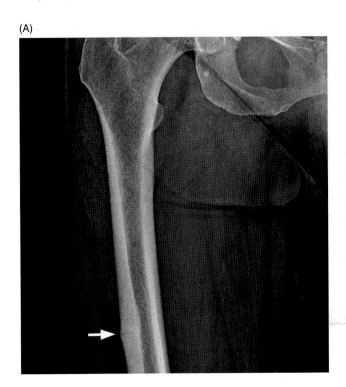

(B)

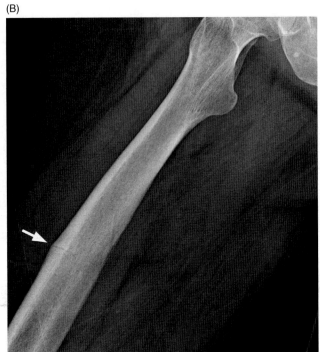

Post-menopausal woman with chronic thigh pain; history of osteoporosis treated with bisphosphonate medications for more than 10 years. AP (A) and frog lateral (B) radiographs of the right femur. There is an incomplete fracture of the lateral femoral cortex (arrows) with heaped up periosteal reaction at the site. Bisphosphonates suppress osteoclast activity and reduce bone resorption and turnover [3]. This in turn may interfere with bone remodeling and fracture healing, increasing the risk of insufficiency fractures in some patients who use bisphosphonates [4–5].

Case 10–16
Total hip replacement femur fracture

(A)

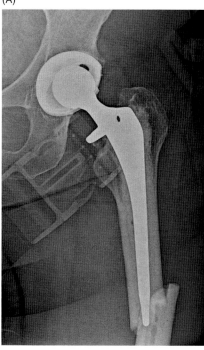

(B)

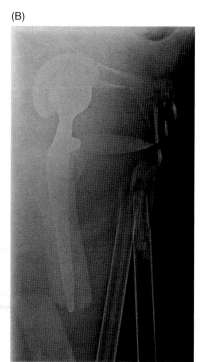

62-year-old woman injured in a ground-level fall. AP (A) and lateral (B) radiographs of the left femur. There is a simple fracture of the proximal femoral shaft at the level of the tip of the stem of a cemented total hip replacement. Interfaces between bone and metal implants act as stress risers, concentrating forces from loading. Fractures of bones with metal implants typically pass through these interfaces.

Case 10–17
Supracondylar femur fracture

(A)

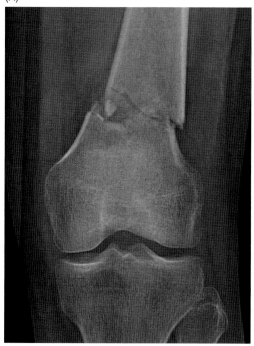

(B)

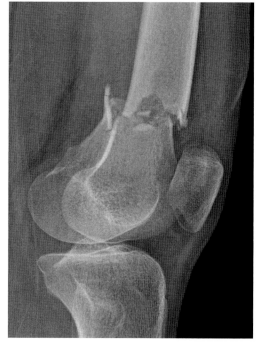

23-year-old woman who crashed during a dirt bike competition. AP (A) and lateral (B) radiographs of the left knee. There is an irregular transverse fracture of the distal femoral shaft, just above the femoral condyles, with a small degree of comminution.

Case 10–18   Supracondylar femur fracture

(A)

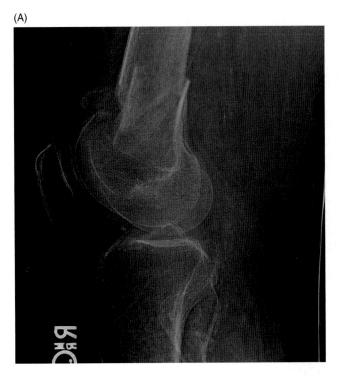

(B)

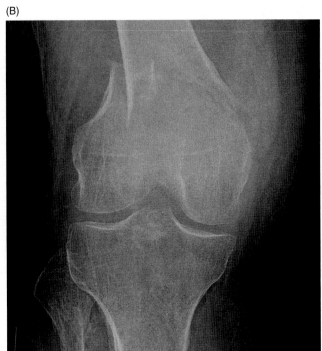

70-year-old man who crashed into a wall with his powered wheelchair. Lateral (A) and AP (B) radiographs of the right knee. There is a comminuted fracture of the distal femoral shaft above the level of the femoral condyles. Fragments of the lateral cortex have been impacted into each other. Osteopenia is present.

Case 10–19   Intercondylar femur fracture

(A)

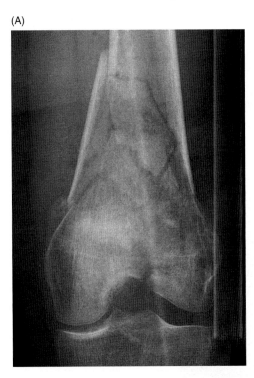

(B)

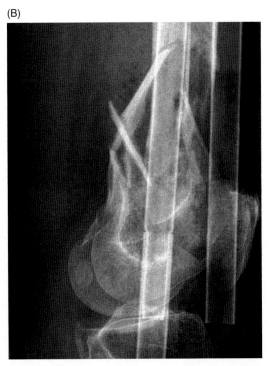

74-year-old man injured in a ground-level fall. AP (A) and lateral (B) radiographs of the left distal femur. There are severely comminuted fractures of the distal femur extending from the metaphysis through the intercondylar notch, with anterior angulation and posterior displacement. There is a fracture through the lateral condyle.

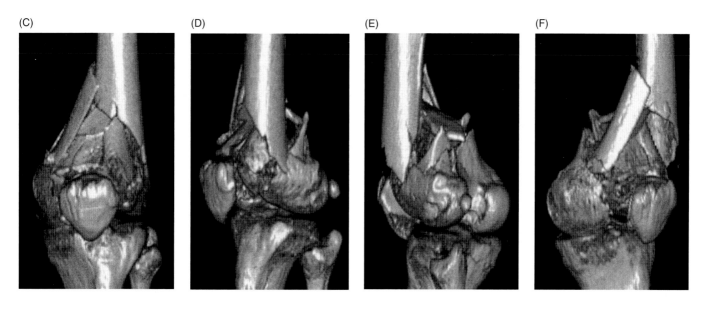

3D surface-rendered CT of the left distal femur (C-F). The high degree of comminution of the distal femur is emphasized by the 3D surface-rendered CT.

Case 10–20
Lateral condyle femur fracture

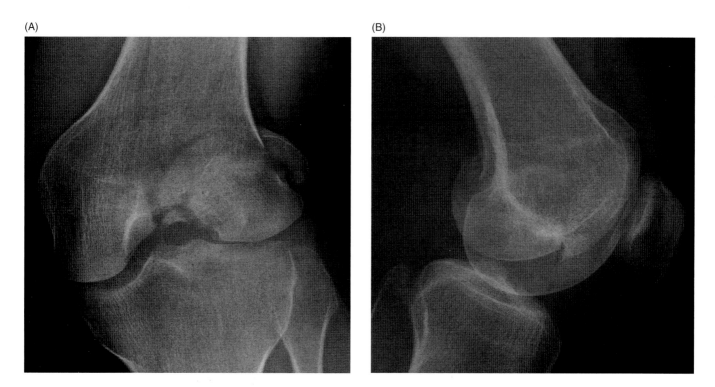

29-year-old man injured after jumping from his skateboard. Oblique (A) and lateral (B) radiographs of the left knee. There is an impacted and mildly displaced fracture of the lateral condyle.

(C)

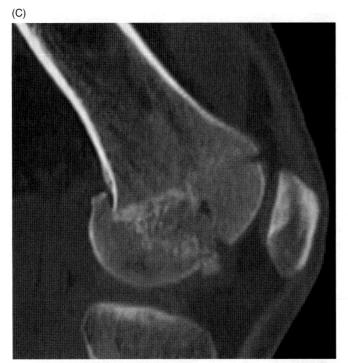

(D)

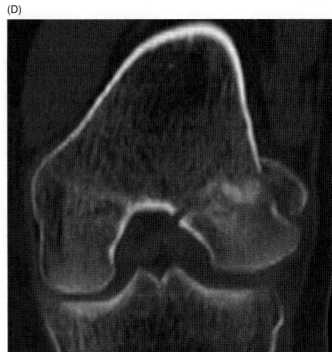

(E)

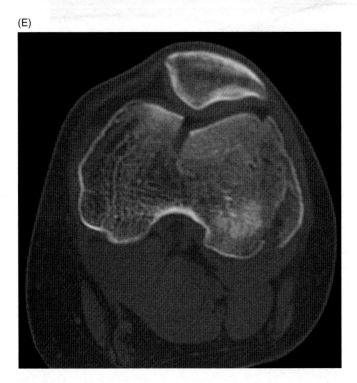

Sagittal (C), coronal (D), and axial CT (E) of the left knee. The fracture (arrows) extends through the base of the lateral condyle and is comminuted. The lateral condyle has been impacted into the metaphysis. The articular surface has been disrupted by a fracture through the lateral condyle in the coronal plane. There is a laterally displaced fracture of the lateral epicondyle. There is a lipohemarthrosis.

Case 10–21
Medial condyle femur fracture (Hoffa fracture)

(A)

(B)

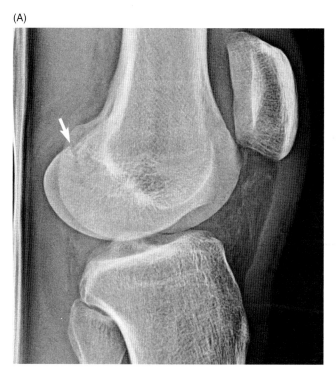

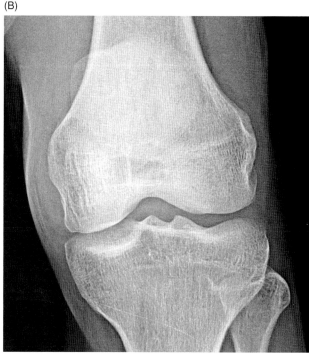

30-year-old man whose leg was pinned by a heavy load during a forklift mishap. Lateral (A) and AP (B) radiograph of the left knee. There is an intra-articular fracture of the posterior portion of the medial femoral condyle, obscured by the overlap with the lateral femoral condyle on the lateral view. The fracture was not apparent on the AP view.

(C)

(D)

(E)

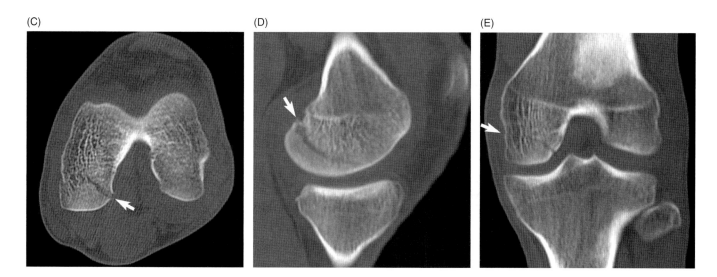

Axial (C), sagittal (D), and coronal (E) CT of the left knee. The fracture extends through the medial condyle in an oblique coronal plane, with minimal displacement and comminution. An isolated femoral condyle fracture in the coronal plane is called a Hoffa fracture, and is thought to be the result of axial loading transmitted through a flexed knee. It is more common on the lateral side.

Case 10–22
Trochlea of femur fracture

(A)

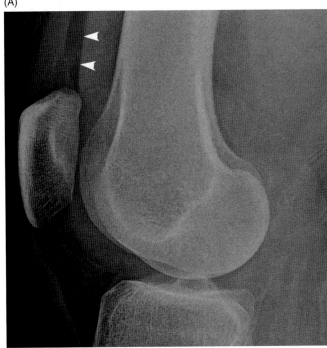

23-year-old female passenger injured in motorcycle crash. Lateral radiograph of the right knee (cross-table). The suprapatellar recess of the knee capsule is distended, with a fat-fluid level. In the setting of trauma, a fat-fluid level is a radiographic sign of an intra-articular fracture. The fracture site bleeds and allows fat from the marrow cavity to spill into the joint cavity, resulting in a lipohemarthrosis [6]. The fat will layer on top of the blood, but can be seen only if the x-ray beam is horizontally oriented (as would be the case in a cross-table lateral).

(B)

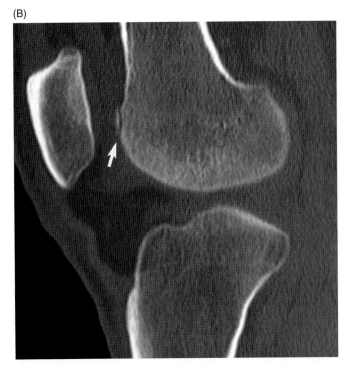

(C)

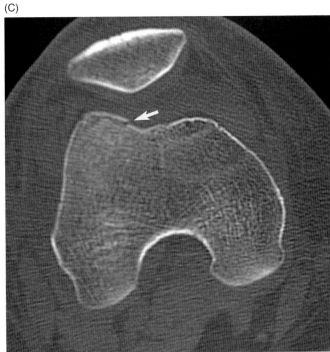

Sagittal (B) and axial (C) CT of the right knee at the level of the lateral facet of the trochlea. There is a minimally displaced fracture of the lateral facet of the femoral trochlea involving the subchondral cortex.

Case 10–23
Medial condyle femur avulsion fracture

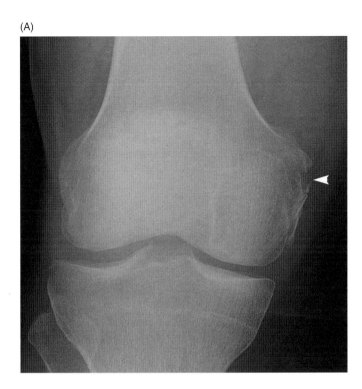

(A)

36-year-old man whose motorcycle collided with a van. AP radiograph of the right knee. There is irregularity along the medial femoral condyle (arrowhead), suspicious for a fracture.

(B)

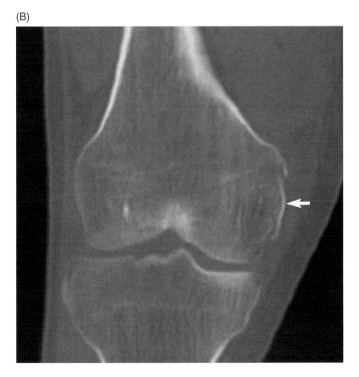

(C)

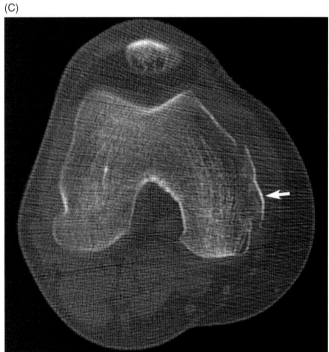

Coronal (B) and axial (C) CT of the right knee. There is a minimally displaced avulsion fracture of the cortex of the medial femoral condyle at the origin of the medial collateral ligament (arrows). This fracture is called a Stieda fracture, and corresponds to an avulsion fracture of the medial collateral ligament at its femoral attachment [7].

Case 10–24
Total knee replacement femur fracture

(A)

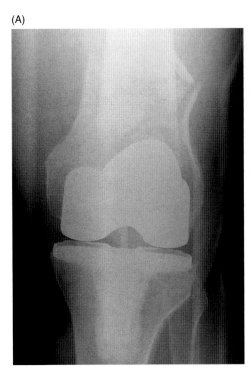

(B)

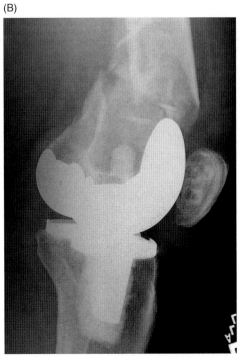

65-year-old man in a motorcycle crash. AP (A) and lateral (B) radiographs of the left knee. There is a comminuted fracture of the distal femoral shaft that extends transversely at the level of a total knee replacement.

(C)

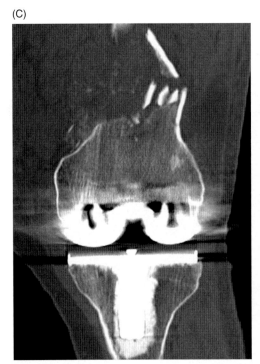

(D)

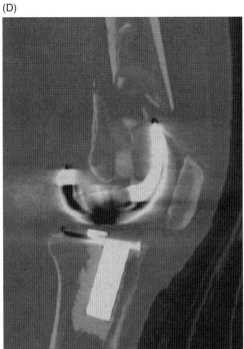

Coronal (C) and sagittal (D) CT of the left knee. CT shows severe comminution. The fracture begins at the anterior superior margin of the femoral component. The bone-metal interface acts as a stress riser, where external loading forces are concentrated. Some periprosthetic fractures after total knee replacement are related to complications of the prosthesis itself, but because of the increasing prevalence of total knee replacements in the elderly segment of the population, the presence of the prosthesis is often incidental. It has been estimated that there are 4.7 million individuals living with total knee replacements in the United States, with a prevalence of 10.38% in the population 80 years or older [8].

References

1. Haleem S, Lutchman L, Mayahi R, Grice JE, Parker MJ. Mortality following hip fracture: Trends and geographical variations over the last 40 years. *Injury*. 2008 Oct;39(10):1157–63. Epub 2008 Jul 24. PMID: 18653186.

2. Massie LK. Treatment of femoral neck fractures emphasizing long term follow-up observations of aseptic necrosis. *Clin Orthop Rel Res*. 1973 May; (92): 147–54. PMID: 4710832.

3. Armamento-Villareal R, Napoli N, Diemer K, Watkins M, Civitelli R, Teitelbaum S, Novack D. Bone turnover in bone biopsies of patients with low-energy cortical fractures receiving bisphosphonates: A case series. *Calcif Tissue Int*. 2009 Jul;85(1):37–44. Epub 2009 Jun 23. PMID: 19548019.

4. Lenart BA, Neviaser AS, Lyman S, Chang CC, Edobor-Osula F, Steele B, van der Meulen MC, Lorich DG, Lane JM. Association of low-energy femoral fractures with prolonged bisphosphonate use: A case control study. *Osteoporos Int*. 2009 Aug;20(8):1353–62. Epub 2008 Dec 9. PMID: 19066707.

5. Schilcher J, Aspenberg P. Incidence of stress fractures of the femoral shaft in women treated with bisphosphonate. *Acta Orthop*. 2009 Jan 1:1–3. PMID: 19568963.

6. Arger PH, Oberkircher PE, Miller WT. Lipohemarthrosis. *Am J Roentgenol Radium Ther Nucl Med*. 1974 May;121(1):97–100. PMID: 4833893.

7. Gottsegen CJ, Eyer BA, White EA, Learch TJ, Forrester D. Avulsion fractures of the knee: Imaging findings and clinical significance. *Radiographics*. 2008 Oct;28(6):1755–70. PMID: 18936034.

8. Maradit Kremers H, Larson DR, Crowson CS, Kremers WK, Washington RE, Steiner CA, Jiranek WA, Berry DJ. Prevalence of Total Hip and Knee Replacement in the United States. *J Bone Joint Surg Am*. 2015 Sep 2;97(17):1386-97. doi: 10.2106/JBJS.N.01141. PMID: 26333733.

Fractures and dislocations of the knee and leg

Felix S. Chew, M.D.

Case 11–1
Quadriceps tendon rupture

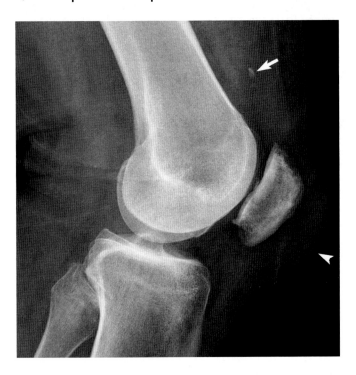

52-year-old man who stumbled and fell to the ground. Lateral radiograph of the left knee. There is marked soft tissue swelling over the patella (arrowhead). There is a proximally distracted avulsion fracture fragment (arrow) from the superior pole of the patella, and the normal quadriceps tendon is not seen. The patella is positioned inferior to its normal position (patella baja). The patella is a sesamoid bone beneath the quadriceps tendon; these findings represent a complete tear of the quadriceps tendon superior to the patella (accounting for the soft tissue swelling) with proximal retraction and avulsion of a small fragment of the superior pole.

Case 11–5 Stellate patella fracture

(A)

(B)

(C)

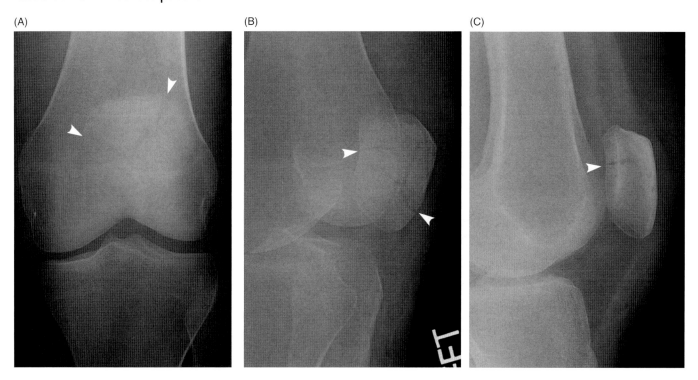

Adult who fell on knee. AP (A), oblique (B), and lateral (C) radiographs of the left knee. There is a stellate fracture (arrowheads) of the patella with minimal displacement. There is a joint effusion and overlying soft tissue swelling. This fracture pattern is the result of direct trauma to the patella; the quadriceps mechanism remains intact.

Case 11–6 Lateral patella dislocation

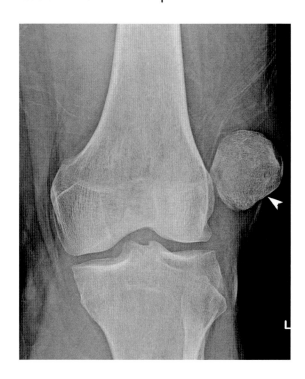

37-year-old man whose patella popped out when he knelt down. AP radiograph of the left knee. The patella (arrowhead) is dislocated to a position just lateral to the femur. The articulation between the femur and tibia is normal. No fracture is seen. Most patellar dislocations occur with non-contact, low-energy flexion-valgus stress. The patella dislocates laterally and may be associated with a variety of soft tissue injuries, especially the medial patellofemoral ligament [2]. MRI may be appropriate to evaluate for concomitant osteochondral injury.

Case 11–7   Posterior knee dislocation

(A)

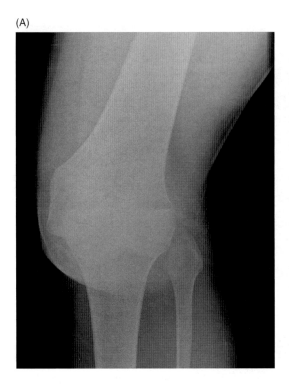

(B)

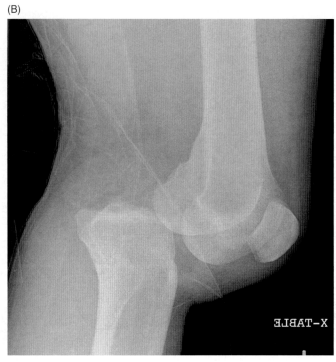

Adult in a high-speed motor vehicle crash. AP (A) and lateral (B) radiographs of the left knee. There is posterior dislocation of the knee. No definite fractures are evident. Severe ligamentous injuries accompany knee dislocations, typically including tears of the anterior and posterior cruciate ligaments [3].

Vascular injuries may also be associated with knee dislocation; a recent meta-analysis found a prevalence of 18% among all acute traumatic knee dislocation patients, with multi-ligament injuries and posterior dislocations as additional risk factors for vascular injuries [4].

Case 11–8   Anterior knee dislocation

(A)

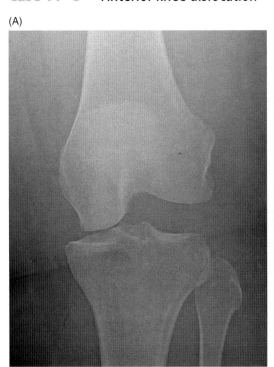

(B)

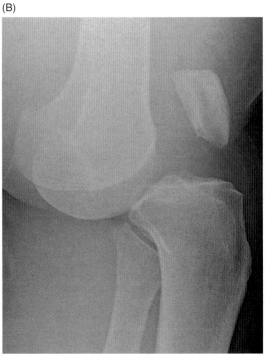

44-year-old woman who tripped on the stairs and fell. AP (A) and lateral (B) radiographs of the left knee. There is anterior dislocation of the knee. No fractures are evident. Subsequent evaluation showed no vascular injuries but tears of anterior and posterior cruciate ligaments and medial and lateral collateral ligaments.

Case 11–9
Lateral knee dislocation

(A)

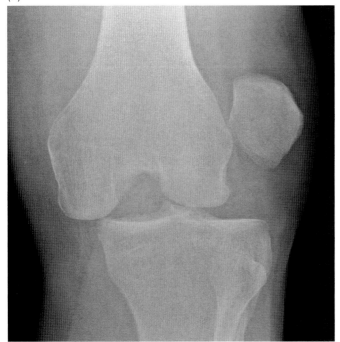

(B)

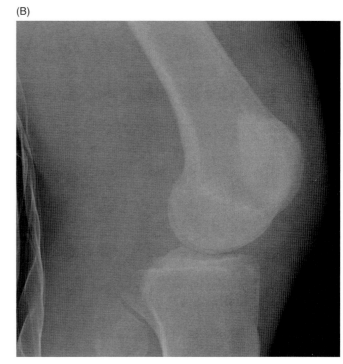

51-year-old man in a sky-diving mishap, losing lift 10 feet above the ground and landing awkwardly. AP (A) and lateral (B) radiographs of the left knee. There is lateral dislocation of the tibia relative to the femur, with the lateral tibial articular surface uncovered and the medial tibial articular surface aligned with the intercondylar notch of the femur. The patella has dislocated laterally with the tibia. The femur and tibia remain aligned in the coronal plane, as shown on the lateral view.

Case 11–10   Medial knee dislocation

(A)

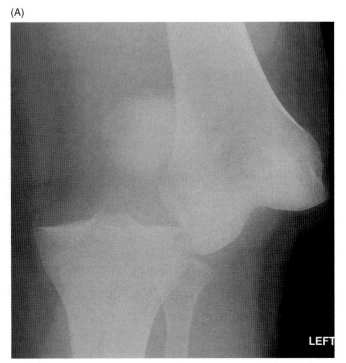

LEFT

(B)

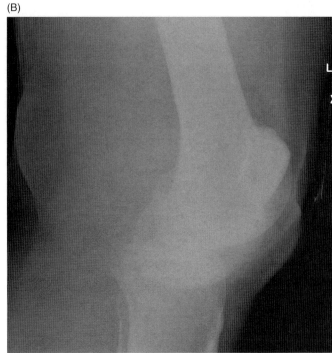

30-year-old man involved in a motorcycle collision. AP (A) and lateral (B) radiographs of the left knee. There is medial dislocation of the tibia relative to the femur. The patella is medially dislocated from the trochlea, but remains aligned with the tibia. Subsequent MRI showed the expected severe multi-ligament injuries.

Case 11–11   Anterior tibial spine fracture

(A)

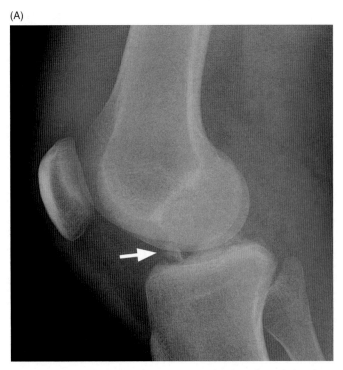

(B)

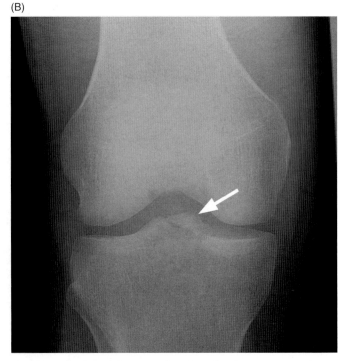

Young adult with a sports injury. Lateral (A) and AP (B) radiographs of the right knee. There is an avulsion fracture of the anterior tibial spine, a component of the median eminence of the tibia, which is indicative of avulsion by the anterior cruciate ligament [5]. There is knee joint effusion.

Case 11–12   Combined ACL-PCL avulsion fractures

(A)

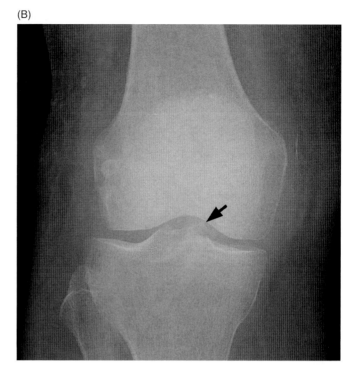

(B)

59-year-old woman in a motorcycle crash. Lateral (A) and AP (B) radiographs of the right knee. There is an avulsion fracture of the anterior tibial spine, indicative of avulsion by the anterior cruciate ligament (short arrow). There is an avulsion fracture of the posterior margin of the tibia (long arrow) suggestive of avulsion by the posterior cruciate ligament. There is extensive soft tissue swelling. There is knee joint effusion.

(C)

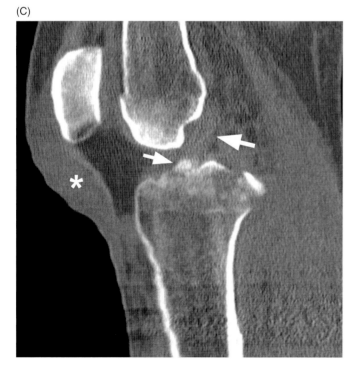

(D)

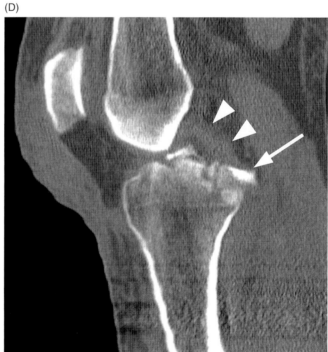

Sagittal CT of the right knee through the median eminence, lateral (C) and medial (D). There is an avulsion fracture of the anterior tibial spine (short arrow). The anterior cruciate ligament (large arrow) is intact and attached to the fragment. There is an avulsion fracture of the posterior margin of the tibia (long arrow). The posterior cruciate ligament (arrowheads) is intact and attached to the fragment. There is extensive soft tissue swelling (*). There is knee joint effusion. In this case, the likely mechanism of injury was hyperextension.

Case 11–13   Segond fracture

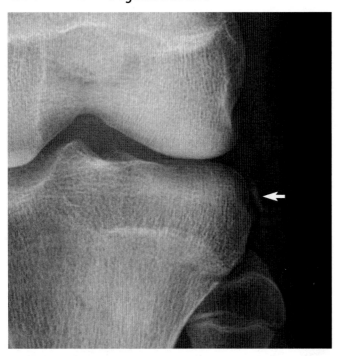

Young adult with a sports injury. AP radiograph of the left knee. There is a small avulsion fragment at the lateral margin of the proximal tibia (arrow). This fracture corresponds to an avulsion of the lateral collateral ligament complex or lateral joint capsule, and is highly associated with tears of the anterior cruciate ligament [5]. A joint effusion is also present. MRI should be obtained to document the ACL tear and to identify additional injuries.

Case 11–14   Fibular styloid avulsion fracture (arcuate sign)

(A)

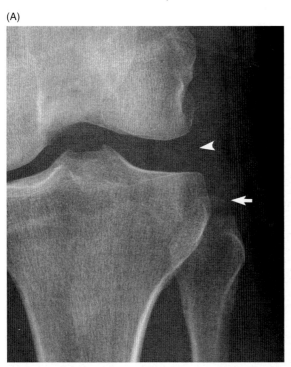

(B)

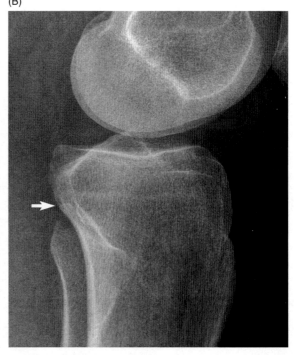

48-year-old woman who was struck by a car as a pedestrian. AP (A) and lateral (B) radiographs of the left knee. There is lateral joint space widening of the knee, indicative of ligamentous injury on the lateral side. There is an avulsion fracture of the styloid process of the head of the fibula, corresponding to an avulsion of the arcuate ligament. The arcuate ligament includes the fibular attachment of the lateral collateral ligament. When a pedestrian is struck in the knee by a car, the car has typically approached from the side and the knee may be forced into valgus or varus, depending on whether the impact is from the lateral or medial side of the knee, respectively.

Case 11–15
Proximal tibiofibular dislocation

(A)

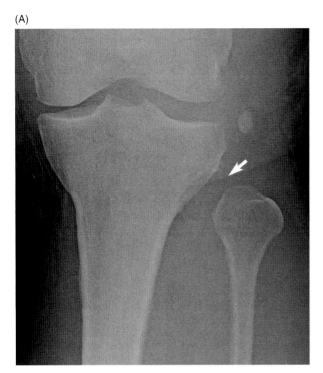

(B)

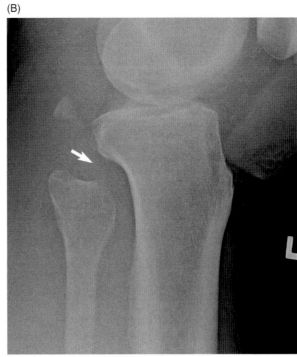

59-year-old man in motorcycle crash. AP (A) and lateral (B) radiographs of the left knee. There is interior and lateral dislocation of the fibula from the proximal tibiofibular joint.

Traumatic disruption of the proximal tibiofibular joint may occur in the setting of high-energy trauma and multi-ligament knee injury as well as in sports activities [6].

Case 11–16

Tibial plateau fracture, Type I

(A)

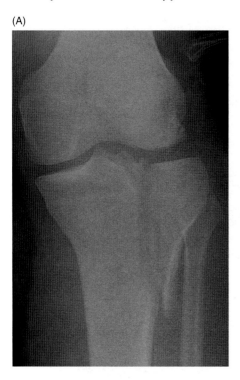

(B)

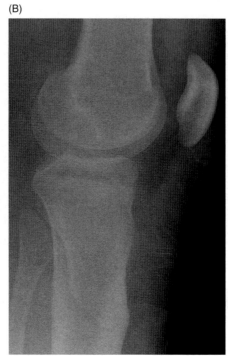

29-year-old man who fell two stories onto concrete. AP (A) and lateral (B) radiographs of the left knee. There is a displaced fracture fragment of the lateral tibial plateau that has split off without depression of the articular surface. There is the expected joint effusion. Tibial plateau fractures may be described according to the Schatzker classification [7–8]: Type I is a split lateral plateau fracture; Type II is a split plateau fracture with depressed fragment; Type III is a depressed lateral plateau fracture (without split fragment); Type IV is a medial plateau fracture; Type V is a bicondylar plateau fracture; Type VI is separation of both plateaus from the metaphysis.

(C)

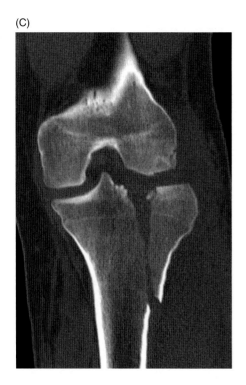

Coronal CT shows the split fracture of the lateral tibial plateau. There is no depression. There is an associated impaction fracture of the lateral femoral condyle. This tibial fracture is a Schatzker Type I fracture (split lateral plateau).

Case 11–17   Tibial plateau fracture, Type II

(A)

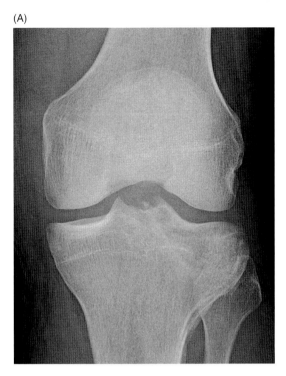

(B)

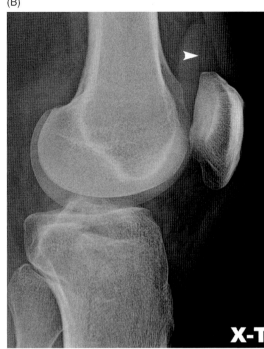

33-year-old man who crashed while snowboarding. AP (A) and lateral (B) radiographs of the left knee. There is a comminuted, depressed lateral tibial plateau fracture with a split lateral fragment. There is a large knee joint effusion with fat-fluid level (arrowhead).

(C)   (D)

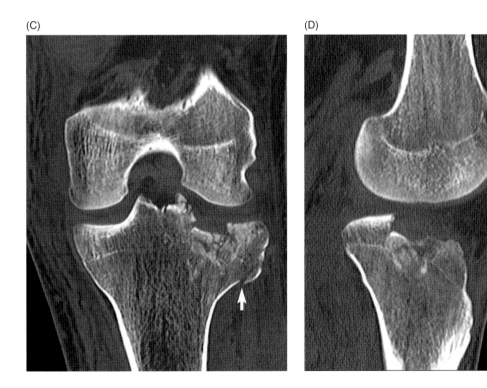

Coronal (C) and sagittal (D) CT of the left knee. The depressed portion involves the central plateau and is highly comminuted. The split fragment involves the anterolateral cortex, and is not depressed. This is a Schatzker Type II fracture.

Case 11–18   Tibial plateau fracture, Type III

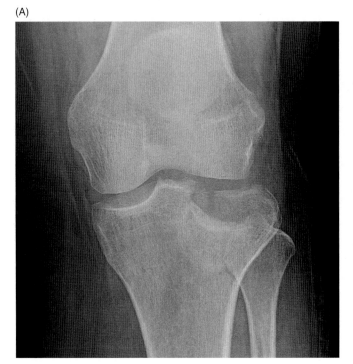

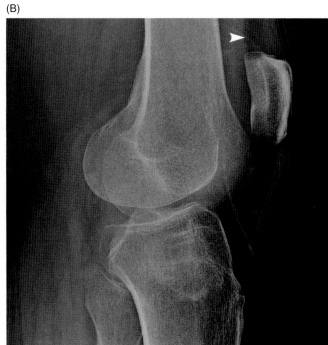

54-year-old woman who tripped and fell. AP (A) and lateral (B) radiographs of the left knee. There is a comminuted, depressed lateral tibial plateau fracture. There is an effusion and fat-fluid level (lipohemarthrosis).

(C)

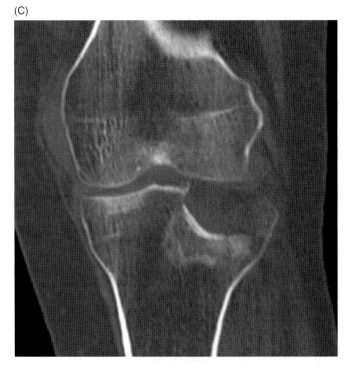

(D)

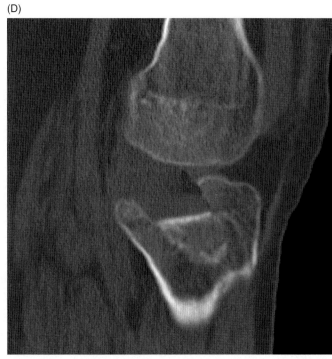

Coronal (C) and sagittal (D) CT of the left knee. There is a depressed lateral tibial plateau fracture, with intact medial plateau. There is no split lateral fragment. This is a Schatzker Type III fracture (depressed lateral plateau).

Case 11–19   Tibial plateau fracture, Type IV

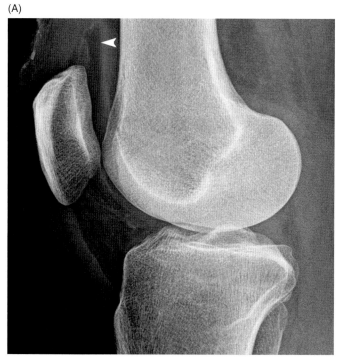

(A)

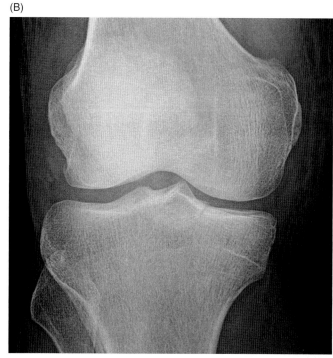

(B)

40-year-old man who was struck by a car as a pedestrian. AP (A) and lateral (B) radiographs of the right knee. There is a minimally impacted medial tibial plateau fracture. The lateral radiograph shows a lipohemarthrosis. The lipohemarthrosis consists of fatty marrow (liquid at body temperature) floating on top of a bloody effusion, indicative of an intra-articular fracture [9]. On radiographs, the lipohemarthrosis will be visible only if the radiograph was obtained with a horizontal x-ray beam; in this case, as should be routine for trauma patients, the radiograph was obtained cross-table with a horizontal beam.

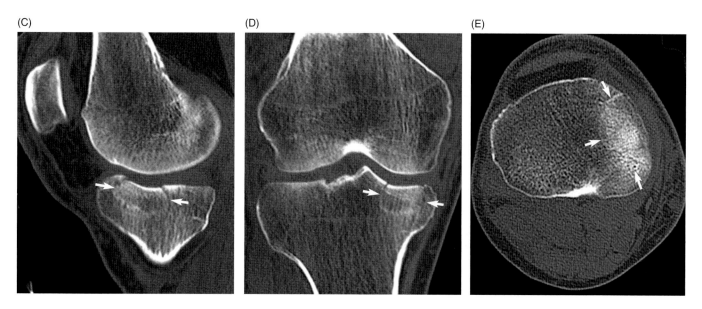

(C)   (D)   (E)

Multiplanar CT of the right knee, sagittal (C), coronal (D), and axial (E). There is a minimally impacted fracture of the medial tibial plateau. This tibial fracture may be classified as a Schatzker Type IV injury (medial plateau fracture).

Case 11–20

Tibial plateau fracture, Type V

(A)

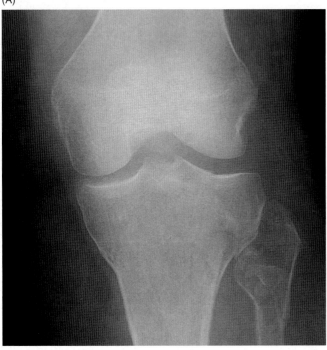

(B)

56-year-old woman in motor vehicle crash. AP (A) and lateral (B) radiographs of the left knee. There are separate fractures of the medial and lateral tibial plateaus; the medial fracture is difficult to see. There is a large joint effusion. There is also a fracture of the proximal fibula.

(C)

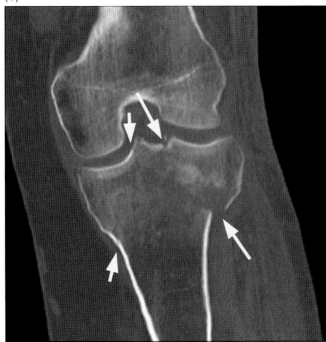

Coronal CT of the left knee. There is a medial fracture with minimal displacement (short arrows), a lateral fracture with greater displacement (long arrows), and an intact central strut that includes the anterior tibial spine. This tibial fracture is relatively uncommon and may be classified as a Schatzker Type V injury (separate bicondylar plateau fractures).

Case 11–21
Tibial plateau fracture, Type VI

(A)

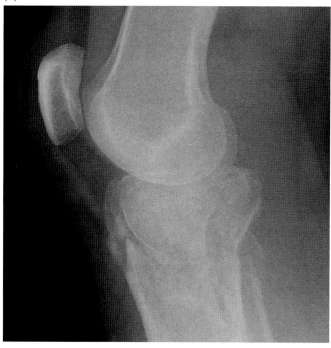

(B)

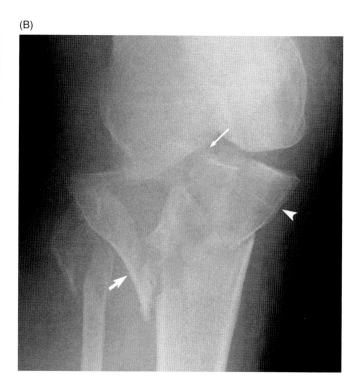

52-year-old woman who fell 12 feet from a ladder. Lateral (A) and AP (B) radiographs of the right knee. There is a bicondylar tibial plateau fracture with separation of the medial (arrowhead) and lateral (arrow) plateaus from the tibial shaft.

There is comminution of the median eminence (long arrow). There is a proximal fibular fracture, and there is a joint effusion with lipohemarthrosis.

(C)

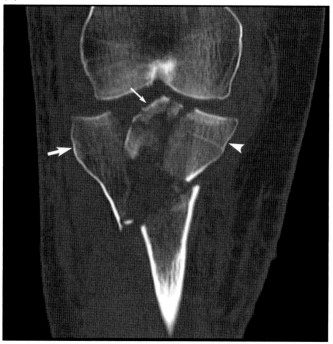

Coronal CT of the right knee. There is a bicondylar tibial plateau fracture with separation of the medial (arrowhead) and lateral (arrow) plateaus from the tibial shaft. There is comminution of the median eminence (long arrow). This tibial fracture may be classified as a Schatzker Type VI fracture.

Case 11–22
Proximal tibial shaft fracture

(A)

(B)

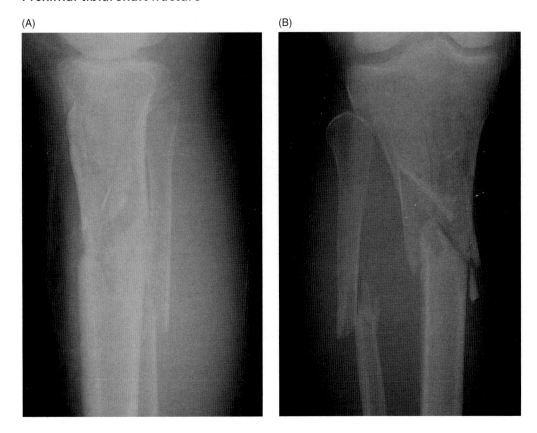

53-year-old woman in motorcycle crash. Lateral (A) and AP (B) radiographs of the right leg. There are severely comminuted fractures of the proximal tibial shaft, with extension to the lateral tibial plateau and spine. There are accompanying fibular shaft fractures.

Case 11–23
Spiral tibial shaft fracture

(A)

(B)

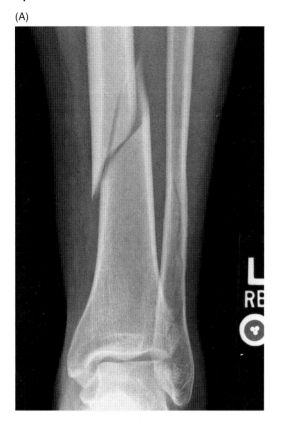

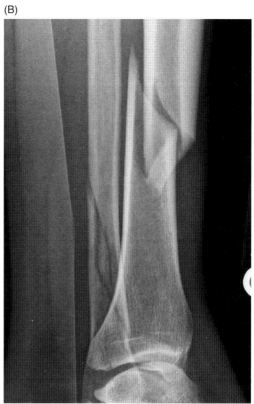

46-year-old man injured walking downhill when he slipped on a pine-cone. AP (A) and lateral (B) radiographs of the left leg. There is a displaced spiral fracture of the distal tibial shaft. There is an accompanying oblique fracture of the proximal fibular shaft. There is also a posterior malleolar fracture.

(C)　　(D)　　(E)　　(F)　　(G)

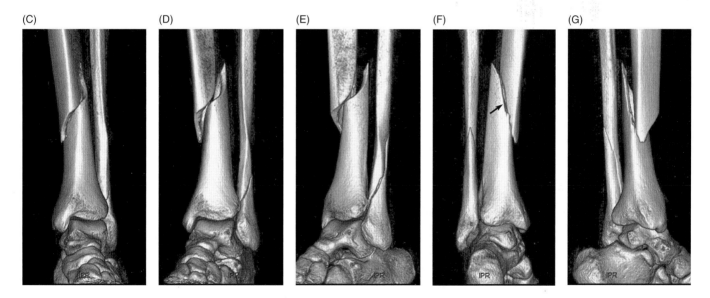

3D surface-rendered CT of the left leg (C-G). The spiral fracture line can be followed circumferentially around the tibial shaft, with a straight fracture line (arrow) connecting the superior and inferior portions of the fracture. There is also an oblique fracture of the distal fibular shaft, running from high posterior to low anterior.

Case 11–24   Segmental tibial and fibular shaft fractures

(A)

(B)

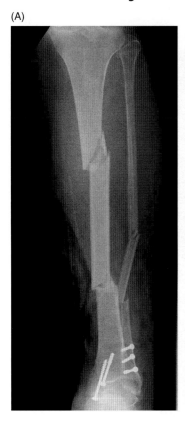
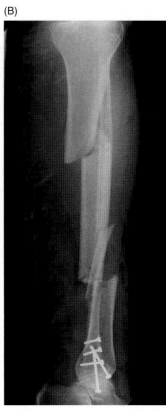

82-year-old woman struck by a car while a pedestrian. AP (A) and lateral (B) radiographs of the left leg. There are segmental fractures of the tibial and fibular shafts. Note that the knee and ankle are pointing in different directions. There is an old, healed ankle fracture with internal fixation. Segmental fractures are the result of high-energy trauma and may be treated by a variety of means, including intramedullary rods, internal fixation, and external fixation [10]. When pedestrians are struck by cars, the level of injury depends on the relative height of the bumper; the severity is related to the speed of the car and the fragility of the victim.

Case 11–25   Open tibia fractures

(A)

(B)

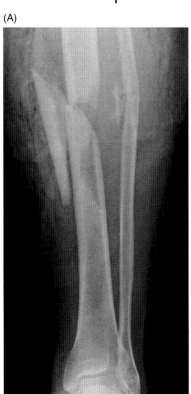
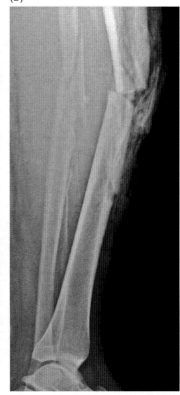

47-year-old man in motorcycle crash. AP (A) and lateral (B) radiographs of the left lower leg. There are comminuted open fractures of the tibial shaft, with gas in the soft tissues. Open fractures carry a significant risk of infection [11].

Case 11–26 Tibial shaft fracture

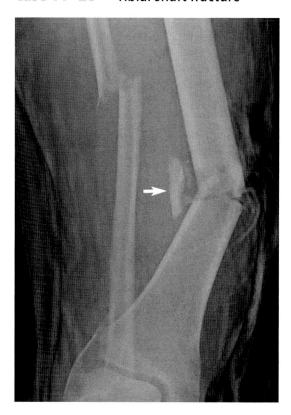

36-year-old woman injured in a fall from horseback. AP radiograph of the right lower leg. There is an open fracture of the distal tibial shaft with lateral angulation of the distal fragment and lateral butterfly fragment. There are also fractures of the fibular shaft and lateral malleolus.

Case 11–27 Tibia stress fracture

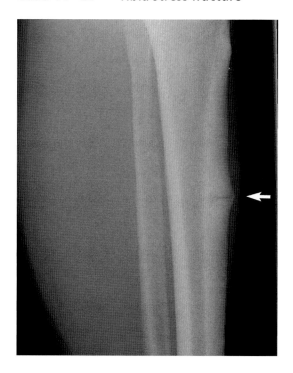

39-year-old man who is an avid soccer player with chronic leg pain. Lateral radiograph of the left lower leg. There is a partially healed stress fracture of the tibia, evident as a transverse line that extends partially across the anterior cortex. Heaped periosteal bone formation adjacent to the fracture line is the result of the healing process. The anterior tibial cortex is hypertrophic from stress remodeling.

Case 11–28
Tibia longitudinal stress fracture

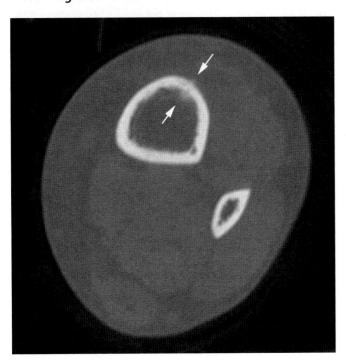

Runner with leg pain. Axial CT slice of the proximal third of the left tibial shaft. There is a longitudinal fracture of the anterior tibial cortex with evidence of periosteal and endosteal healing (arrows). Longitudinal stress fractures are relatively uncommon and may require CT, MRI, or radionuclide bone scan for demonstration [12–14]. (Source: Chew FS. Skeletal Radiology: The Bare Bones. 3rd Edition. Copyright © 2010 by Felix Chew.)

Case 11–29
Multiple tibia stress fractures

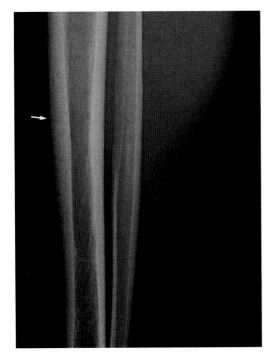

35-year-old man with chronic leg pain. Lateral radiograph of the right lower leg. There are multiple stress fractures in the anterior tibial cortex seen as short horizontal lines extending partway across the cortex. One of the fractures is indicated by an arrow, but more are present. Most stress fractures may be managed by rest and activity modification; in some circumstances, intramedullary rod placement may be appropriate for a more rapid return to activity [15].

References

1. Della Rocca GJ. Displaced patella fractures. *J Knee Surg*. 2013 Oct;26(5):293–9. doi: 10.1055/s-0033-1353988. Epub 2013 Aug 21. PMID: 23966286.

2. Duthon VB. Acute traumatic patellar dislocation. *Orthop Traumatol Surg Res*. 2015 Feb;101(1S):S59–S67. doi: 10.1016/j.otsr.2014.12.001. Epub 2015 Jan 12. PMID: 25592052.

3. Robertson A, Nutton RW, Keating JF. Dislocation of the knee. *J Bone Joint Surg Br*. 2006 Jun;88(6):706–11. PMID: 16720759.

4. Medina O, Arom GA, Yeranosian MG, Petrigliano FA, McAllister DR. Vascular and nerve injury after knee dislocation: A systematic review. *Clin Orthop Relat Res*. 2014 Sep;472(9):2621–9. doi: 10.1007/s11999-014-3511-3. PMID: 24554457; PMCID: PMC4117866.

5. Gottsegen CJ, Eyer BA, White EA, Learch TJ, Forrester D. Avulsion fractures of the knee: Imaging findings and clinical significance. *Radiographics*. 2008 Oct;28(6):1755–70. PMID: 18936034.

6. Porrino JP, Richardson ML, Mulcahy H, Chew FS, Twaddle B. Disruption of the proximal tibiofibular joint in the setting of multi-ligament knee injury. *Skeletal Radiol*. 2015 Aug;44(8):1199. doi: 10.1007/s00256-015-2170-0. PMID: 25975186.

7. Schatzker J, McBroom R, Bruce D. The tibial plateau fracture. The Toronto experience 1968–1975. *Clin Orthop Relat Res*. 1979 Jan–Feb;(138):94–104. PMID: 445923.

8. Markhardt BK, Gross JM, Monu JU. Schatzker classification of tibial plateau fractures: Use of CT and MR imaging improves assessment. *Radiographics*. 2009 Mar–Apr;29(2):585–97. PMID: 19325067.

9. Pierce CB, Eaglesham DC. Traumatic lipo-hemarthrosis of the knee. *Radiology* 1942;39(6):655–62.

10. French B, Tornetta P III. High-energy tibial shaft fractures. *Orthop Clin North Am*. 2002 Jan;33(1):211–30, ix. PMID: 11832322.

11. Olson SA, Schemitsch EH. Open fractures of the tibial shaft: An update. *Instr Course Lect*. 2003;52:623–31. PMID: 12690887.

12. Daunt N, Gribbin D, Slater GS. Longitudinal tibial stress fractures. *Australas Radiol*. 1998 Aug;42(3):188–90. PMID: 9727238.

13. Craig JG, Widman D, van Holsbeeck M. Longitudinal stress fracture: Patterns of edema and the importance of the nutrient foramen. *Skeletal Radiol*. 2003 Jan;32(1):22–7. Epub 2002 Nov 23. PMID: 12525940.

14. Pozderac RV. Longitudinal tibial fatigue fracture: An uncommon stress fracture with characteristic features. *Clin Nucl Med*. 2002 Jul;27(7):475–8. PMID: 12072771.

15. Young AJ, McAllister DR. Evaluation and treatment of tibial stress fractures. *Clin Sports Med*. 2006 Jan;25(1):117–28, x. PMID: 16324978.

Fractures and dislocations of the ankle

Felix S. Chew, M.D.

Pilon fracture of tibia

(A)

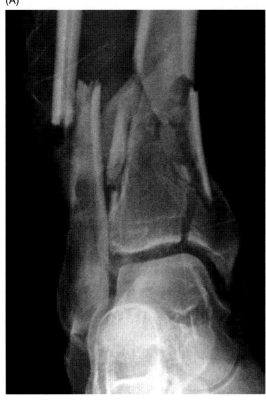

47-year-old man with polytrauma. AP radiograph of the right distal tibia and fibula. There is a comminuted fracture of the tibia that extends from the joint line of the ankle proximally into the shaft. There is an accompanying distal fibular shaft fracture.

(B)

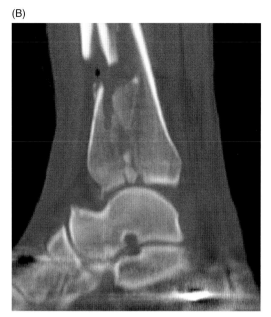

(C)

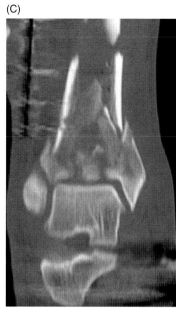

Sagittal (B) and coronal (C) CT of the right distal tibia and fibula. There is severe comminution and the involvement of the articular surface and distal metaphysis of the tibia.

(D)

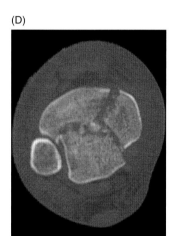

Axial CT at the right distal tibia and fibula, just superior to the tibial plafond. The characteristic fracture pattern is present, with anterior, posterior, and medial major fragments, and central comminution. This injury is called a pilon fracture, and is the result of severe axial compression that is transmitted through the foot and ankle joint to the distal tibia [1–2]. A common circumstance for this fracture is an automobile crash where the feet are braced against the floorboard at the moment of impact.

Case 12–2
Pilon fracture of tibia

(A)

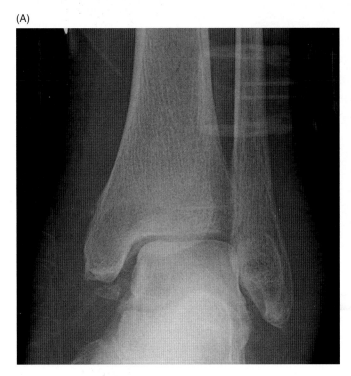

(B)

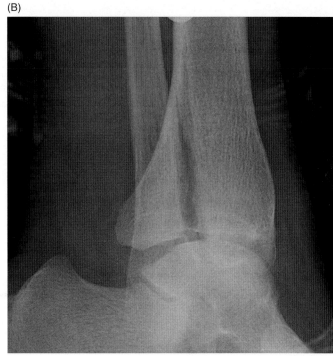

85-year-old woman injured in a high-speed motor vehicle crash. AP (A) and lateral (B) radiographs of the left ankle. There is an intra-articular fracture of the distal tibia in the coronal plane.

There is an avulsion fracture of the tip of the medial malleolus, and the medial ankle mortise is widened. There is extensive soft tissue swelling.

(C)

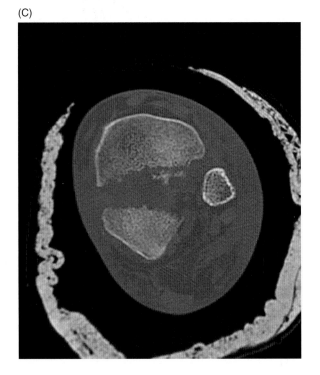

Axial CT at the left distal tibia. There is a displaced intra-articular fracture of the tibia in the coronal plane and dislocation of the distal tibio-fibular joint.

Case 12–3
Distal tibial shaft fracture

(A)

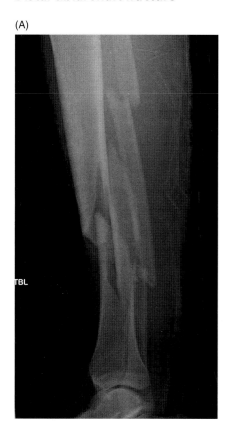

(B)

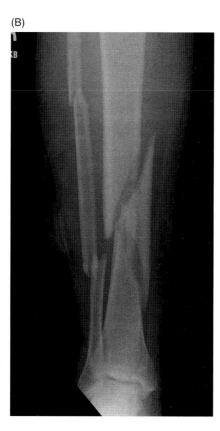

35-year-old man injured as a pedestrian struck by a car. Lateral (A) and AP (B) radiographs of the right distal tibia and fibula. There is a comminuted fracture of the distal tibial shaft with an intra-articular component extending to the ankle joint.

(C)

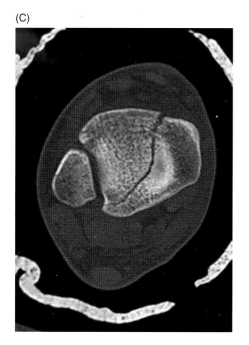

Axial CT of the right distal tibia. There is a mildly displaced intra-articular fracture of the tibial plafond dividing it into anterolateral and posteromedial fragments.

(D)

(E)

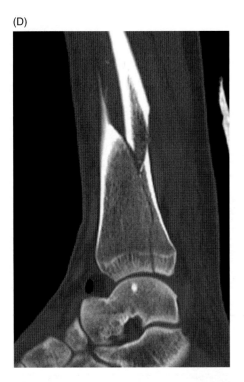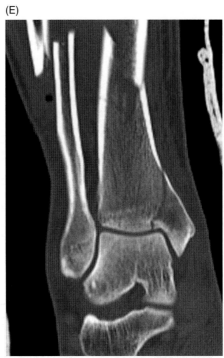

Sagittal (D) and coronal (E) CT of the right distal tibia. The distal intra-articular fracture does not have a step-off at the articular surface.

Case 12–4 Lateral ankle sprain

(A)

(B)

(C)

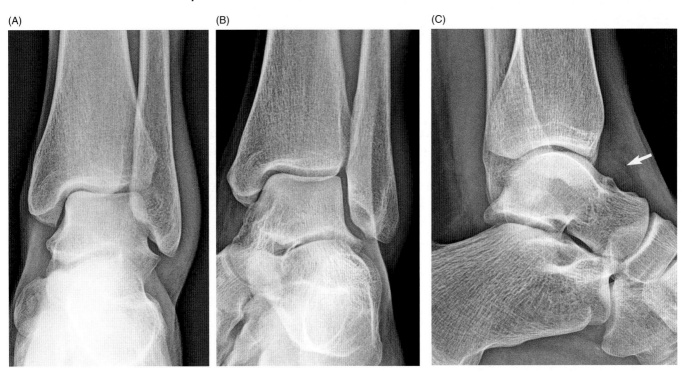

32-year-old woman who injured her ankle at the gym. AP (A), mortise (B), and lateral (C) radiographs of the left ankle. There is soft tissue swelling over the lateral malleolus, more evident when the medial and lateral sides are compared. No fracture is present. This appearance indicates a lateral ankle sprain, and usually corresponds to a tear of the anterior talofibular ligament. There is also an ankle effusion that is evident on the lateral radiograph (arrow).

Lateral malleolar fracture

(A)   (B)   (C)

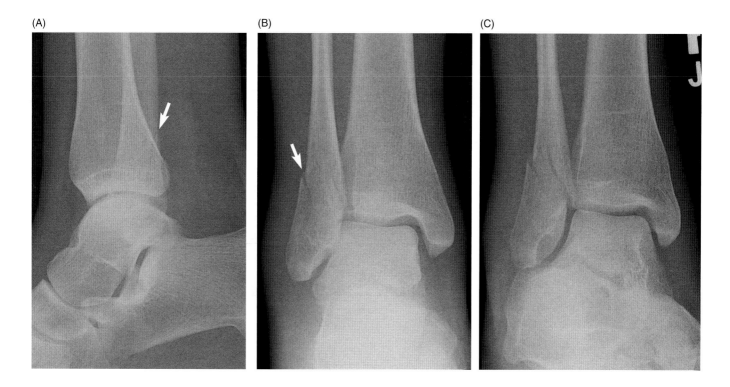

23-year-old woman who twisted her ankle. Lateral (A), AP (B), and mortise (C) radiographs of the right ankle. There is an oblique fracture of the distal fibula (arrow), extending from the posterior cortex inferiorly to the anterior cortex. The fracture extends to the level of the tibio-fibular syndesmosis. There is overlying soft tissue swelling. The distal fragment is only mildly displaced. This is the most common type of ankle fracture. The Danis-Weber system focuses exclusively on the level of the fibular fracture [3–5]. An ankle fracture in which the fibular fracture is entirely below the syndesmosis classified as a Weber A. If a portion of the fibular fracture extends to the level of the syndesmosis, it is a Weber B. If the fibular fracture is entirely above the syndesmosis, it is a Weber C. If there is no fibular fracture, the classification system does not apply. This case would be classified as a Weber B.

Case 12–6 Lateral malleolar fracture

(A)

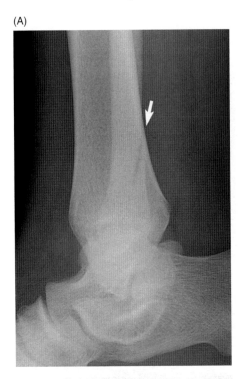

(B)

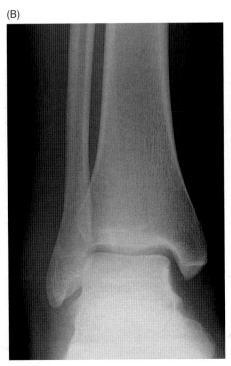

(C)

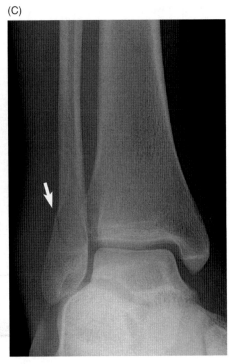

30-year-old man injured his ankle playing soccer. Lateral (A), AP (B), and mortise (C) radiographs of the right ankle. There is an oblique fracture of the distal fibula (arrow) with minimal displacement. The fracture extends from the posterior cortex inferiorly to the level of the syndesmosis. The overlying soft tissues are swollen, but the ankle mortise appears intact. This injury is a Weber B. Based on cadaver studies, Lauge-Hansen [6–10] described four mechanisms for ankle fractures. Each mechanism is a combination of foot position and direction of force, with multiple stages of severity: Supination-Adduction (S-A),

Supination External Rotation (S-ER), Pronation-Abduction (P-A), and Pronation-External Rotation (P-ER). The most common stage is S-ER, with four stages of severity: anterior tibiofibular ligament tear (Stage 1), oblique fracture of the lateral malleolus extending distally to the level of the plafond (anteroinferior to posterosuperior; Stage 2), posterior malleolar avulsion fracture or posterior tibial-fibular ligament tear (Stage 3), and transverse medial malleolar avulsion fracture or deltoid ligament rupture (classic trimalleolar; Stage 4). This case fits the S-ER mechanism.

(D)

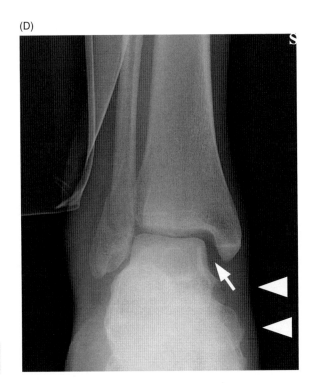

AP passive stress radiograph of the right ankle. The passive stress radiograph is obtained by laying the patient on the injured side and placing a cushion underneath the leg. The foot and ankle dangle over the end of the cushion, and the weight of the foot provides passive stress on the fracture site. The arrowheads indicate the direction of the stress. A horizontal x-ray beam is used to expose the radiograph. There is lateral displacement of the distal fibula fragment, lateral shift of the talus within the ankle mortise, and widening of the space (arrow) between the talus and the medial malleolus. This widening indicates that the deltoid ligament, which attaches the medial malleolus to the talus and calcaneus, is torn, and that the ankle is unstable. This case fits Lauge-Hansen S-ER, Stage 4.

Case 12–7
Distal fibular shaft fracture

(A)   (B)   (C)

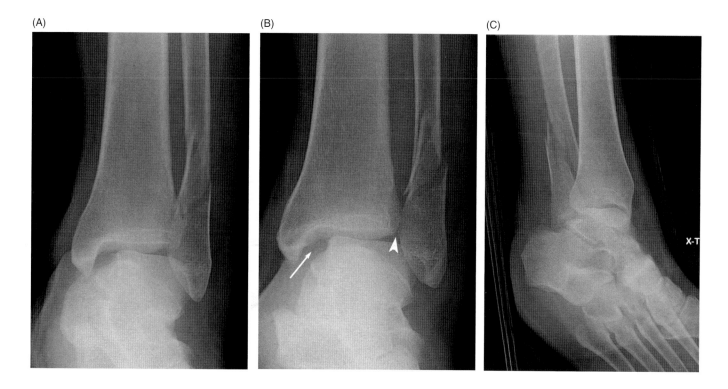

50-year-old woman with ground-level fall. AP (A), mortise (B), and lateral (C) radiographs of the left ankle. There is a laterally displaced oblique fracture of the distal fibular shaft that is entirely above the level of the distal tibio-fibular syndesmosis. The syndesmosis itself is widened (arrowhead). There is an abnormally large space between the medial malleolus and the talus (long arrow), consistent with deltoid ligament disruption, and the talus is shifted laterally with respect to the tibia. This fracture would be classified as a Weber C. Under

the Lauge-Hansen system, this injury would be classified as Pronation-External Rotation (P-ER), which has the following stages: medial malleolar fracture or deltoid ligament rupture (Stage 1), anterior tibio-fibular ligament disruption (Stage 2), fibular fracture above syndesmosis (Stage 3), and posterior malleolar fracture or posterior tibio-fibular ligament disruption (Stage 4). In this case, the displacement of the talus and lateral malleolus indicate that the posterior tibio-fibular ligament has been disrupted, making this P-ER, Stage 4.

Case 12–8
Lateral malleolar avulsion fracture

(A)

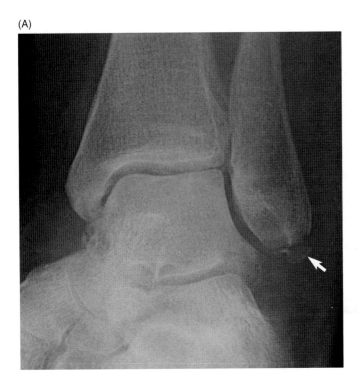

(B)

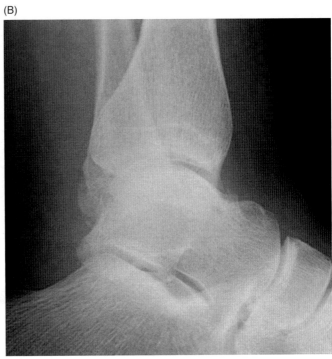

55-year-old woman injured in a motor vehicle crash. Mortise (A) and lateral (B) radiographs of the left ankle. There is a transverse fracture at the tip of the lateral malleolus, indicative of an avulsion by the lateral collateral ligament. The fragment is only mildly displaced. The overlying soft tissues are swollen. This fracture could be classified as a Weber A, because the fibular fracture is entirely below the syndesmosis. This fracture would be classified under Lauge-Hansen as Supination-Adduction (S-A), Stage 1. In S-A, Stage 2, the medial malleolus also would be fractured vertically. The practical application of the Lauge-Hansen system is that the stages occur in sequence, guiding one's search for the components of each stage.

Case 12–9

Lateral malleolar avulsion fracture

(A)

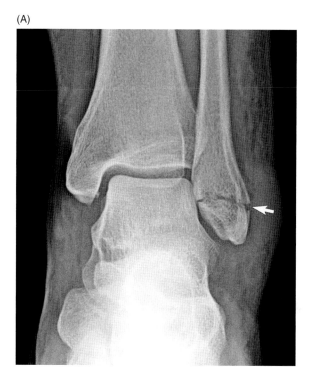

(B)

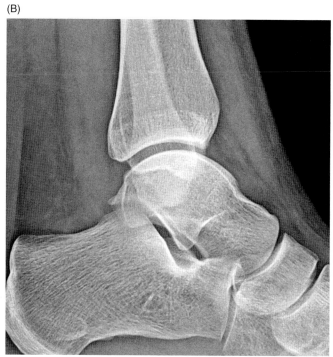

25-year-old woman who inverted and twisted her ankle while walking on flat ground. Mortise (A) and lateral (B) radiographs of the left ankle. There is a transverse fracture of the lateral malleolus, indicative of an avulsion by the lateral collateral ligament. The fragment is only mildly displaced. The overlying soft tissues are swollen. This fracture could be classified as a Weber A, because the fibular fracture is entirely below the syndesmosis.

Case 12–10
Medial malleolar fracture

(A)

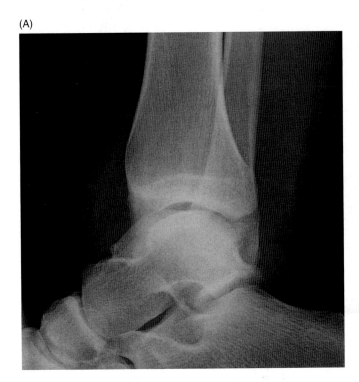

(B)

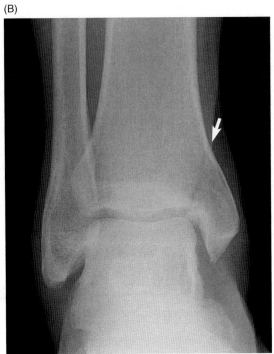

(C)

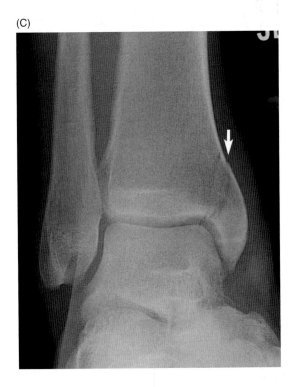

33-year-old man who fell. Lateral (A), AP (B), and mortise (C) radiographs of the right ankle. There is an oblique fracture (arrow) of the medial malleolus extending proximally and laterally from the tibial plafond. Without a fibular fracture, the Weber classification cannot be used. This case would match the Lauge-Hansen Supination-Adduction (S-A) mechanism, which consists of a transverse avulsion fracture of the lateral malleolus or lateral collateral ligament tear (Stage 1), and a vertical medial malleolus fracture (Stage 2). With a vertical medial malleolar fracture present and a lateral malleolar fracture absent, the lateral collateral ligament must have been ruptured for the injury to have passed through Stage 1 and on to Stage 2.

Case 12–11   Ankle fracture-dislocation

(A)

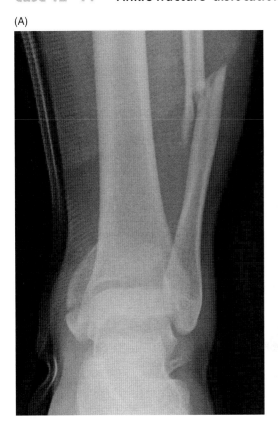

(B)

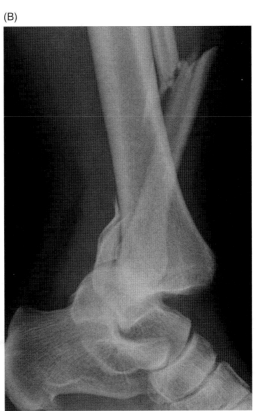

36-year-old woman injured in motorcycle accident. AP (A) and lateral (B) radiographs of the left ankle. There is ankle fracture-dislocation with transverse avulsion fracture of the medial malleolus, comminuted fibular shaft fracture above the syndesmosis, and posterior malleolar fracture.

(C)

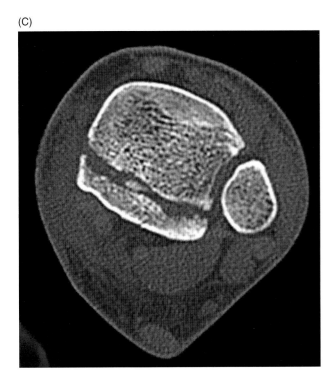

(D)

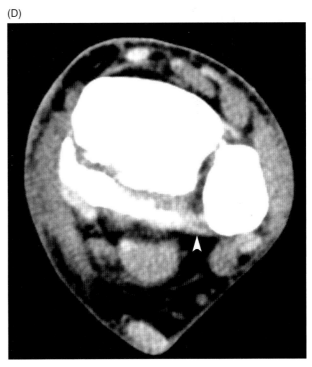

Axial CT of the left ankle following closed reduction, bone (C) and soft tissue (D) reconstructions at the same anatomic level. The posterior malleolus fracture is mildly displaced, with intact posterior tibio-fibular ligament visible on soft tissue setting. This injury would fit the Lauge-Hansen Pronation-External Rotation (P-ER) mechanism, which consists of a transverse avulsion fracture of the medial malleolus or deltoid ligament tear (Stage 1), disruption of the anterior tibiofibular ligament or avulsion fracture at its insertion sites (Stage 2), spiral fracture of the distal fibula at or above the syndesmosis (anterosuperior to posteroinferior; Stage 3), and posterior malleolar avulsion fracture or rupture of the posterior tibiofibular ligament (Stage 4).

Case 12–12

Medial malleolar fracture

(A)　　　　　　　　　　(B)　　　　　　　　　　(C)

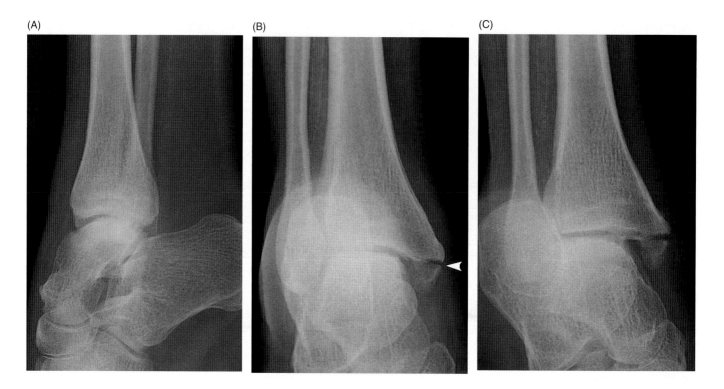

41-year-old man who twisted his ankle. Lateral (A), AP (B), and mortise (C) radiographs of the right ankle. There is a transverse fracture through the medial malleolus (arrowhead) at the level of the tibial plafond. The fracture is mildly displaced.

Without a fibular fracture, the Danis-Weber classification cannot be used. In the Lauge-Hansen system, this could be classified as a Pronation-Abduction, Stage 1 or 2.

Case 12–13
Trimalleolar fracture

(A)

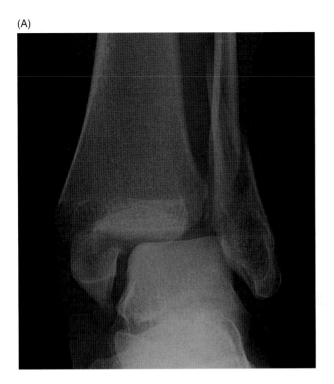

(B)

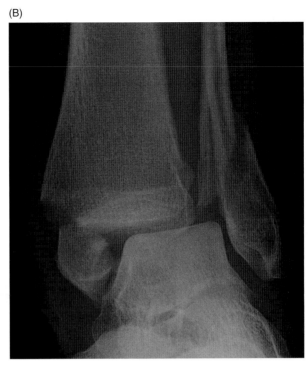

(C)

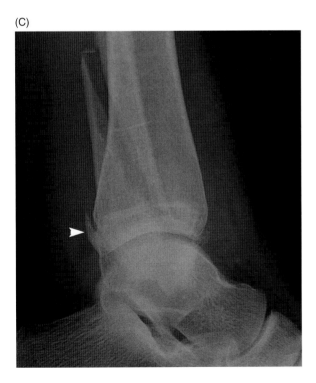

34-year-old woman who fell. AP (A), mortise (B), and lateral (C) radiographs of the left ankle. There is a transverse fracture of the medial malleolus at the level of the syndesmosis with lateral displacement; the malleolar fragment is apposed to the talus, which is shifted laterally, indicating that the deltoid ligament is intact. There is a lateral displaced and angulated fracture of the distal fibula extending from the posterior aspect of the shaft distally and anteriorly to the level of the tibial plafond. The lateral malleolar fragment is apposed to the talus, indicating that the lateral collateral ligaments are intact. The lateral radiograph shows a small posterior malleolar fragment that has displaced with the lateral malleolar fragment. The syndesmosis is widened. This injury could be classified as Weber B and S-ER, Stage 4.

Case 12–14
Ankle fracture-dislocation

(A)

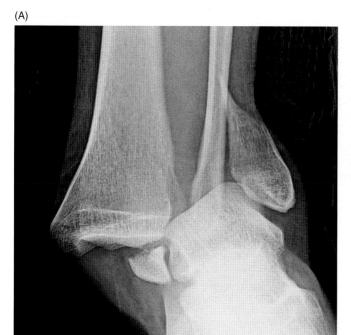

(B)

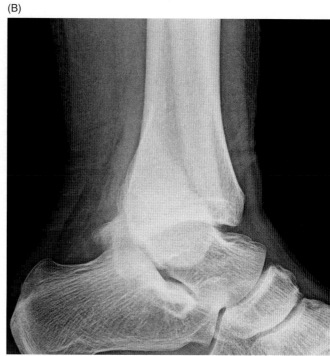

45-year-old man injured in a motorcycle crash. AP (A) and lateral (B) radiographs of the left ankle. There is a lateral fracture-dislocation of the talus (with attached foot). There is a transverse fracture of the medial malleolus and an oblique fracture of the distal fibular shaft, above the syndesmosis. This case would fit the Lauge-Hansen Pronation-Abduction (P-A) mechanism, which consists of a transverse avulsion fracture of the medial malleolus or deltoid ligament tear (Stage 1), disruption of the anterior tibio-fibular ligament (Stage 2), and fibular shaft fracture above the level of the syndesmosis (Stage 3). It could also be classified as a Weber C. Note the severe abduction of the foot, pulling off the medial malleolus and pushing off the distal fibula.

Case 12–15
Adult Tillaux fracture

(A)

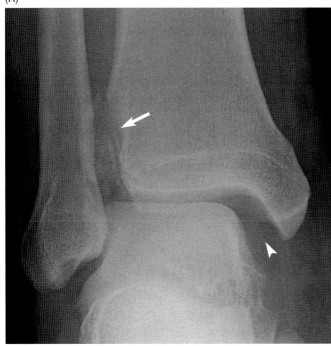

49-year-old man who was a pedestrian struck by a car. Mortise radiograph of the right ankle. There is lateral displacement of the fibula with an accompanying avulsion fracture of the lateral aspect of the tibia (arrow). There is lateral subluxation of the talus within the ankle mortise, and the medial clear space is widened (arrowhead). These findings indicated disruption of the deltoid ligament and the syndesmosis, consistent with a Lauge-Hansen P-A mechanism of injury.

(B)

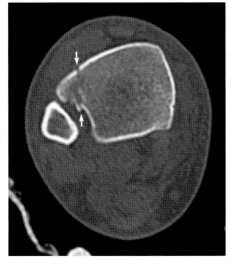

Axial CT of the right ankle at the level of the syndesmosis. There is an avulsion fracture of the anterolateral margin of the distal tibia (arrow). The Tillaux fracture is an avulsion fracture of the anterolateral tibia at the attachment of the anterior tibio-fibular ligament (Chaput's tubercle) [11] and may occur in isolation as S-ER stage 1, or in combination with other injuries as higher stages of the S-ER, P-ER, and P-A mechanisms.

Case 12–16   Maisonneuve fracture

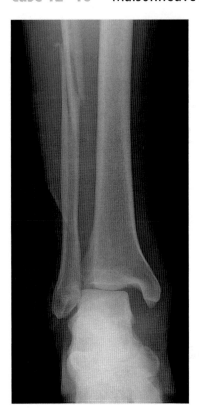

27-year-old man who was crushed under a falling object. AP radiograph of the right ankle. There is a high fibular shaft fracture. There is lateral displacement and dislocation of the distal tibio-fibular syndesmosis, consistent with ligamentous rupture of the anterior and posterior tibiofibular ligaments and tear of the interosseous membrane from the syndesmosis proximally to the level of the fibular fracture. The talus has shifted laterally within the ankle mortise, indicative of rupture of the deltoid ligament. This injury complex is called a Maisonneuve fracture. This could have the Lauge-Hansen classification of P-ER stage 4, or Weber C. Correlation of the Weber and Lauge-Hansen classifications is as follows: Weber A may occur with S-A; Weber B may occur with S-ER; Weber C may occur with P-ER and P-A.

Case 12–17   Open ankle dislocation

(A)

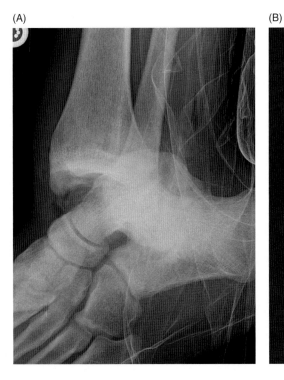

(B)

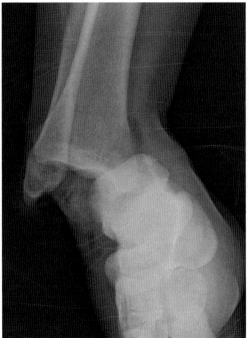

18-year-old man injured playing basketball. Lateral (A) and AP (B) radiographs of the right ankle. There is posteromedial dislocation of the tibio-talar joint. There is a lateral soft tissue injury with the lateral malleolus protruding through. Gas is present within the ankle joint and adjacent soft tissues. No fracture is present.

Case 12–18
Ankle fracture-dislocation

(A)

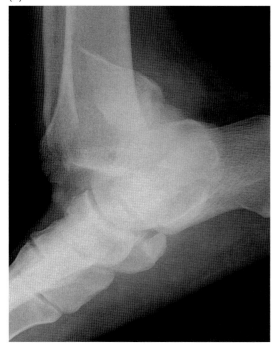

(B)

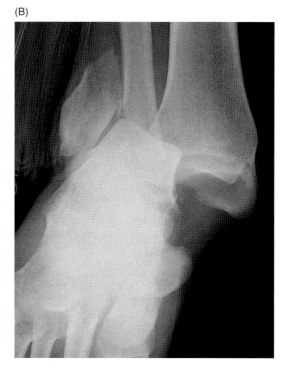

54-year-old man injured in ground-level fall. Lateral (A) and AP (B) radiographs of the right ankle. There is a grossly displaced fracture of the distal fibula with posterolateral dislocation of the talus from the ankle mortise.

References

1. Helfet DL, Koval K, Pappas J, Sanders RW, DiPasquale T. Intraarticular "pilon" fracture of the tibia. *Clin Orthop Relat Res.* 1994 Jan;(298):221–8. PMID: 8118979.

2. Barei DP, Nork SE. Fractures of the tibial plafond. *Foot Ankle Clin.* 2008 Dec;13(4):571–91. PMID: 19013397.

3. Danis R, ed. *Theorie et pratique de l'osteosynthese.* Paris, France: Masson & Cie, 1949.

4. Muller ME, Allgower M, Schneider R, Willenegger H. *Manual of internal fixation.* 3rd ed. Bern, Switzerland: Springer, 1991; 595–612.

5. Weber BG. *Die verletzungen des oberen sprunggelenkes.* 2nd ed. Bern, Switzerland: Huber, 1972.

6. Lauge-Hansen N. Ligamentous ankle fractures; diagnosis and treatment. *Acta Chir Scand.* 1949 Mar 23;97(6):544–50. PMID: 18129346.

7. Lauge-Hansen N. Fractures of the ankle. II. Combined experimental-surgical and experimental-roentgenologic investigations. *Arch Surg.* 1950 May;60(5):957–85. PMID: 15411319.

8. Lauge-Hansen N. Fractures of the ankle. III. Genetic roentgenologic diagnosis of fractures of the ankle. *Am J Roentgenol Radium Ther Nucl Med.* 1954 Mar;71(3):456–71. PMID: 13124631.

9. Lauge-Hansen N. Fractures of the ankle. IV. Clinical use of genetic roentgen diagnosis and genetic reduction. *AMA Arch Surg.* 1952 Apr;64(4):488–500. PMID: 14902249.

10. Lauge-Hansen N. Fractures of the ankle. V. Pronation-dorsiflexion fracture. *AMA Arch Surg.* 1953 Dec;67(6):813–20. PMID: 13103952.

11. Duchesneau S, Fallat LM. The Tillaux fracture. *J Foot Ankle Surg.* 1996 Mar–Apr;35(2):127–33; discussion 189. PMID: 8722880.

Fractures and dislocations of the tarsal bones

Felix S. Chew, M.D., and Hyojeong Mulcahy, M.D.

Case 13–1
Talar neck fracture

(A)

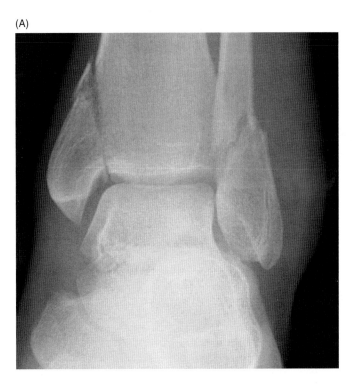

(B)

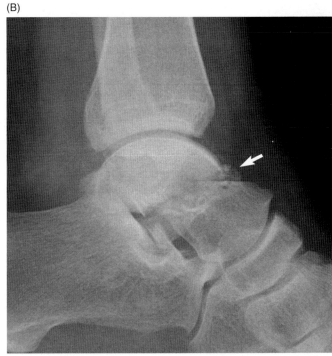

30-year-old man injured in motor vehicle crash. AP (A) and lateral (B) radiographs of the left ankle. There are bimalleolar ankle fractures. There is a talar neck fracture (arrow) with a small amount of comminution. The fracture enters the posterior facet of the subtalar joint. Talar neck fractures may be described using the Hawkins classification: Type I is a non-displaced fracture; Type II is associated with subtalar subluxation or dislocation; Type III is associated with subtalar and ankle dislocation.

Case 13–2   Talar extrusion

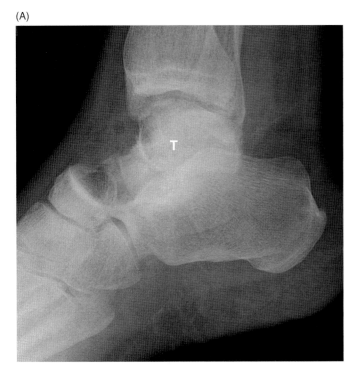

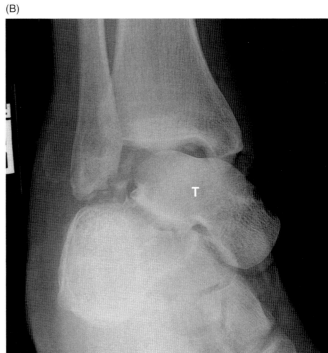

46-year-old man in 30-foot fall. Lateral (A) and AP (B) radiographs of the right ankle. The talus (T) is extruded in the medial direction from the ankle. This injury represents simultaneous

medial dislocation of the ankle and lateral subtalar dislocation of the foot.

(C)

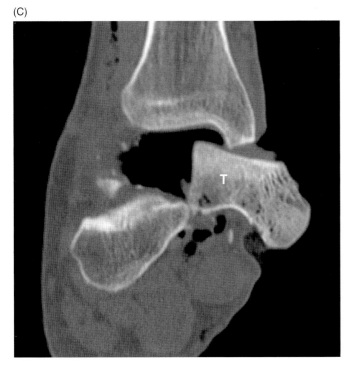

(D)

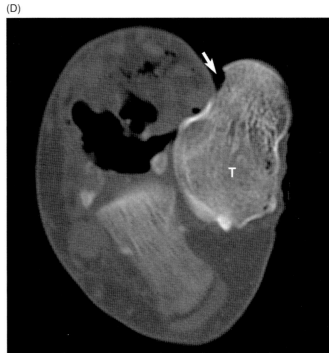

Coronal (C) and axial (D) CT images of the right hindfoot. There is moderate internal rotation and medial displacement of talus (T). The anterior medial aspect of the talus extrudes through an open wound in the soft tissues and skin (arrow). Accordingly, there is large amount of air within the ankle joint. There are multiple small bone fragments about the injury site, and an osteochondral fracture donor site on the lateral aspect of the head of the talus (arrow). Open talar fractures with extrusion of the talar body or even the entire talus are typically the result of high-energy trauma and are frequently associated with markedly displaced fractures, severe soft-tissue injury, contamination, and disruption of the talar blood supply [1–4].

Case 13–3
Talar extrusion

(A)

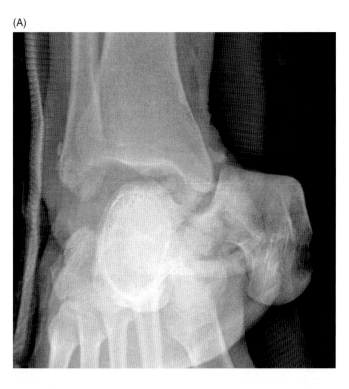

(B)

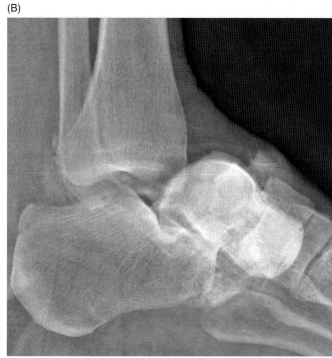

61-year-old woman in motor vehicle crash. AP (A) and lateral (B) radiographs of the right ankle. There has been complete medial extrusion of the talus, simultaneous medial dislocation of the ankle, and lateral subtalar dislocation of the foot. Talar extrusion is a rare injury. The talus can be extruded anteromedially, as in this case, or anterolaterally [5].

Case 13–4

Talar dome osteochondral fracture

(A)

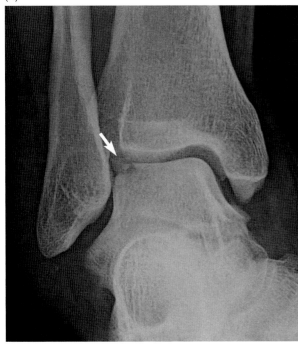

24-year-old man in high-speed motor vehicle crash. Mortise radiograph of the right ankle. There is a mildly displaced fracture of the lateral corner of the talar dome (arrow). The lateral or medial corner of the dome of the talus may be compressed against the ankle mortise during the traumatic event [4]. These fractures may require CT or MR for visualization.

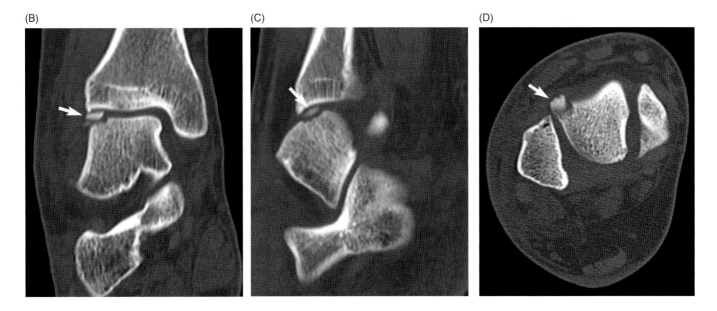

(B)

(C)

(D)

Multiplanar CT of the right ankle in coronal (B), sagittal (C), and axial (D) planes. The anterolateral corner of the talar dome is fractured with a small displaced fragment. The fragment includes the articular cartilage overlying the subchondral bone.

Case 13–5

Lateral process of talus fracture

(A)

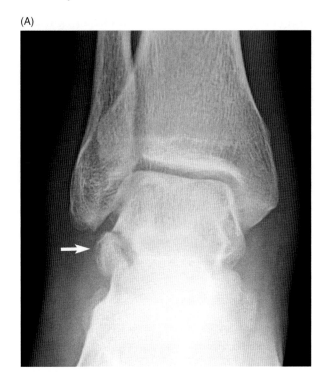

(B)

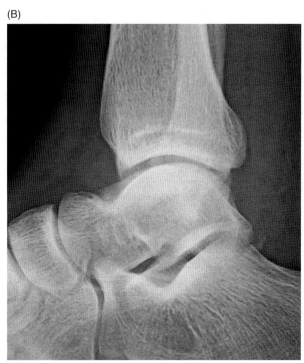

Man injured in 20-foot fall. AP (A) and lateral (B) radiographs of the right ankle. There is a comminuted lateral process of talus fracture (arrow). There is diffuse soft tissue swelling.

(C)

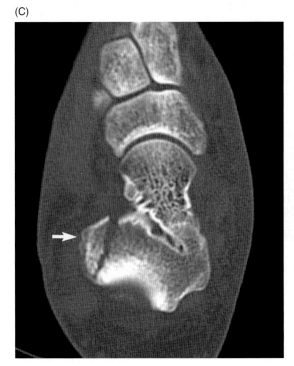

(D)

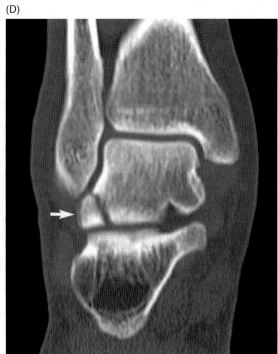

Axial (C) and sagittal (D) CT of the ankle. There is a comminuted fracture of the lateral process of the talus (arrows), extending into the anterior medial aspect of the posterior facet. The lateral process of the body of the talus is a broad-based wedge-shaped prominence that articulates dorsolaterally with the fibula and inferomedially with the calcaneus, thereby forming the lateral part of the subtalar joint. Fracture of the lateral process is seen frequently in snowboarders [6]. Before the development of this sport, these fractures were rare and generally associated with motor vehicle accidents, falls from a height, or simple inversion injuries [7]. With the increasing popularity of snowboarding, fractures of the lateral process of the talus occur more frequently and account for 2.3% of snowboarding injuries.

Case 13–6
Dorsal avulsion talus fracture

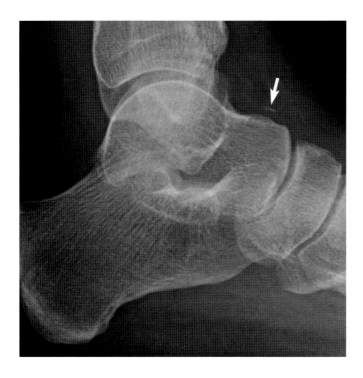

52-year-old woman who twisted her ankle. Lateral radiograph of the left ankle. There is an avulsion fracture dorsal to the head of the talus (arrow), corresponding to the attachment of the dorsal talonavicular ligament.

Case 13–7

Talus avulsion fractures

(A)

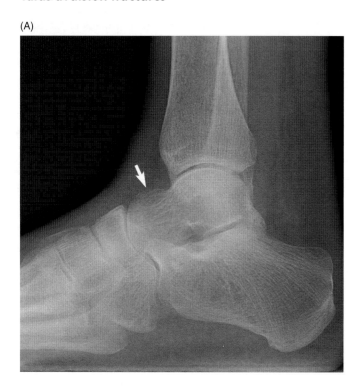

57-year-old woman with twisting injury to foot in motor vehicle crash. Lateral radiograph of the right ankle. There is a subtle dorsal avulsion fracture of talar neck (arrow).

(B)   (C)   (D)

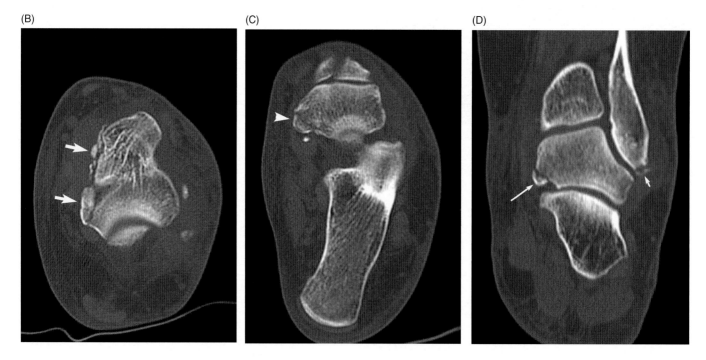

Axial (B-C) and coronal (D) CT of the right ankle. There is a mildly comminuted fracture involving the medial margin of the talus with minimal displacement (large arrows). There is a minimally displaced fracture of the medial aspect of the navicular (arrowhead) and a small accessory navicular. There is a talar medial process avulsion fractures (long small arrow) and an avulsion fracture at the tip of the lateral malleolus (short small arrow).

Case 13–8

Medial subtalar dislocation

(A)

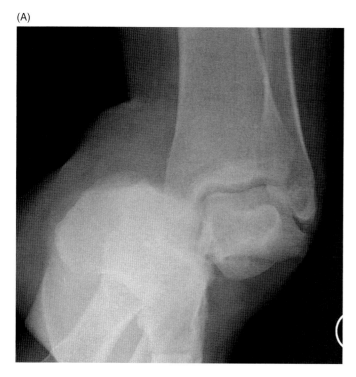

(B)

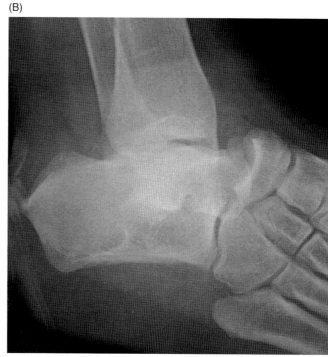

28-year-old woman sustained a twisting injury while play-ing basketball. AP (A) and lateral (B) radiographs of the right ankle. There has been gross medial dislocation of the foot from the talus. There are simultaneous dislocations of the talocalca-neal and talonavicular joints, an injury referred to as subtalar or peritalar dislocation. Following reduction, CT showed a few small avulsion fractures. Most subtalar dislocations are medial and may occur with low energy inversion or twisting, as in this case [8].

Case 13–9

Lateral subtalar dislocation

(A)

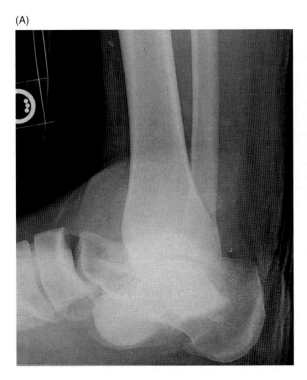

(B)

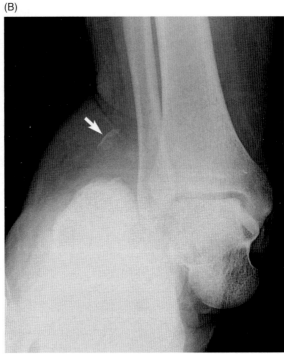

36-year-old woman injured in motor vehicle crash. Lateral (A) and AP (B) radiographs of the right ankle. The lateral view shows full overlap of the talus and the calcaneus. The AP view confirms that the talus and calcaneus are side-by-side rather than over-and-under, with the foot dislocated laterally. No more than 25% of subtalar dislocations are lateral [8]. The

displaced bone fragment lateral to the distal fibula (arrow) is an avulsion fracture of the peroneal tendon sheath. The peroneal tendons were dislocated from their normal location along the posterior aspect of the distal fibula when the foot dislocated laterally, taking with them their sheath and its bony attachment.

(C)

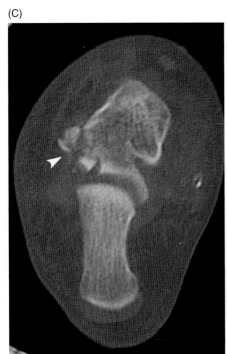

(D)

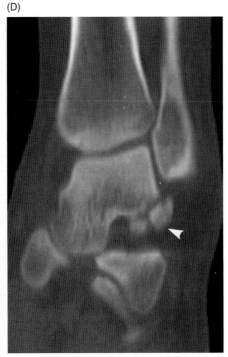

Axial (C) and coronal (D) CT of the right ankle. CT scan following reduction shows comminuted fractures of the talus at the lateral aspect of the posterior facet of the subtalar joint (arrowheads). CT should be obtained following reduction to identify fractures that might be radiographically occult [9]. The patient subsequently had open reduction and internal fixation of her fractures.

Case 13–10

Intra-articular calcaneal compression fracture, centrolateral depression type

(A)

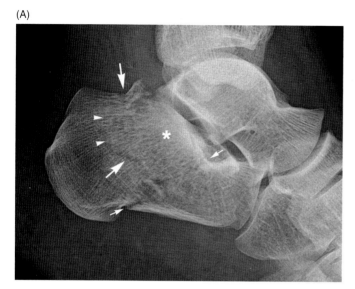

(B)

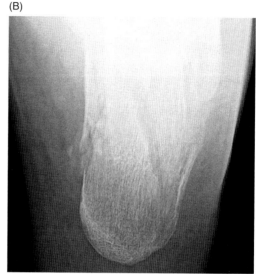

38-year-old man who fell from a height of 6 feet, landing on his feet. Lateral (A) and axial (B) radiographs of the left calcaneus. There is a comminuted calcaneal fracture with the primary fracture line extending through the posterior subtalar facet to the plantar surface (small arrows) and a secondary fracture line exiting vertically just posterior to the posterior subtalar facet (large arrows). The major posterior facet fragment (asterisk) is impacted into the calcaneal tuberosity resulting in a zone of sclerosis where the trabecular bone has been crushed together (arrowheads). Calcaneal fractures may be divided into those that involve the posterior facet of the subtalar joint (intra-articular) and those that do not (extra-articular). Accordingly, extra-articular calcaneal fractures may involve articular surfaces that are not the posterior subtalar facet.

(C)

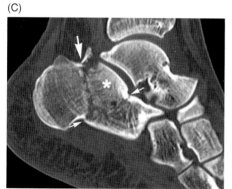

(D)

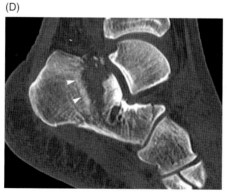

(E)

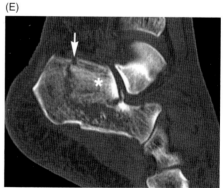

Sagittal CT of the left calcaneus, medial (C) to lateral (E). The primary fracture line (small arrows) begins at the angle of Gissane (also called critical angle) and extends to the plantar surface at the calcaneal tuberosity. A secondary fracture line extends posterior to the posterior subtalar facet (large arrows). There are two major posterior subtalar facet fragments (asterisks). Depression of the posterior facet fragments into the body of the calcaneus has crushed the trabecular bone (arrowheads).

(F)   (G)   (H)

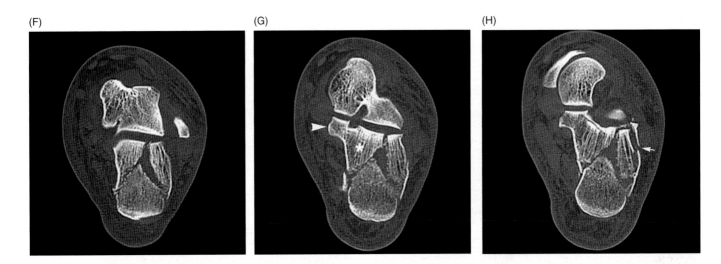

Axial CT of the left calcaneus, superior (F) to inferior (H). Comminuted fractures separate the posterior subtalar facet of the calcaneus into a medial fragment (asterisk) that includes the sustentaculum tali (arrowhead) and a lateral fragment. There is further comminution of the lateral fragment (small arrow). In the classification of Essex-Lopresti for intra-articular fractures [10–11], compression of the talus into the calcaneus splits the calcaneus through the posterior facet into an anteromedial fragment that includes the sustentaculum and a posterior tuberosity fragment. A secondary fracture may appear posterior to the facet (centrolateral compression type) or may appear in the posterior tuberosity (tongue type). This case is an example of a centrolateral compression type intra-articular calcaneal fracture.

Case 13–11   Intra-articular calcaneal compression fracture, tongue type

(A)   (B)

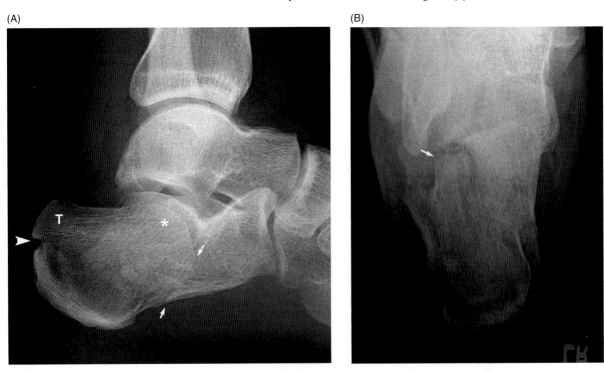

47-year-old man who fell from an 8-foot height. Lateral (A) and axial (B) radiographs of the left calcaneus. There is an impacted calcaneal fracture with the fracture line vertically extending to the posterior facet (arrows), and horizontally extending to the tuberosity (arrowhead). The principal fragment of the posterior facet (asterisk) contains the upper portion of the tuberosity, and this fragment is called the tongue fragment (T). This intra-articular fracture is designated as a tongue type calcaneal fracture.

(C)

(D)

(E)

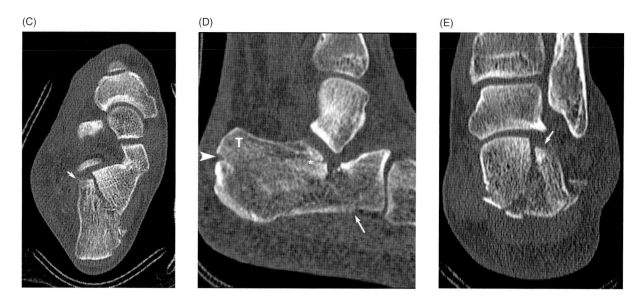

Multiplanar CT of the left calcaneus, axial (C), sagittal (D), and coronal (E). There is a comminuted intra-articular fracture (arrows) of the calcaneus. There is a tongue fragment (T) extending posteriorly from the posterior subtalar facet (asterisk). The Sanders classification of intra-articular calcaneal fractures uses the number and displacement of fractures of the posterior subtalar facet as shown on axial CT [12]. Type 1 has nondisplaced (less than 2 mm) fractures; if there is 2 mm or more of displacement of the articular fracture(s), it is Type 2 or higher. Type 2 has one primary intra-articular fracture, Type 3 has two primary intra-articular fractures, and Type 4 has three or more primary intra-articular fractures. There are subtypes of Types 2 and 3. In Type 2a, the fracture is lateral; in Type 2b, the fracture is central; in Type 2c, the fracture is medial. In Type 3ab the fractures are lateral and central; in Type 3ac, the fractures are lateral and medial; in Type 3bc, the fractures are central and medial. This case could be classified as Sanders Type 2b.

Case 13–12   Calcaneal fracture-dislocation

(A)

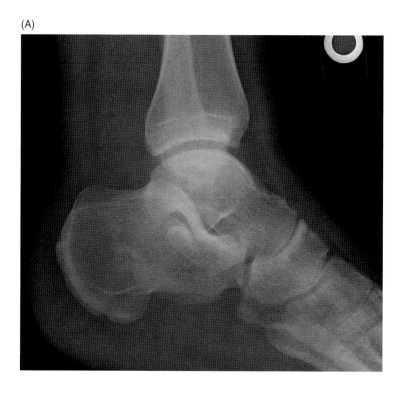

(B)

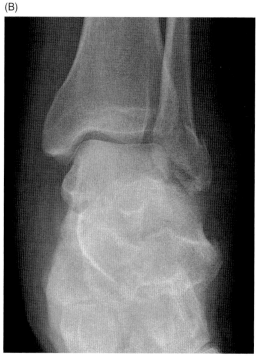

(C)

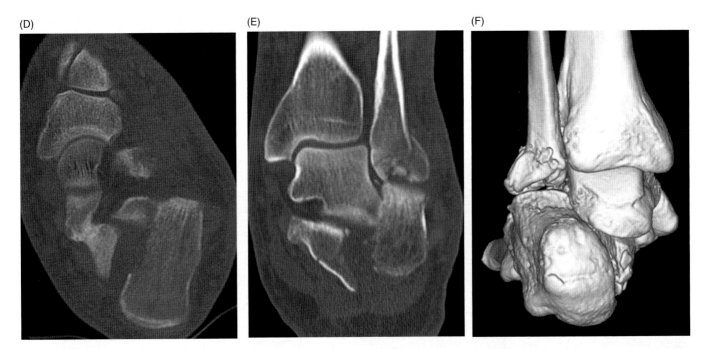

31-year-old man who tripped and fell. Lateral (A), AP (B), and oblique (C) radiographs of the left ankle. There is a comminuted intra-articular fracture of the calcaneus. A major displaced fragment has dislocated from the posterior facet of the subtalar joint and is positioned inferior to the lateral malleolus, which is also fractured.

(D)   (E)   (F)

Axial (D), coronal (E), and 3-D surface-rendered (F) CT of the left ankle. The axial image shows a comminuted intra-articular fracture of the calcaneus. The sustentaculum is a separate fragment that has an intact articulation at the middle subtalar facet, but a major fragment of the body of the calcaneus has displaced laterally and dislocated from the posterior subtalar facet, resulting in an uncovered articular surface. The coronal image shows the lateral displacement and dislocation of the calcaneal body fragment to a position inferior to the lateral malleolus, which is also fracture. The sustentaculum fragment includes a small portion of the posterior facet articulation. The 3D surface-rendered CT shows the ankle from behind, with the uncovered posterior facet of the talus and the calcaneal body impacted beneath the lateral malleolus.

Case 13–13   Calcaneus anterior process fracture

(A)

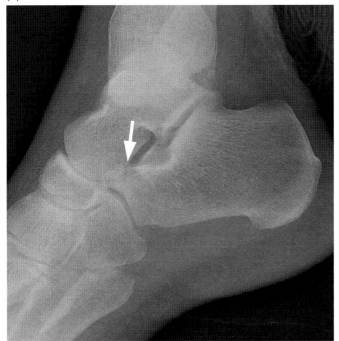

(B)

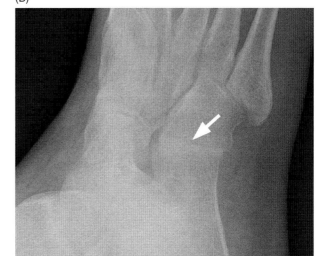

27-year-old man who fell from a 75-foot height. Lateral (A) and oblique (B) radiographs of the right foot. There is a minimally displaced fracture at the anterior process of calcaneus (arrows). Fractures of the anterior process are the most common form of avulsion fracture of the calcaneus. The anterior process serves as the attachment of the bifurcate ligament. This ligament extends from the anterior process in two limbs, one attaching to the lateral portion of the navicular bone and the other to the adjoining surface of the cuboid bone. The fracture is best seen on oblique views and may not be visible on AP and lateral views.

Case 13–14   Achilles avulsion fracture

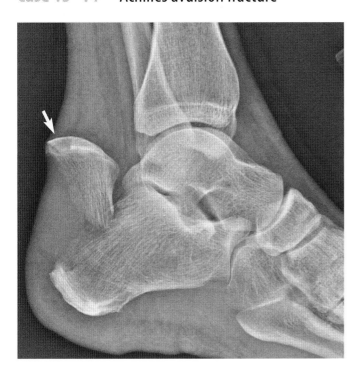

64-year-old woman who slipped on the stairs. Lateral radiograph of the left calcaneus. There is an extra-articular fracture of the superior portion of the body of the calcaneus with proximal distraction. The fracture fragment includes the insertion of the Achilles tendon (arrow).

Case 13–15

Calcaneal tuberosity fracture

(A)

(B)

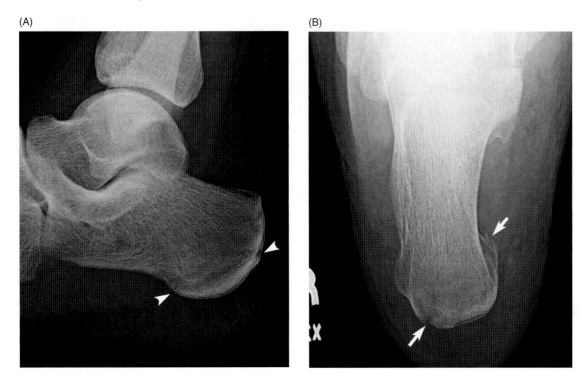

23-year-old man who was hit by a bus. Lateral (A) and axial (B) radiographs of the right calcaneus. There is a mildly impacted fracture (arrows and arrowheads) of the calcaneal tuberosity, seen more easily on the axial radiograph.

(C)

(D)

(E)

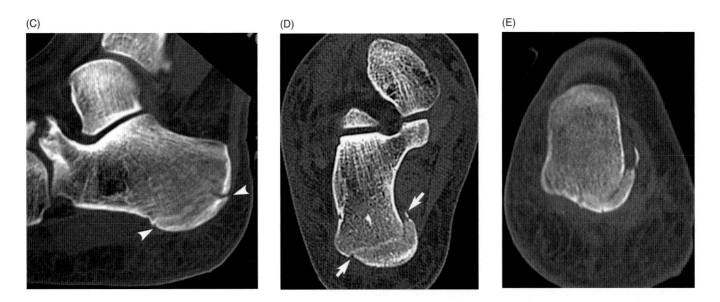

Multiplanar CT of the right calcaneus, sagittal (C), axial (D), and coronal (E) images. The fracture (arrows and arrowheads) is extra-articular and does not involve any of the articular surfaces nor the insertion of the Achilles tendon.

Case 13–16   Chopart joint fracture-dislocation

(A)

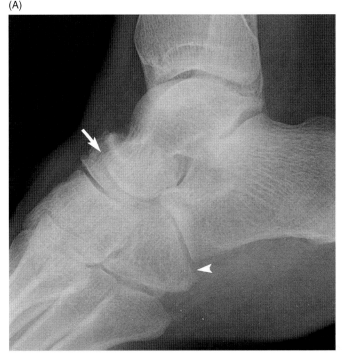

(B)

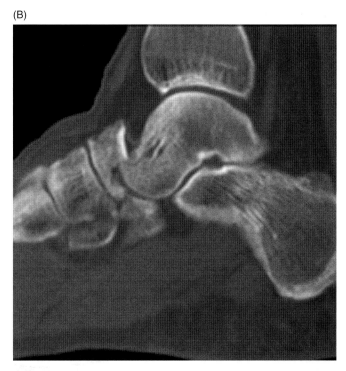

34-year-old man in motor vehicle crash. Lateral radiograph (A) and sagittal CT (B) of the right foot. The lateral radiograph shows overlapping of the head of the talus and the proximal navicular (arrow). There is subluxation of the calcaneal cuboid joint, and there is a fracture of the inferior cuboid (arrowhead). The sagittal CT shows the head of the talus has impacted into the navicular, which sustained comminuted fractures. There is dorsal dislocation of the navicular.

(C)

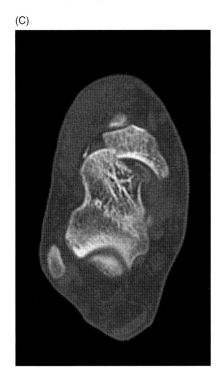

(D)

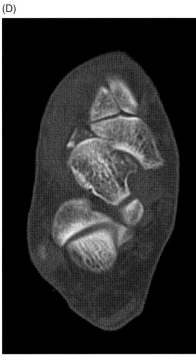

(E)

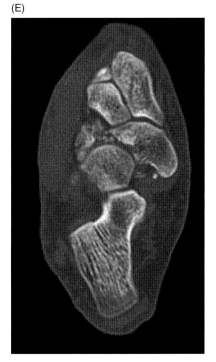

Axial CT of the foot, superior (C) to inferior (E). The axial images show the medial aspect of the navicular is impacted into the medial aspect of the head of the talus, which is fractured. There is reciprocal impaction of the lateral aspect of the head of the talus into the lateral navicular, which has also fractured with severe comminution. The findings are that of a Chopart fracture-dislocation from high-energy axial loading. The joint between the hindfoot, and the midfoot, composed of the talonavicular and calcaneocuboid joints, is referred to as the Chopart joint. Chopart joint injuries are considered to be very rare and generally require surgical treatment unless non-displaced and stable [13].

Case 13–17
Chopart joint fracture-dislocation

(A)

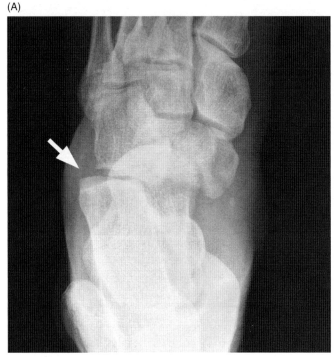

(B)

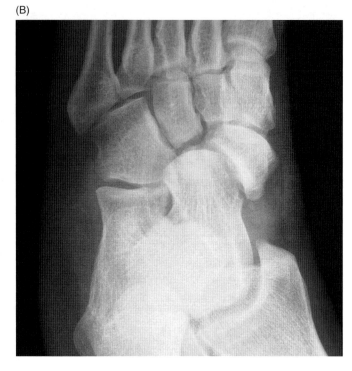

(C)

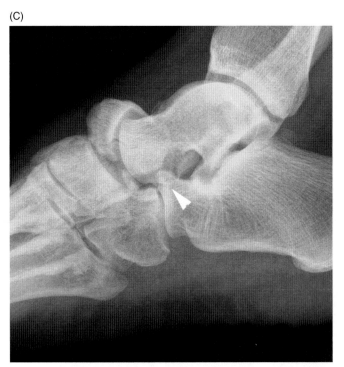

41-year-old man injured in a 40-foot fall while washing windows. AP (A), oblique (B), and lateral (C) radiographs of the foot. There is severe misalignment of the midfoot. The navicular is medially and dorsally subluxated relative to the head of the talus as well as relative to the cuneiforms. The cuboid and lateral cuneiform no longer articulate with the displaced navicular. There is widening of the calcaneal-cuboid joint and medial subluxation of the cuboid (short arrow). The normal space between the navicular and calcaneus has been grossly widened and there is an anterior process of the calcaneus fracture (arrowhead). There are multiple fractures of the navicular. There is mild posterior subluxation of the subtalar joint, with protusion of the talar head into the gap between the cuboid and navicular. The socket that receives the head of the talus, called the acetabulum pedis, is formed by the concave articular surface of the navicular, the anterior and middle subtalar facets of the calcaneus, the spring (calcaneonavicular) ligament, and the bifurcate ligament [13]. In this case, the acetabulum pedis has been severely disrupted.

Case 13–18   Navicular stress fracture

(A)

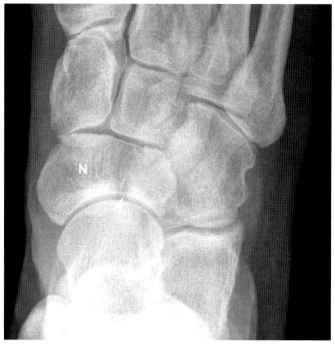

(B)

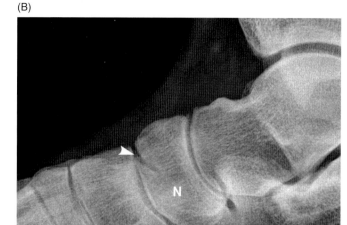

52-year-old woman with foot pain for three months. AP (A), and lateral (B) radiographs of the foot. There is an isolated navicular fracture (arrowhead) in an oblique sagittal plane extending between the naviculocuneiform and talonavicular joints, separating the navicular into medial and lateral fragments. There is minimal displacement. N=navicular medial fragment.

(C)

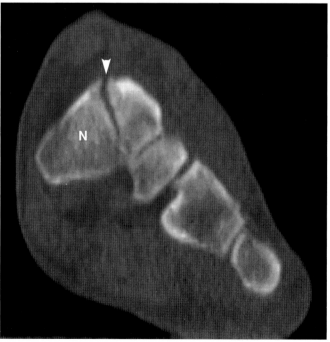

(D)

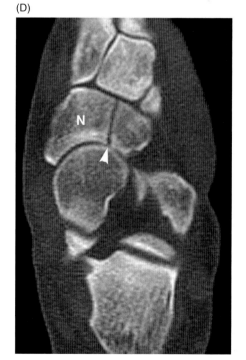

Coronal (C) and axial (D) CT of the foot. The minimally displaced navicular fracture (arrowheads) shows sclerosis of the fracture margins, but no definite bridging callus. The fracture may progress to nonunion without intervention. Navicular body fractures can be divided into three types according to the Sangeorzan classification: Type I has a horizontal fracture plane with dorsal and plantar fragments; Type II has a sagittal fracture plane with medial and lateral fragments; Type III has comminution and significant displacement of the medial and lateral poles [13–14]. This is a Type II navicular fracture. N=navicular medial fragment.

Case 13–19
Navicular body fracture

(A)

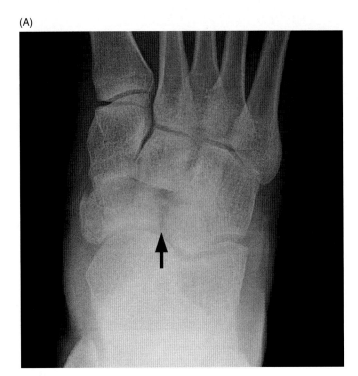

(B)

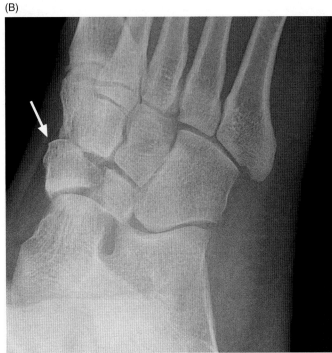

(C)

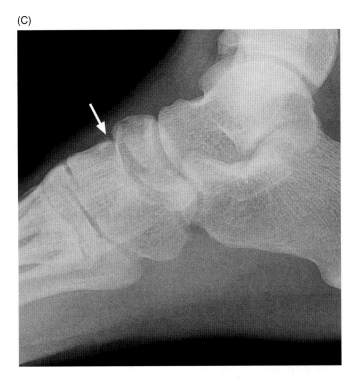

26-year-old man who fell down the stairs. AP (A), oblique (B), and lateral (C) radiographs of the foot. There is a comminuted fracture of the body of the navicular (black arrow). The fracture extends into the talonavicular joint as well as into the naviculocuneiform joint. There is dorsal subluxation of the medial fragment at the naviculocuneiform joint (white arrows), and separation of the medial and lateral fragments. This may be considered a (Sangeorzan) Type III navicular body fracture.

Case 13–20
Navicular avulsion fracture

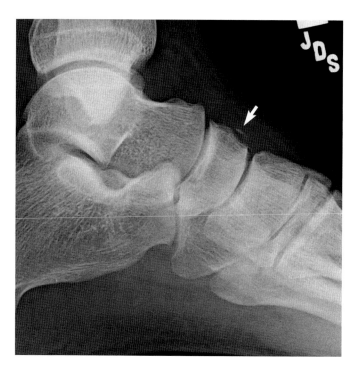

17-year-old man who slipped on the ice and fell. Lateral radiograph of the left foot. There is a thin fragment of bone (arrow) just dorsal to the navicular with soft tissue swelling. The fracture is adjacent to the naviculocuneiform joint and involves the naviculocuneiform ligament. An avulsion fracture involving the talonavicular ligaments would be closer to the talus. Avulsion fractures may also involve the insertion of the tibialis posterior insertion at the navicular tuberosity [13–14].

Case 13–21   Cuboid fracture

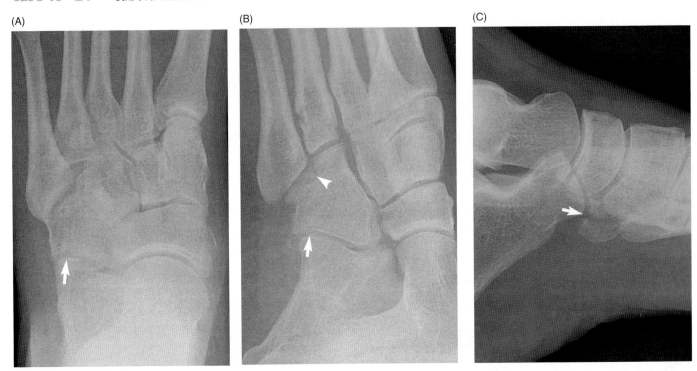

(A)   (B)   (C)

30-year-old woman injured in motor vehicle crash. AP (A), oblique (B), and lateral (C) radiographs of the left foot. The AP and oblique radiographs show subtle irregularity of the distal and proximal (arrows) articular surfaces of the cuboid. The lateral view shows a cuboid fracture extending from proximal to distal articular surfaces.

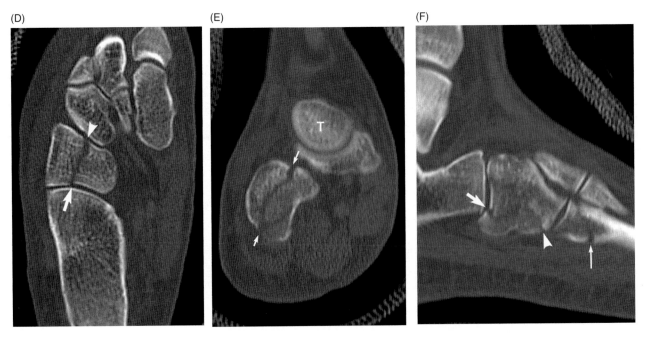

(D)   (E)   (F)

Multiplanar CT of the midfoot in axial (D), coronal (E), and sagittal (F) planes. The cuboid fracture is clearly demonstrated by CT. The cuboid fracture extends from the calcaneal-cuboid joint surface (arrow) across to the fifth TMT joint surface (arrowhead). On the axial view, the major fracture plane is curved (small arrows). There is also a fracture of the proximal shaft of the fifth metatarsal (long arrow). Cuboid fractures may occur with abduction of the forefoot, compressing it between the metatarsal bases and the calcaneus; this has been called the nutcracker mechanism. T=talus.

Case 13–22
Medial cuneiform fracture

(A)

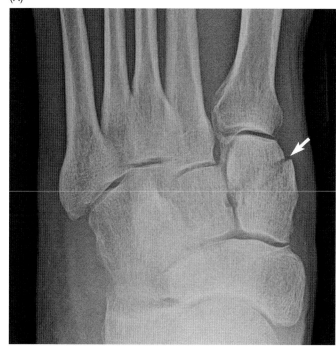

56-year-old man whose foot was run over by a car. AP radiograph of the left foot. There is a mildly displaced fracture (arrow) of the medial cuneiform.

(B)

(C)

(D)

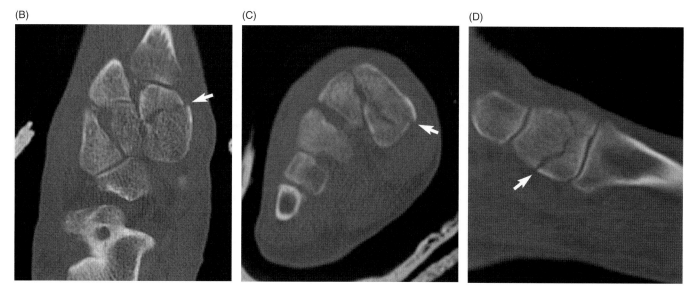

Multiplanar CT of the left midfoot in axial (B), coronal (C), and sagittal (D) planes. The fracture (arrows) is mildly comminuted and extends to the first TMT and the medial-middle cuneiform articulations. The small avulsion fracture at the lateral base of the first metatarsal and widening of the first and second metatarsal bases suggest Lisfranc injury.

Case 13–23
Medial cuneiform fracture

(A)

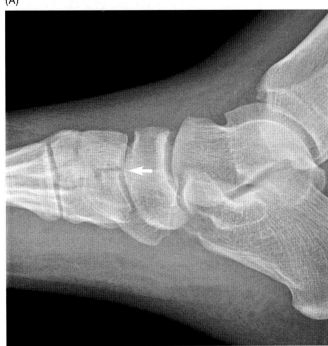

44-year-old man with plantar hyperflexion injury sustained while bicycling. Lateral radiograph of the right foot. There is a possible fracture line with horizontal orientation (arrow) overlying the cuneiform bones. Complex anatomy with overlapping tarsal bones makes it difficult to be sure.

(B)

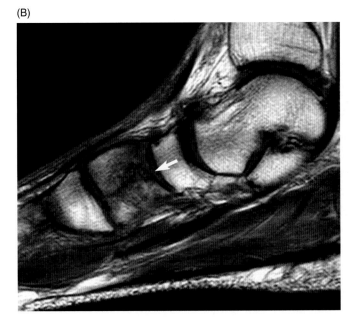

(C)

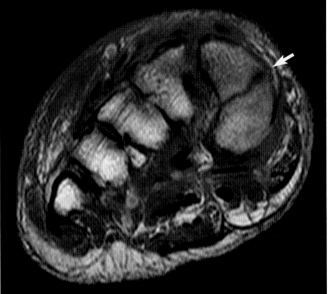

T1 MRI of the midfoot in sagittal (B) and coronal (C) planes. Because of continued pain, MRI was performed several days after the incident. There is a non-displaced fracture (arrow) extending through the medial cuneiform involving the first TMT and naviculocuneiform articular surfaces and dividing the bone into dorsal and plantar fragments.

Case 13–24

Os peroneum fracture

(A)

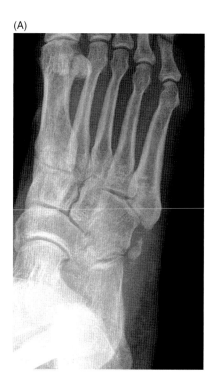

(B)

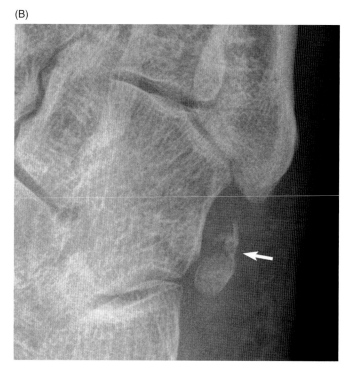

66-year-old man with pain near the base of the fifth meta-tarsal. Oblique radiograph (A) of the right foot and magnification detail (B). There is an avulsed and distracted fracture of the os peroneum (arrow). The os peroneum is a sesamoid bone located within the peroneus longus tendon in the region of the cuboid tunnel. It is present in its fully ossified form in up to 20% of adults and is bilateral in approximately 60% of these. A bipartite appearance is a frequent finding, occurring in approximately 30% of adults with an os peroneum. A fracture of an os peroneum can occur after trauma and may be associated with a peroneus longus tendon tear. Radiographic differentiation between a fractured os peroneum and a multipartite os peroneum may be problematic. In an acute setting, the fracture margins appear non-sclerotic and the bone fragments typically fit together like pieces of a puzzle. Conversely, a rounded, smooth, sclerotic margin is consistent with multipartite os peroneum. It is conceivable that remodeling of fracture fragments over time could give the appearance of a multipartite os peroneum [15].

References

1. Lduc S, Clare MP, Laflamme GY, Walling AK. Posttraumatic avascular necrosis of the talus. *Foot Ankle Clin.* 2008 Dec;13(4):753–65. PMID: 19013407.

2. Smith CS, Nork SE, Sangeorzan BJ. The extruded talus: Results of reimplantation. *J Bone Joint Surg Am* 2006;88:2418–24. PMID: 17079399.

3. Halvorson JJ, Winter SB, Teasdall RD, Scott AT. Talar neck fractures: A systematic review of the literature. *J Foot Ankle Surg.* 2013 Jan–Feb;52(1):56–61. doi: 10.1053/j. jfas.2012.10.008. Epub 2012 Nov 13. PMID: 23153783.

4. Dale JD, Ha AS, Chew FS. Update on talar fracture patterns: A large level I trauma center study. *AJR Am J Roentgenol.* 2013 Nov;201(5):1087–92. doi: 10.2214/AJR.12.9918. PMID: 24147480.

5. Van Opstal N, Vandeputte G. Traumatic talus extrusion: Case reports and literature review. *Acta Orthop Belg.* 2009 Oct;75(5):699–704. PMID: 19999887.

6. von Knoch F, Reckord U, von Knoch M, Sommer C. Fracture of the lateral process of the talus in snowboarders. *J Bone Joint Surg Br.* 2007 Jun;89(6):772–7. PMID: 17613502.

7. Hawkins LG. Fracture of the lateral process of the talus. *J Bone Joint Surg Am.* 1965 Sep;47:1170–5. PMID: 14337775.

8. Bohay DR, Manoli A II. Subtalar joint dislocations. *Foot Ankle Int.* 1995 Dec;16(12):803–8. PMID: 8749354.

9. Bohay DR, Manoli A II. Occult fractures following subtalar joint injuries. *Foot Ankle Int* 1996;17:164–9. PMID: 8919622.

10. Epstein N, Chandran S, Chou L. Current concepts review: Intra-articular fractures of the calcaneus. *Foot Ankle Int.* 2012 Jan;33(1):79–86. doi: 10.3113/FAI.2012.0079. PMID: 22381241.

11. Badillo K, Pacheco JA, Padua SO, Gomez AA, Colon E, Vidal JA. Multidetector CT. Evaluation of calcaneal fractures. *Radiographics.* 2011 Jan–Feb;31(1):81–92. doi: 10.1148/rg.311105036. PMID: 21257934.

12. Sanders R, Fortin P, DiPasquale T, Walling A. Operative treatment in 120 displaced intraarticular calcaneal fractures. Results using a prognostic computed tomography scan classification. *Clin Orthop Relat Res.* 1993 May;(290):87–95. PMID: 8472475.

13. Benirschke SK, Meinberg EG, Anderson SA, Jones CB, Cole PA. Fractures and dislocations of the midfoot: Lisfranc and Chopart injuries. *Instr Course Lect.* 2013;62:79–91. PMID: 23395016.

14. Rosenbaum AJ, Uhl RL, DiPreta JA. Acute fractures of the tarsal navicular. *Orthopedics.* 2014 Aug;37(8):541–6. doi: 10.3928/01477447-20140728-07. PMID: 25102497.

15. Brigido MK, Fessell DP, Jacobson JA, et al. Radiography and US of os peroneum fractures and associated peroneal tendon injuries: Initial experience. *Radiology* 2005;237:235–41. PMID: 16183934.

Fractures and dislocations of the metatarsals and toes

Hyojeong Mulcahy, M.D., and Felix S. Chew, M.D.

Case 14–1

Lisfranc fracture-dislocation (homolateral type)

(A)

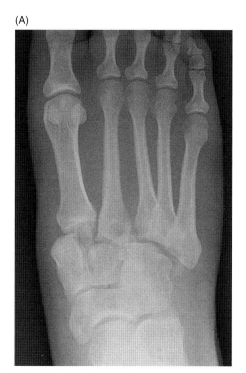

(B)

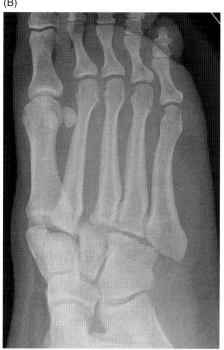

(C)

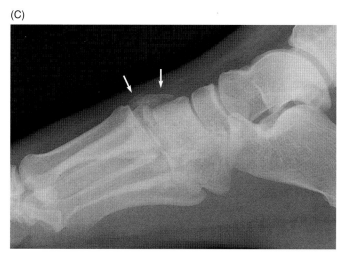

20-year-old woman who had a twisting foot injury on a trampoline. AP (A), oblique (B), and lateral (C) radiographs of the right foot. There is lateral subluxation of the first through fifth metatarsals at the tarsometatarsal (TMT) joints. The entire forefoot has been laterally displaced such that the first metatarsal is now aligned with the medial-middle cuneiform joint, and all the metatarsals are dorsally subluxated as a unit with respect to the tarsals. Small avulsed fragments are noted at the metatarsal bases on the lateral view (arrows). There is dorsal and medial soft tissue swelling around the midfoot. The Lisfranc injury is a dislocation of the TMT joints. There are three basic patterns of injury according to the Ouenu and Kuss classification [1–2]: the homolateral type is dislocation of all the metatarsals together; the divergent type is dislocation of metatarsals in separate directions; the isolated type is dislocation of some but not all the metatarsals. This case is a homolateral type, with lateral dislocation.

Case 14–2

Lisfranc fracture-dislocation (divergent type)

(A)

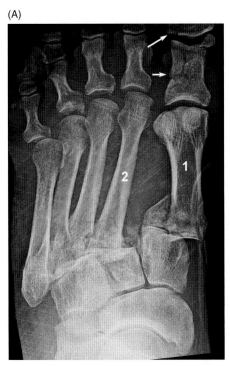

(B)

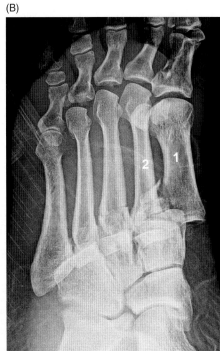

53-year-old woman injured in a motor vehicle crash. AP (A), oblique (B), and lateral (C) radiographs of the left foot. There are lateral fracture-dislocations of the second through fifth TMT joints. There is a fracture-dislocation of the first TMT joint and the metatarsal has been displaced medially and dorsally (large arrow). There are also fractures of the proximal (short arrow) and distal (long arrow) phalanges of the great toe. This case is an example of the divergent type of Lisfranc injury. The Lisfranc injury is named for a military surgeon from the Napoleonic wars who described forefoot fracture-dislocations that occurred in cavalrymen who had been unhorsed and dragged with a foot still in a stirrup. The contemporary bicyclist with feet strapped or clipped to the pedals may suffer the analogous injury.

(C)

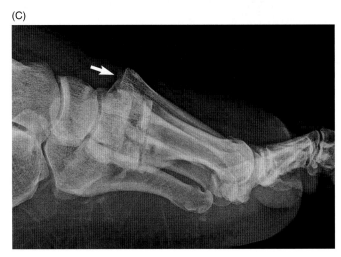

Case 14–3

Lisfranc fracture-dislocation (homolateral type)

(A)

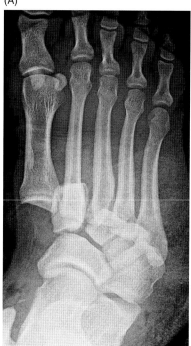

(B)

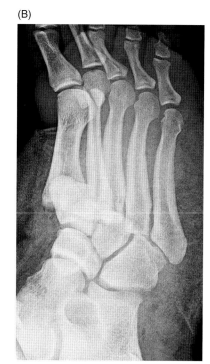

(C)

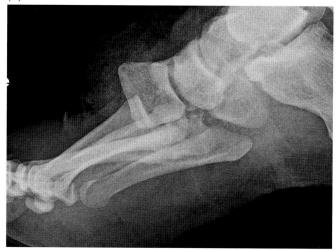

40-year-old man injured in motorcycle crash. AP (A), oblique (B), and lateral (C) radiographs of the right foot. There is plantar dislocation of all five TMT joints, with extensive degloving injury of the dorsal soft tissues. Plantar dislocation of the forefoot is unusual. This is a homolateral type of Lisfranc dislocation, but in the plantar direction rather than the lateral direction.

Case 14-4   Occult Lisfranc fracture-dislocation

(A)   (B)   (C)

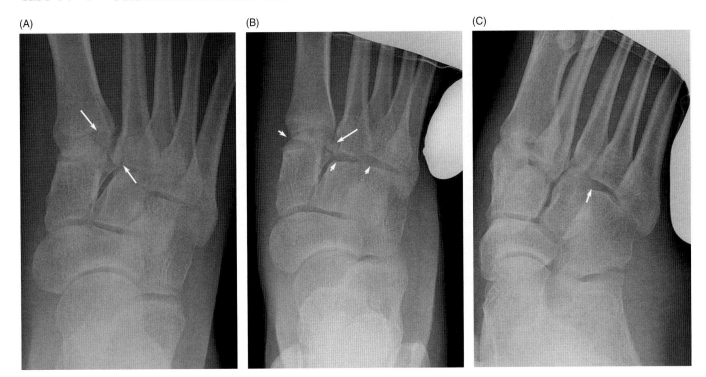

40-year-old man injured in motor vehicle crash. AP (A) and valgus stress (B-C) radiographs of the right foot. There are fracture fragments between the first and second TMT joints (long arrows) that are easy to overlook, but the joint spaces appear normal. With valgus stress, the Lisfranc joints subluxate (short arrows) and fracture fragments are more evident at the first and second TMT joints. The joint spaces should not widen under stress.

(D)   (E)

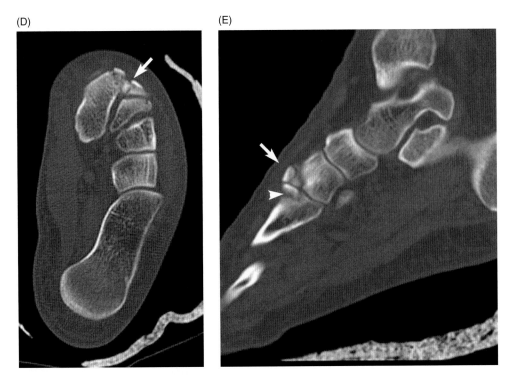

Multiplanar CT through the right midfoot, axial (D) and sagittal (E) images. There are small avulsion fractures at the TMT joints involving the medial and middle cuneiforms (arrows) and the bases of the first and second metatarsals (arrowhead).

Isolated Lisfranc injury at first TMT joint

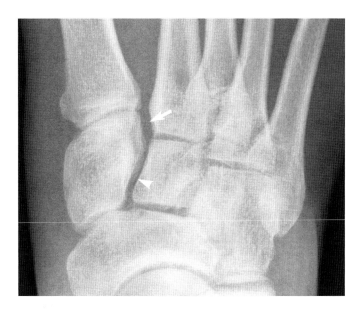

41-year-old woman who tripped on the hose at a gas station. AP radiograph of the right foot. There is widening of the space between the first and second metatarsal bases (arrow), and between the medial and middle cuneiforms (arrowhead). The first and second TMT joints appear properly aligned. The first ray was unstable on clinical exam. This case is an example of the isolated type of Lisfranc injury.

Case 14–6
Fifth metatarsal tuberosity fracture

(A)

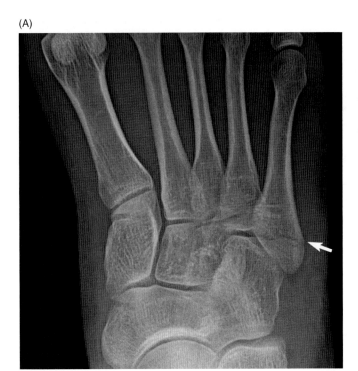

(B)

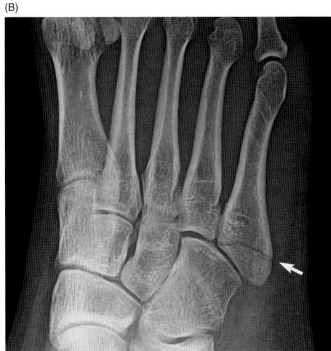

(C)

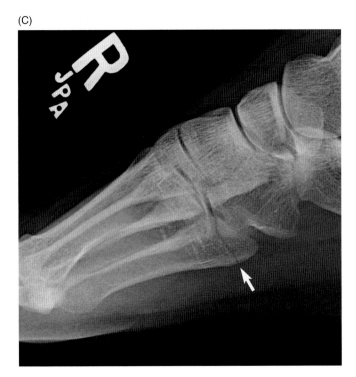

19-year-old woman who fell while walking. AP (A), oblique (B), and lateral (C) radiographs of the right foot. There is a non-displaced fracture of the base of the fifth metatarsal tuberosity (arrows). The fracture extends into the TMT joint. The fifth metatarsal is the most frequently fractured bone in the foot; the majority of fifth metatarsal fractures involve the proximal end [3–4]. The classification of proximal fifth metatarsal fractures is related to the location of the fracture relative to the fifth TMT and the fourth-fifth intermetatarsal joints [5]. The tuberosity fracture involves or is more proximal than the fifth TMT articular surface and is sometimes called a Zone 1 fracture. The size of the fracture fragment may range from one that involves the entire TMT joint to a tiny cortical avulsion fragment. These fractures generally heal well with symptomatic treatment, even when displaced [5–6]. These appear to be avulsion fractures of the lateral cord of the plantar aponeurosis [7–8].

Case 14–7
Fifth metatarsal Jones fracture

(A)

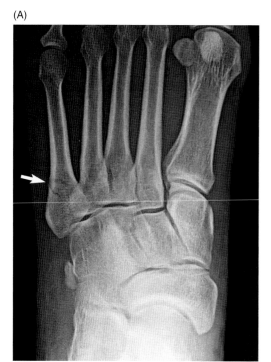

(B)

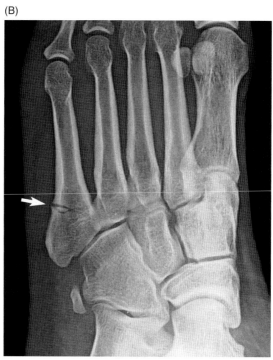

(C)

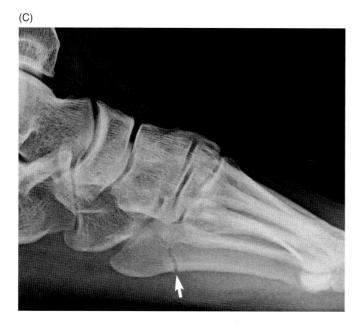

38-year-old man with a twisting injury to the left foot. AP (A), oblique (B), and lateral (C) radiographs of the left foot. There is a minimally displaced transverse fracture (arrow) of the proximal fifth metatarsal at the junction of the metaphysis and diaphysis, extending transversely into the fourth-fifth intermetatarsal joint. A fracture that involves this joint is a Jones fracture, sometimes called a Zone 2 fracture. The original description of Jones fractures designates fractures that occur 0.75 inch (2 cm) from the proximal tip of the metatarsal. There is evidence that more-proximal Jones fractures may be lumped with tuberosity fractures in terms of treatment and outcome, and perhaps be simply called metaphyseal fractures [6]. However, distal Jones fractures are at risk for complications of healing.

Case 14–8

Fifth metatarsal meta-diaphyseal fracture

(A)

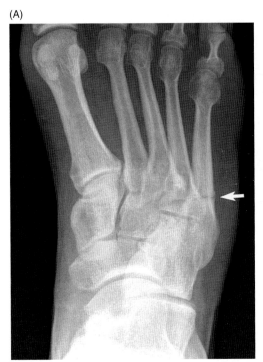

(B)

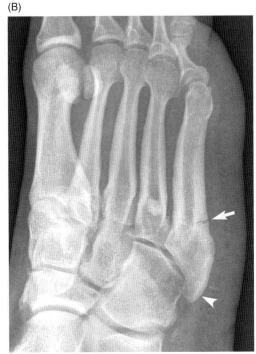

(C)

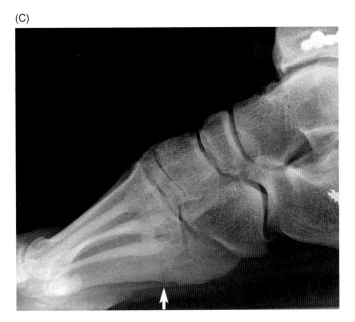

34-year-old man who sustained an injury to the lateral side of his right foot playing basketball. AP (A), oblique (B), and lateral (C) radiographs of the right foot. There is an incomplete transverse fracture (arrow) at the junction of the diaphysis and metaphysis involving the inferolateral cortex of the fifth metatarsal. This fracture was treated with internal fixation by an intramedullary screw. The elongated styloid process of the base of the fifth metatarsal (arrowhead) is likely the sequel of remote trauma. Fifth diaphyseal stress fractures, sometimes called Zone 3, are located in a vascular watershed region and are at risk for complications of healing. They typically present with pain but a fracture line may not become apparent on radiographs until weeks after onset. Polzer et al. [6], who suggested combining tuberosity avulsion fractures with proximal Jones fractures, also advocate combining distal Jones fractures with diaphyseal stress fractures, calling them meta-diaphyseal fractures [6]. Unfortunately, the exact borderline does not appear to have an obvious radiographic landmark.

Case 14–9

Fifth metatarsal shaft fracture

(A)

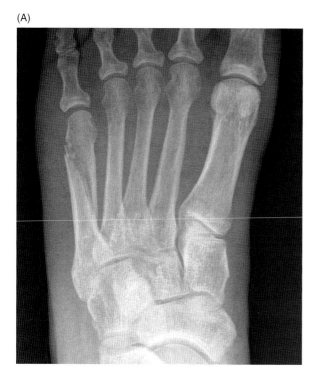

(B)

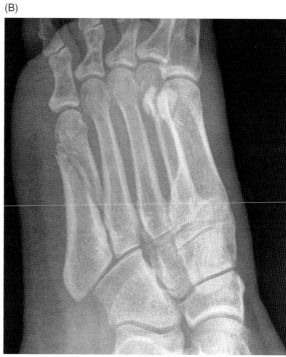

(C)

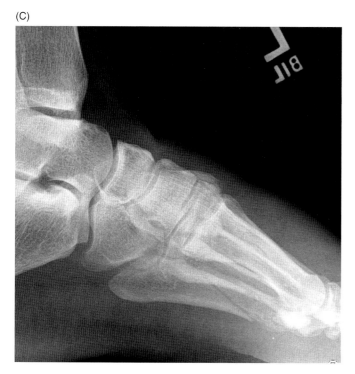

49-year-old woman who fell while standing barefoot on furniture. AP (A), oblique (B), and lateral (C) radiographs of the left foot. There is a minimally displaced oblique fracture (arrows) at the fifth distal metatarsal shaft and neck. The morphology of the fracture suggests axial compression as the mechanism.

Case 14–10
Metatarsal shaft fractures

(A)

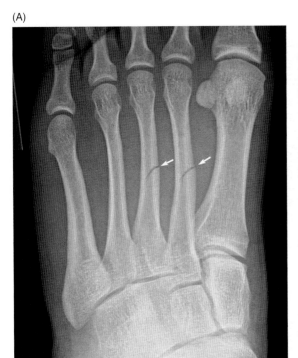

(B)

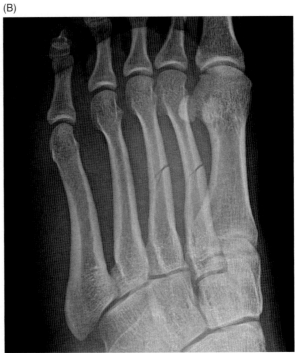

(C)

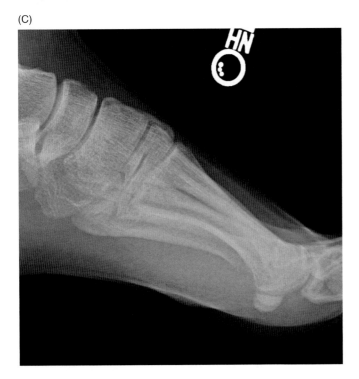

19-year-old man injured his foot playing soccer. AP (A), oblique (B), and lateral (C) radiographs of the left foot. There are transverse, incomplete fractures at the second and the third metatarsal mid-shafts (arrows). Fractures of the shaft and neck of the metatarsal bones and phalanges are often the result of heavy objects falling on the foot. Less commonly, the phalanges may be fractured as the foot strikes furniture or other objects. These fractures are transverse, oblique, or comminuted. Rarely a longitudinal linear fracture is encountered.

Case 14–11

Metatarsal shaft fractures

(A)

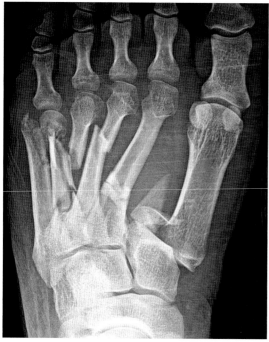

(B)

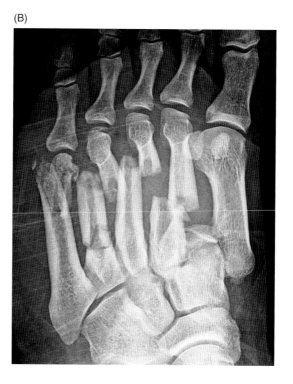

(C)

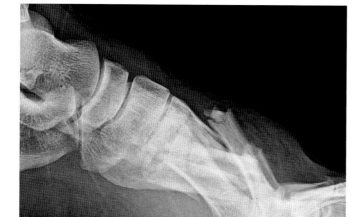

26-year-old man who injured his foot in a motorcycle crash. AP (A), oblique (B), and lateral (C) radiographs of the left foot. There is a fracture-dislocation of the first TMT joint with medial dislocation of the first metatarsal. There is a comminuted transverse fracture of the second metatarsal shaft. There is a transverse fracture of the third metatarsal shaft. There is a segmental fracture of the fourth metatarsal shaft and an osteochondral fracture of the fourth metatarsal head. There is a comminuted oblique fracture of the fifth metatarsal shaft and neck.

Case 14–12   Lateral sesamoid fracture

(A)

(B)

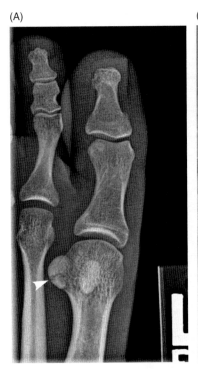
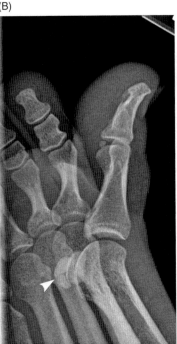

23-year-old woman with great toe pain the morning after marching many miles in a military reenactment. AP (A) and lateral (B) radiographs of the left great toe. There is a non-displaced transverse fracture of the lateral sesamoid of the great toe (arrows). A fracture may be distinguished from the more common bipartite sesamoid by the sharpness of the fracture line and the lack of cortical margins. In addition, the fracture fragments usually look as if they could fit back together perfectly, while the separate ossifications of a bipartite (or multipartite) bone typically do not. Most fractures of the sesamoids of the great toe are stress injuries [9–10].

Case 14–13   Medial sesamoid fracture

(A)

(B)

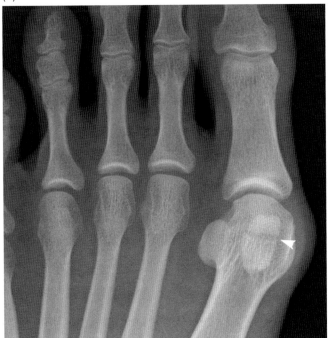

32-year-old woman who has had pain below the first metatarsophalangeal joint for 6 weeks. AP (A) and lateral (B) radiographs of the left great toe. There is a non-displaced transverse fracture of the medial sesamoid of the great toe (arrows).

Bipartite or multipartite sesamoids are common findings, with one study reporting a prevalence of 14% and a preponderance of 82% on the medial side [11].

Case 14–14
First metatarsophalangeal dislocation

(A)

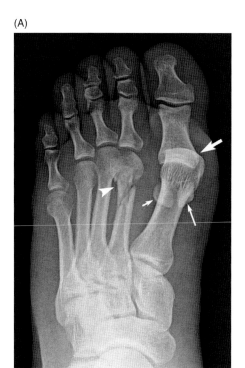

(B)

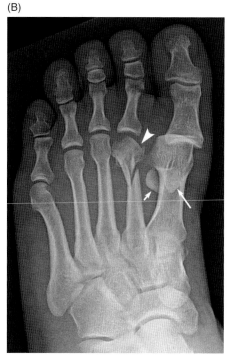

(C)

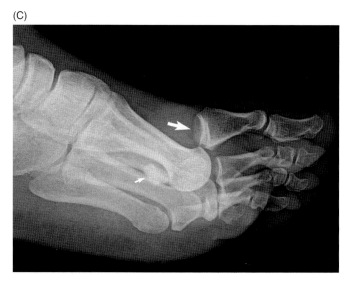

50-year-old man injured mountain climbing when large chunk of ice fell on his foot. AP (A), oblique (B), and lateral (C) radiographs of the left foot. On AP view, there is overlapping of the first metatarsophalangeal joint (arrow), indicating that they are no longer in the same plane and are therefore dislocated. The medial (long arrow) and lateral (short arrow) sesamoids are positioned more proximally than anatomic, and there is a comminuted fracture of the second metatarsal head and neck (arrowhead). On the oblique view, it is more apparent that the great toe is dislocated dorsally and that the sesamoids are on the plantar side of the metatarsal, findings confirmed on the lateral view. Traumatic dislocations of the first MTP joints are considered rare [12–13]. Based on case reports, the prevailing view is that the dislocations are caused by severe hyperextension, dislocating the proximal phalanx dorsally and disrupting the sesamoid mechanism. In the cases reported and classified by Jahss [13], the sesamoids were split apart from each other and retracted to either side of the metatarsal. Giannikas [12] reported similar cases as Jahss, as well as a case identical to the one presented here, in which the sesamoids remained together but were apparently detached from the proximal phalanx. Variations have continued to appear as case reports [14–17].

Case 14–15   Fifth metatarsophalangeal joint dislocation

(A)

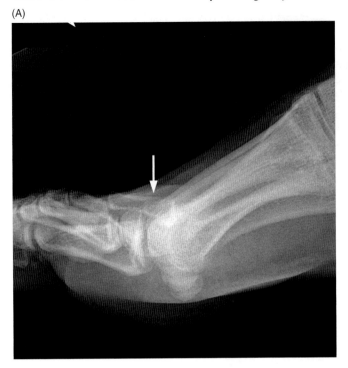

(B)

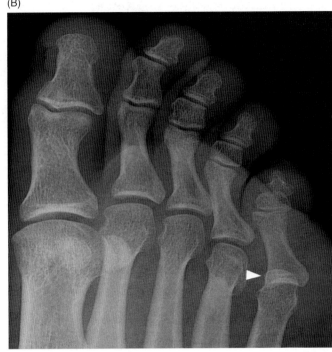

26-year-old man injured in a 30-foot fall. Lateral (A) and oblique (B) radiographs of the right foot. On AP view, there is lateral dislocation of the fifth proximal phalanx with respect to the fifth metatarsal. On lateral view, the fifth proximal phalanx is dorsally dislocated (arrow). There is no fracture. An oblique view demonstrates overlapping of the fifth metatarsophalangeal joint (arrowhead). Dorsal dislocation may be hard to detect on the oblique view.

Case 14–16   Great toe (proximal phalanx) fracture

(A)

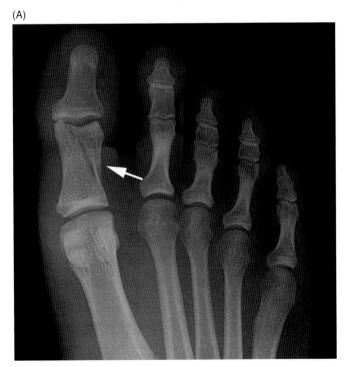

(B)

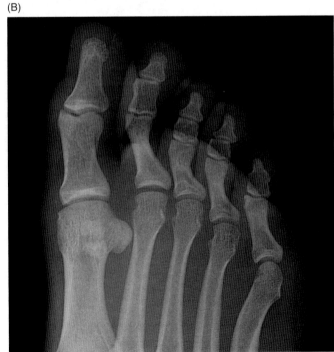

21-year-old woman who injured her foot when she landed on another player while playing basketball. AP (A) and oblique (B) radiographs of the right foot. There is a minimally displaced oblique fracture of the first proximal phalanx extending in to the first interphalangeal joint, distally (arrow). The fracture is not clearly seen on the oblique view.

Case 14–17 Fourth and fifth toe (proximal phalanges) fractures

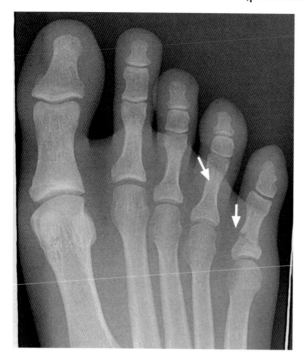

26-year-old woman who stubbed her toes into a banister while running down stairs. AP radiograph of the right foot. There are minimally displaced oblique fractures of the fourth and fifth proximal phalanges (arrows).

Case 14–18 Second toe (proximal phalanx) fracture

(A)

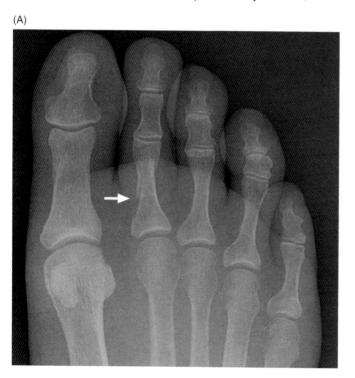

(B)

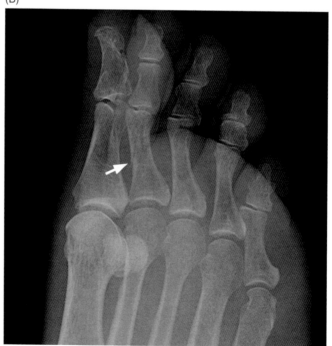

A 70-year-old woman stumbled at home. AP (A) and oblique (B) radiographs of the right foot. There is an oblique fracture through the proximal second phalanx (arrows). There is mild displacement of the fracture fragments. There is adjacent soft tissue swelling.

Case 14–19

Fifth toe (proximal phalanx) fracture

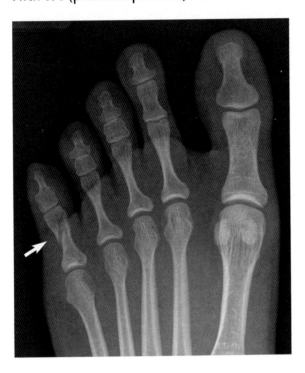

41-year-old woman who stubbed her little toe. AP radiograph of the right foot. There is an oblique, displaced fracture of the fifth proximal phalanx with mild lateral angulation (arrow). The oblique fracture morphology is indicative of axial loading of the phalanx along its long axis as a result of stubbing the toe.

Case 14–20

Fifth toe (proximal phalanx) fracture

(A)

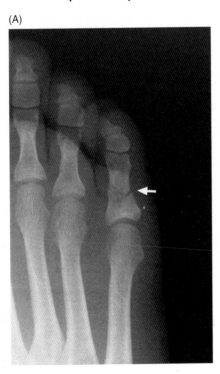

(B)

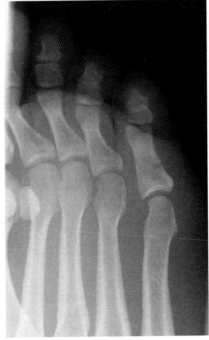

30-year-old man dropped a stereo speaker on the foot. AP (A) and oblique (B) radiographs of the right foot. There is a non-displaced transverse fracture through the shaft of the fifth proximal phalanx (arrow). There is soft tissue swelling around the fracture site. The transverse fracture morphology is typical of an injury caused by a dropped object. Because of its vulnerable position at the lateral margin of the foot, the fifth toe is the most commonly fractured lesser toe [18].

Case 14–21

Fifth proximal interphalangeal joint dislocation

(A)

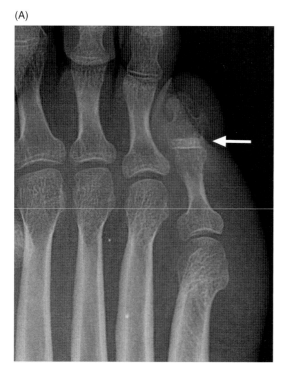

(B)

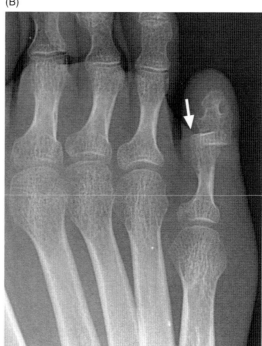

(C)

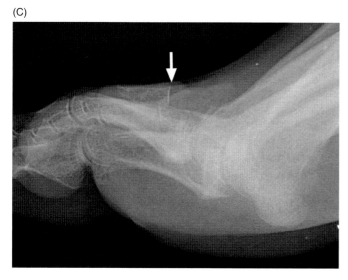

49-year-old man stubbed his fifth toe. AP (A), oblique (B), and lateral (C) radiographs of the right foot. There is dorsal dislocation of the fused fifth distal and middle phalanges at the proximal interphalangeal (PIP) joint. The fifth PIP joint is narrowed and overlapped on AP and oblique radiographs (arrows); however, there is complete dislocation on the lateral radiograph (arrow). A PIP dislocation that is irreducible may require surgery to remove interposed soft tissues such as the flexor tendon or the volar plate [19].

Case 14–22
Great toe avulsion fracture

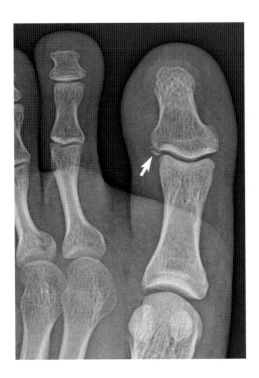

35-year-old man who slipped and fell, hitting his great toe against the pavement. AP radiograph of the left great toe. There is a minimally displaced avulsion fracture (arrow) at the lateral margin of the distal phalanx of the great toe at the interphalangeal joint, representing an avulsion fracture at the lateral collateral ligament. The presumptive mechanism of injury was varus loading of the great toe.

Case 14–23
Third toe (distal phalanx) fracture

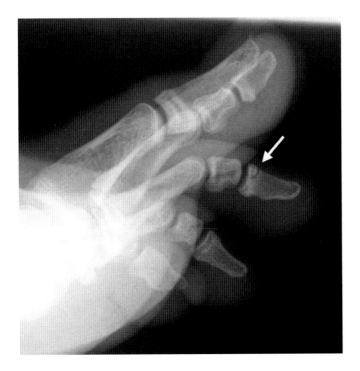

17-year-old man who stubbed his toe. Lateral radiograph of the left third toe. There is a subtle fracture at the dorsal margin of the base of the distal phalanx of the third toe. There is minimal displacement (arrow). Soft tissue swelling is present around the distal interphalangeal joint.

Case 14–24
Fifth toe distal (phalanx) fracture

(A)

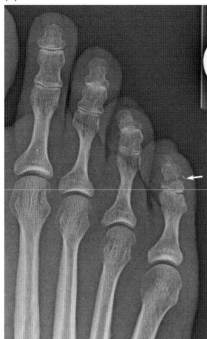

(B)

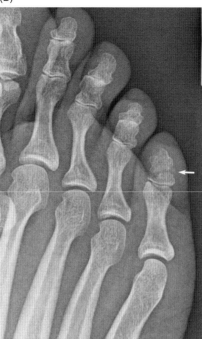

57-year-old man whose toe was stepped on. AP (A) and oblique (B) radiographs of the right toes. The fifth toe has two phalanges and one IP joint, a common anatomic variant resulting from interphalangeal coalition. There is a transverse, minimally displaced fracture of the distal phalanx (arrow). Fractures through an interphalangeal coalition have been reported to heal more slowly than expected [20].

Case 14–25
Multiple toe fractures

(A)

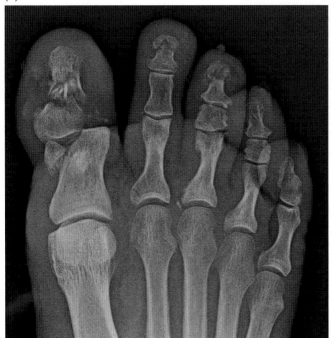

(B)

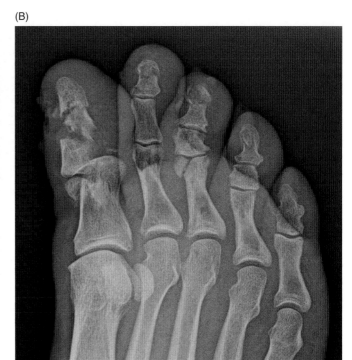

52-year-old man who was struck by a car while walking. AP (A) and oblique (B) radiographs of the right foot. There are multiple injuries of the toes. At the great toe, there is a displaced intra-articular fracture of the medial condyle of the proximal phalanx with medial dislocation of the IP joint and a comminuted transverse fracture of the distal phalanx; there are small avulsion fragments at the lateral aspect of the distal phalanx. At the second toe, there is a comminuted fracture of the tuft of the distal phalanx and a non-displaced fracture of the base of the proximal phalanx at the MTP joint. At the third toe, there is a comminuted fracture of the tuft of the distal phalanx, medial condylar fracture of the proximal phalanx at the PIP joint, and avulsion fractures of the proximal phalanx at the lateral aspect of the PIP joint and at the medial aspect of the MTP joint. At the fourth toe, there is a comminuted fracture of the distal phalanx.

Case 14–26
Multiple toe fractures, dislocations, and degloving injuries

(A)

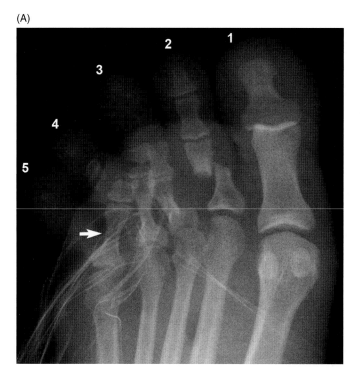

(B)

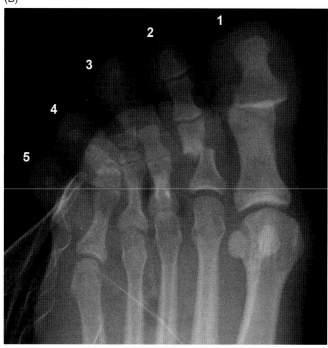

(C)

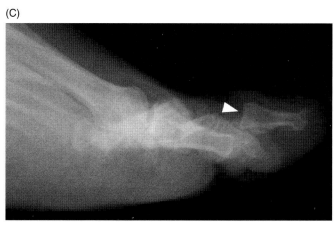

29-year-old woman whose toes were run over by a commuter bus. AP (A) and oblique (B) radiographs of the left foot. The IP joint of the great toe is dislocated, with overlap of the proximal and distal phalanges at the joint. The second toe has sustained a transverse fracture of the proximal phalanx with one shaft width displacement. There is lateral dislocation of the DIP joint of the third toe. In addition, there is a fracture of the tip of the distal phalanx with degloving of the distal soft tissues from the remaining bones of the toe. At the fourth toe, there are fractures of the distal and middle phalanges with degloving. At the fifth toe, there is a fracture of the distal phalanx with degloving. There has been complete degloving of the fourth and fifth toes, with the soft tissues squeezed off of the bones by the bus tire as it ran over the foot. Lateral radiograph of the foot. There is dorsal dislocation of the first proximal phalanx at the interphalangeal joint (arrowhead). Gas in the soft tissue surrounding the toes is consistent with open fractures. Detachment of the unbroken skin from the underlying bone is an injury called internal degloving. At its more familiar site in the lower limb, it may lead to a Morel-Lavallee lesion. In the toe, it is a rare lesion that has been called empty toe. Caused by compressive and shearing forces, empty toe may ultimately require amputation [21–22].

Case 14–27
Mangled foot

(A)

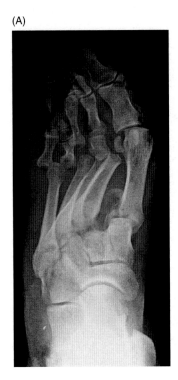

(B)

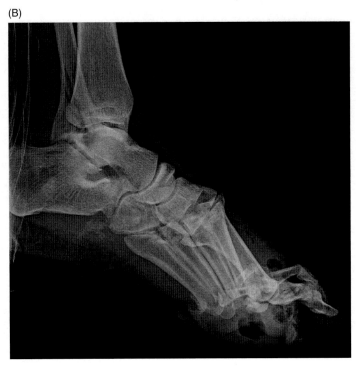

44-year-old man injured in motorcycle crash. AP (A) and lateral (B) radiographs of the left foot. There are multiple fracture-dislocations at the Lisfranc joint involving both metatarsal bases and tarsal bones. There are multiple injuries at the MTP joints, including dislocations of the third, fourth, and fifth toes, displaced fracture of the second metatarsal neck, and fracture-subluxation of the first MTP joint. There are multiple toe fractures. There is extensive soft tissue loss and gas within the soft tissues. There is also an open ankle fracture. The foot could not be saved because of the extensive bone, muscle, tendon, and neurovascular injuries. Unlike the hand, where the aesthetic restoration of function by replantation of amputated or near-amputated digits may be crucial to the rehabilitation of the patient, replantation of the toes is generally not considered. Amputation is often necessary when function cannot be restored [23].

References

1. Thompson MC, Mormino MA. Injury to the tarsometatarsal joint complex. *J Am Acad Orthop Surg*. 2003 Jul–Aug;11(4):260–7. PMID: 12889864.

2. Desmond EA, Chou LB. Current concepts review: Lisfranc injuries. *Foot Ankle Int*. 2006 Aug;27(8):653–60. PMID: 16919225.

3. Armagan OE, Shereff MJ. Injuries to the toes and metatarsals. *Orthop Clin North Am*. 2001 Jan;32(1):1–10. PMID: 11465121.

4. Petrisor BA, Ekrol I, Court-Brown C. The epidemiology of metatarsal fractures. *Foot Ankle Int*. 2006 Mar;27(3):172–4. PMID: 16539897.

5. Lawrence SJ, Botte MJ. Jones' fractures and related fractures of the proximal fifth metatarsal. *Foot Ankle*. 1993 Jul–Aug;14(6):358–65. PMID: 8406253.

6. Polzer H, Polzer S, Mutschler W, Prall WC. Acute fractures to the proximal fifth metatarsal bone: Development of classification and treatment recommendations based on the current evidence. *Injury*. 2012 Oct;43(10):1626–32. doi: 10.1016/j.injury.2012.03.010. Epub 2012 Mar 30. PMID: 22465516.

7. DeVries JG, Taefi E, Bussewitz BW, Hyer CF, Lee TH. The fifth metatarsal base: Anatomic evaluation regarding fracture mechanism and treatment algorithms. *J Foot Ankle Surg*. 2015 Jan–Feb;54(1):94–8. doi: 10.1053/j.jfas.2014.08.019. Epub 2014 Oct 16. PMID: 25441854.

8. Richli WR, Rosenthal DI. Avulsion fracture of the fifth metatarsal: Experimental study of pathomechanics. *AJR Am J Roentgenol*. 1984 Oct;143(4):889–91. PMID: 6332501.

9. Van Hal ME, Keene JS, Lange TA, Clancy WG Jr. Stress fractures of the great toe sesamoids. *Am J Sports Med*. 1982 Mar–Apr;10(2):122–8. PMID: 7081526.

10. Cohen BE. Hallux sesamoid disorders. *Foot Ankle Clin*. 2009 Mar;14(1):91–104. PMID: 19232995.

11. Favinger JL, Porrino JA, Richardson ML, Mulcahy H, Chew FS, Brage ME. Epidemiology and imaging appearance of the normal Bi-/multipartite hallux sesamoid bone. *Foot Ankle Int*. 2015 Feb;36(2):197–202. doi: 10.1177/1071100714552484. Epub 2014 Sep 18. PMID: 25237171.

12. Giannikas AC, Papachristou G, Papavasiliou N, Nikiforidis P, Hartofilakidis-Garofalidis G. Dorsal dislocation of the first metatarso-phalangeal joint. Report of four cases. *J Bone Joint Surg Br*. 1975 Aug;57(3):384–6. PMID: 1158954.

13. Jahss MH. Classic article: Foot & ankle 1:15, 1980 traumatic dislocations of the first metatarsophalangeal joint. *Foot Ankle Int*. 2006 Jun;27(6):401–6. PMID: 16764794.

14. Lantor H, Borovoy MA. A new classification of first metatarsophalangeal joint dislocations (type I B). *J Foot Surg*. 1987 Jan–Feb;26(1):75–7. PMID: 3559046.

15. Copeland CL, Kanat IO. A new classification for traumatic dislocations of the first metatarsophalangeal joint: Type IIC. *J Foot Surg*. 1991 May–Jun;30(3):234–7. PMID: 1874996.

16. Hall RL, Saxby T, Vandemark RM. A new type of dislocation of the first metatarsophalangeal joint: A case report. *Foot Ankle*. 1992 Nov–Dec;13(9):540–5. PMID: 1478586.

17. Tondera EK, Baker CC. Closed reduction of a rare type III dislocation of the first metatarsophalangeal joint. *J Manipulative Physiol Ther*. 1996 Sep;19(7):475–9. PMID: 8890029.

18. Van Vliet-Koppert ST, Cakir H, Van Lieshout EM, De Vries MR, Van Der Elst M, Schepers T. Demographics and functional outcome of toe fractures. *J Foot Ankle Surg*. 2011 May–Jun;50(3):307–10. doi: 10.1053/j.jfas.2011.02.003. Epub 2011 Mar 25. PMID: 21440463.

19. Veen M, Schipper IB. Irreducible fracture of the proximal interphalangeal joint of the fifth toe. *J Emerg Med*. 2013 Jan;44(1):e63–5. doi: 10.1016/j.jemermed.2011.09.002. Epub 2012 Jan 4. PMID: 22221984.

20. Sammarco GJ, Hockenbury RT. Fracture of an interphalangeal coalition: A report of two cases. *Foot Ankle Int*. 2000 Aug;21(8):690–2. PMID: 10966370.

21. Tarleton AA, Faust KC, Davis JA. Empty toe phenomenon: A big problem for a little toe. *Skeletal Radiol*. 2014 Jan;43(1):71–4. doi: 10.1007/s00256-013-1690-8. Epub 2013 Aug 2. PMID: 23907280.

22. Tang CL, Lee SS, Lin TY, Lin YK, Yeh YS, Lin HL, Lee WC, Chen CW. Empty toe: A unique type of closed degloving injury with dismal outcome. *Am J Emerg Med*. 2013 Jan;31(1):263.e1-3. doi: 10.1016/j.ajem.2012.03.031. Epub 2012 Jul 12. PMID: 22795410.

23. Hallock GG. The mangled foot and ankle: Soft tissue salvage techniques. *Clin Podiatr Med Surg*. 2014 Oct;31(4):565–76. doi: 10.1016/j.cpm.2014.06.006. Epub 2014 Aug 5. PMID: 25281516.

Fractures and dislocations of the face

Christin M.B. Foster,* M.D., CDR, MC, USN, and Felix S. Chew, M.D.

The views expressed in this chapter are those of the authors and do not reflect the official policy or position of the Department of the Navy, Department of Defense, or the U.S. Government.

Case 15–1

Tripod fracture

(A)

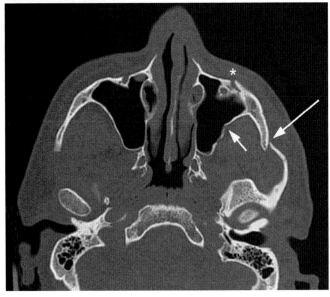

44-year-old man who fell. Axial CT of the face. The tripod fracture is the most common zygomatico-orbital fracture. The most common cause is being struck in the face during an altercation. As might be expected, mandibular fractures often occur in association with tripod fractures [1]. Three fractures comprise the tripod fracture pattern as shown. Fractures of the left zygomatic arch (long white arrow), anterior (*), and lateral walls (short white arrow) of the left maxillary sinus are seen in the axial CT image through the level of the maxillary sinuses.

* "I am a military service member (or an employee of the U.S. Government). This work was prepared as part of my official duties. Title 17, USC, section 105 provides that 'Copyright protection under this article is not available for any work of the United States Government.' Title 17, USC, section 101 defines U.S. Government work as work prepared by a military service member or employee of the U.S. Government as part of that person's official duties."

(B)

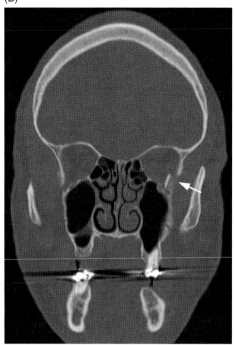

Coronal CT of the face. Coronal CT image through the orbits shows a fracture of the lateral wall of the left orbit (arrow).

Case 15–2

Le Fort fracture, Type I

(A)

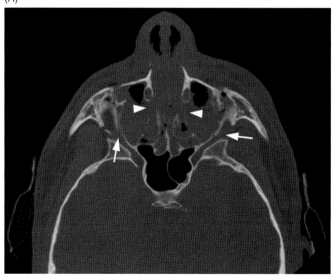

Adolescent male who fell off his bicycle. Axial CT of the face. Le Fort I fractures separate the palate from the maxilla [2–3]. In the axial CT, the medial walls (arrowheads) and lateral walls (short white arrows) of both maxillary sinuses are fractured.

(B)

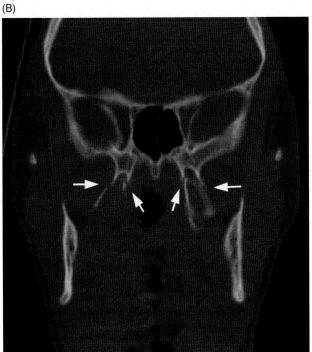

Coronal CT of the face. Bilateral pterygoid plate fractures are shown in the coronal CT (arrows). The teeth of the maxilla would move relative to the rest of the face on physical exam.

Case 15–3

Le Fort fracture, Type II

(A)

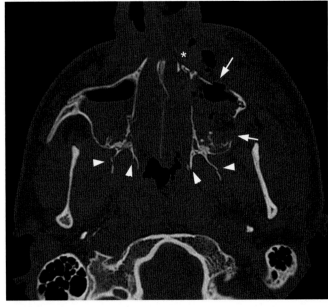

Facial injuries sustained in a motorbike crash. Axial CT of the face. In Le Fort II, or pyramidal fractures, the fractures form a pyramid around the nose. In the axial CT image through the maxillary sinuses, fracture lines pass across the left nasal bone (*), through the left anterior and posterolateral maxillary sinus walls (white arrows) and bilateral pterygoid plates (arrowheads).

(B)

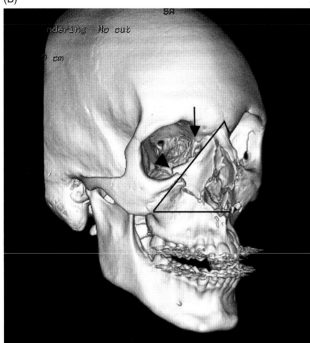

3D surface-rendered CT of the face. Oblique 3D CT of the right side of the face shows the pyramidal nature of the fracture (black line) and the involvement of the medial (arrow) and inferior orbital rims (arrowheads). In these fractures, the nose and teeth would move as a unit relative to the rest of the face [2–3]. Le Fort fractures may be asymmetric, with different types of fractures on each side of the face.

Case 15–4

Le Fort fracture, Type III

(A)

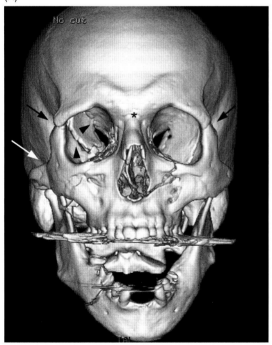

Multiple facial fractures sustained in a fall. 3D surface-rendered CT of the face. Instead of passing inferiorly through the front of the face, Le Fort III fractures continue to extend laterally through the lateral orbital wall, zygomaticofrontal suture and zygomatic arch [2–3]. This is usually a high-energy injury, and fractures will also pass through the ethmoid, vomer, and pterygoid plates. These fractures result in complete separation of the face from the rest of the skull. In this frontal 3D CT reconstruction, fractures are seen across the nasofrontal suture (*), right posterior and lateral orbit (black arrowheads), bilateral zygomaticofrontal sutures (black arrows) and right zygomatic arch (white arrow).

(B)

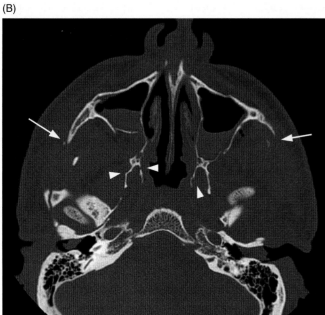

Axial CT of the face. Image through the maxillary sinuses shows fractures through both zygomatic arches (white arrows) and pterygoid plates (arrowheads).

(C)

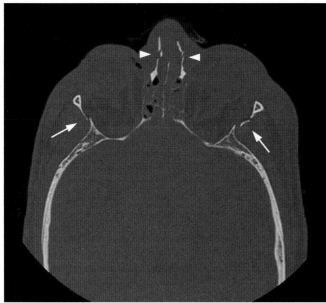

Axial CT of the face. Image through the orbits shows bilateral lateral orbital wall fractures (arrows) to advantage. Comminuted nasal fractures are also seen (arrowheads).

Case 15–5

Isolated zygomatic arch fracture

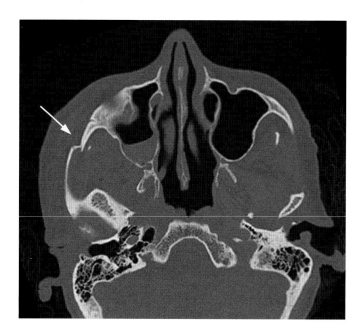

Elderly woman who fell. Axial CT of the face. Usually from a direct blow to the cheek, a zygomatic arch fracture causes flattening of the cheek contour and may affect masseter muscle activity or impinge the temporalis muscle [1]. In this axial CT through the level of the right zygomatic arch, a comminuted zygoma fracture with mild depression is demonstrated (arrow).

Case 15–6

Orbital blowout fracture

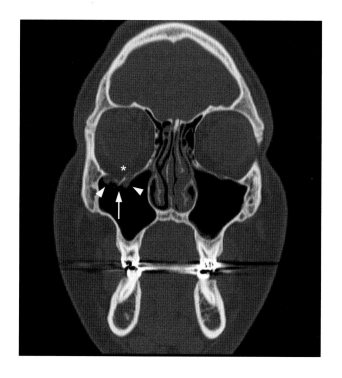

Impact injury to the right eye. Coronal CT of the face. In the orbital blowout fracture, pressure increases in the orbit and decompresses through the orbital floor. Fat often herniates into the maxillary sinus, but if the inferior rectus muscle is involved with the fracture fragments, it may become trapped and cause diplopia [4]. This patient also sustained a non-displaced right nasal bone fracture (not shown). In this coronal CT through the orbits, a comminuted fracture of the right orbital floor is shown (white arrow). Small amounts of orbital fat herniate (arrowheads) into the right maxillary sinus without additional herniation of the nearby inferior rectus muscle (*).

Case 15–7
Orbital blowin fracture

(A)

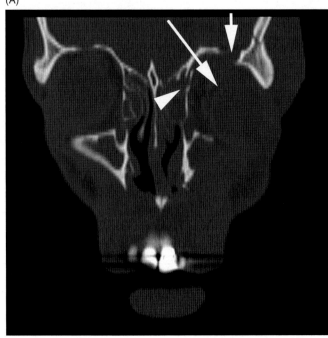

Coronal CT of the face. Orbital blowin fractures push fragments into the postseptal orbit, the opposite of the orbital blowout fracture. Characteristics include decreased orbital volume, proptosis and displacement of the globe in the orbital plane. Common complicating features of the orbital blowin fracture include restricted globe mobility (24%) and diplopia (32%). Less common complications include globe rupture, superior orbital fissure syndrome and optic nerve injury [5]. On this coronal CT image, fractures of the orbital roof (short arrow) and medial orbital wall (arrowhead) decrease the volume of the orbit, displacing the globe inferolaterally (long arrow).

(B)

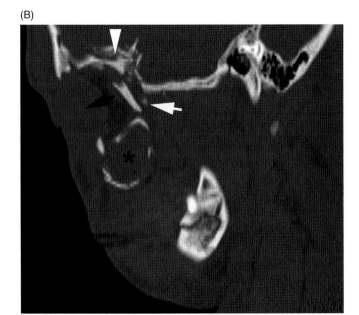

Sagittal CT of the face. Sagittal CT image shows fracture fragments from the posterolateral orbit (white arrow) and orbital roof (arrowhead) causing anterior globe displacement and proptosis (black arrow). Maxillary sinus full of hemorrhage also shown (*). This case demonstrates a so-called pure fracture involving only the roof, floor, or walls. Impure fractures also involve the orbital rim.

Orbital roof fracture

(A)

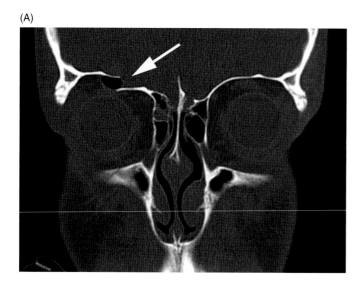

Blunt trauma to the face. Coronal CT of the face. Similar in mechanism to the orbital blowout fracture, orbital roof fractures occur with blunt force to the globe and orbit [6]. In this coronal CT, discontinuity of the orbital roof with a small focus of air (arrow) is identified.

(B)

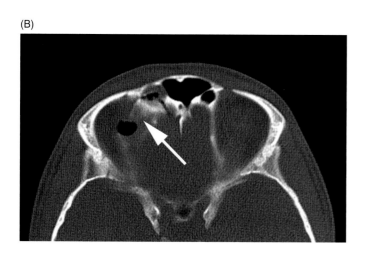

Axial CT of the face. Superior ethmoid air cell origin of the air is identified on the axial CT (arrow).

Facial smash fracture

(A)

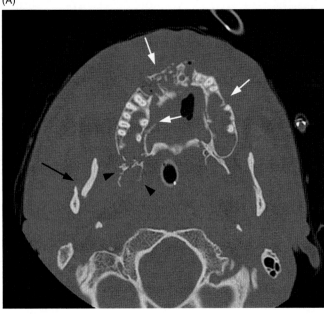

High speed motor vehicle crash. Axial CT of the face. As a result of high-energy trauma such as a motor vehicle crash, comminution of most of the facial structures results. Axial CT through the maxilla. Fractures of the alveolar ridge (white arrows), right pterygoid plates (black arrowheads) and right mandible (black arrow) are present.

(B)

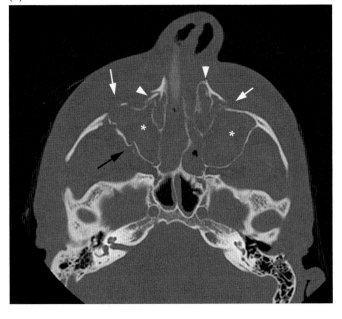

Axial CT of the face. Axial CT through the maxillary sinuses. The sinuses are opacified with blood (*) as a result of the fractures through the right lateral maxillary sinus wall (black arrow), bilateral anterior maxillary sinus walls (white arrows) and nasolacrimal ducts (arrowheads).

(C)

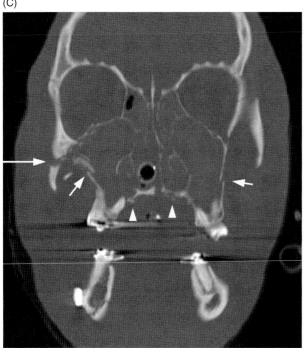

Coronal CT of the face. Coronal CT through the midface. Fractures of the lateral maxillary sinus walls (short white arrows), hard palate (arrowheads), and right zygomaticomaxillary suture (long white arrow) are present.

(D)

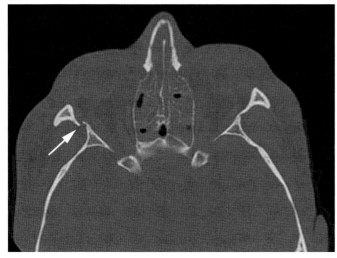

Axial CT of the face. Axial CT through the orbits. A right lateral orbital wall fracture is present (arrow). This patient's injuries follow the central facial smash pattern [7–8].

Case 15–10

Nasal fracture

(A)

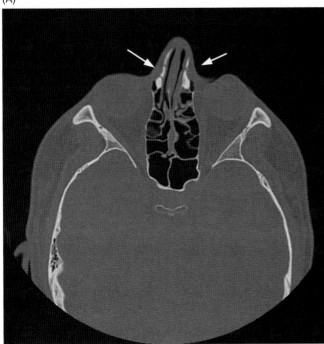

Young man with facial trauma. Axial CT of the face. Nasal fracture is a common result of assault or sporting injuries. For anything more than a mild, closed unilateral fracture, open reduction is frequently necessary [9]. Axial CT through the nasofrontal suture shows non-displaced right and left nasal fractures (arrows).

(B)

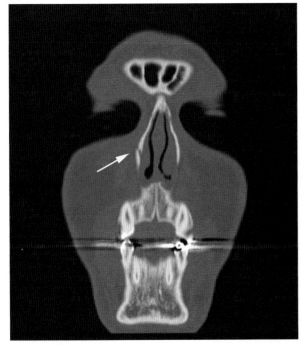

Coronal CT of the face. Coronal CT shows a non-displaced anterior right nasal fracture (arrow).

Case 15–11
Comminuted nasal fracture

(A)

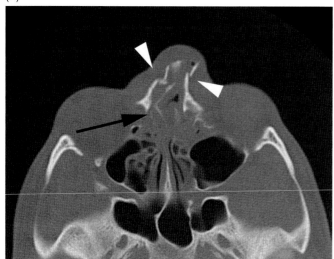

Struck in the face by a baseball. Axial CT of the face. In the axial CT image, bilateral comminuted, displaced nasal bone (white arrowheads) and bony nasal septum fractures (black arrow) result from a high-energy impact by a baseball.

(B)

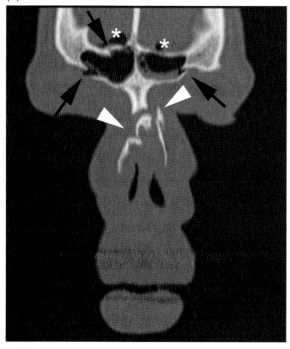

Coronal CT of the face. Comminuted, mildly displaced nasal fractures (white arrowheads). Additional fractures of the frontal sinus (black arrows) are seen with small foci of pneumocephalus (*) on the coronal CT.

Case 15–12
Frontal sinus fracture

(A)

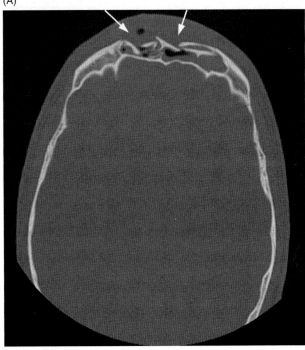

Blunt trauma to the face. Axial CT of the face. Axial CT shows a comminuted fracture of the anterior wall of the frontal sinus (arrows).

(B)

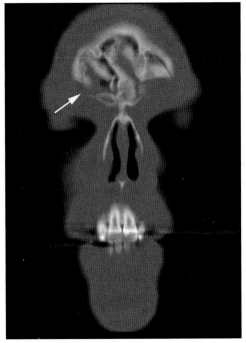

Coronal CT of the face. Coronal CT shows a comminuted fracture of the anterior wall of the frontal sinus (arrows). Fortunately, in this case, the risk of intracranial infection is low as the posterior wall of the frontal sinus remains intact [10].

Case 15–13
Naso-orbitoethmoid (NOE) fracture

(A)

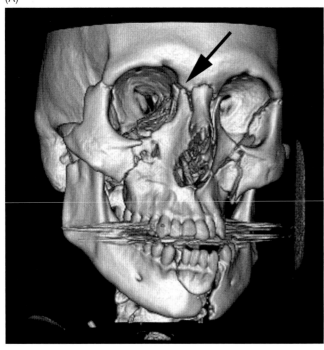

Blunt trauma to the face. 3D surface-rendered CT of the face. Naso-orbitoethmoid (NOE) fractures fall into the facial smash pattern of fractures. As shown on this coronal 3D CT reconstruction, there are numerous fractures of the maxillofacial structures. The NOE fracture (arrow) is important because it can involve the insertion of the medial canthal ligament. Should this fracture not be reduced properly, there may be increased distance between the inner eye corners (telecanthus) and globe malposition [11].

(B)

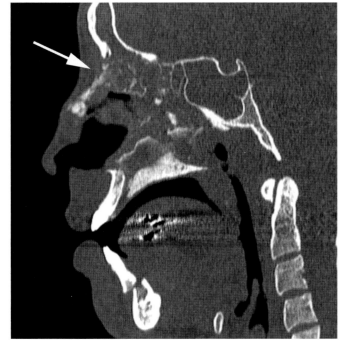

Sagittal CT of the face in midline. The NOE fractures extend from nasal bones (white arrow) posterior into the anterior ethmoid air cells. The frontal and sphenoid sinuses are opacified with blood.

(C)

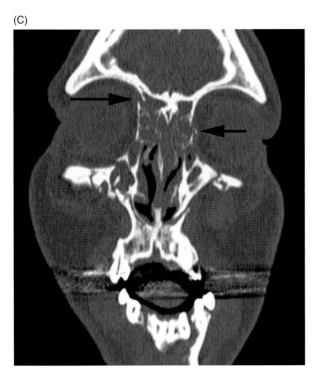

(D)

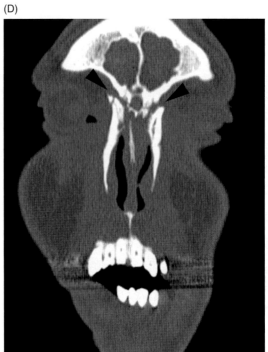

Coronal CT of the face, posterior (C) to anterior (D). The NOE fractures extend transversely through the nasal bones into the anterior ethmoid air cells (black arrows) and involve both medial orbital walls (black arrowheads).

Case 15–14

Symphyseal mandible fracture

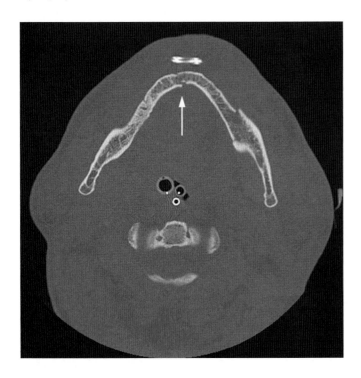

High-speed motor vehicle crash. Axial CT of the mandible. This patient sustained significant facial trauma when his car was rear-ended and pushed into an intersection and then struck by another vehicle traveling at high speed. Axial CT through the mandible shows a non-displaced symphyseal mandible fracture (arrow), one of many fractures this patient incurred. Symphyseal fractures comprise 7–15% of mandible fractures [12, 13].

Case 15–15
Parasymphyseal mandible fracture

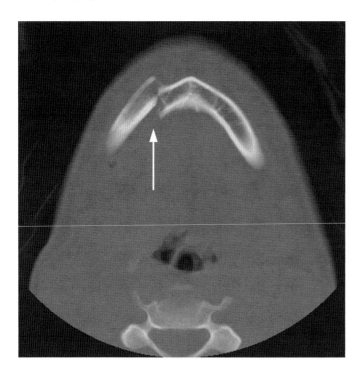

Young man who was beaten about the face, with clinically visible tooth fracture. Axial CT of the mandible. Axial CT through the mandible. In this mildly displaced vertical fracture (arrow), muscles tend to displace the fragments in the horizontal plane.

Case 15–16
Body of mandible fracture

(A)

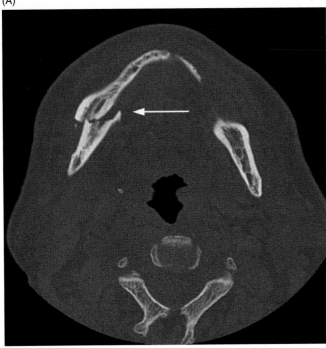

Man with multiple facial fractures after assault. Axial CT of the mandible. The body is the most common mandible fracture site, comprising approximately 30% of mandible fractures [12]. Axial CT through the mandible shows a mildly displaced right mandibular body fracture (arrow).

(B)

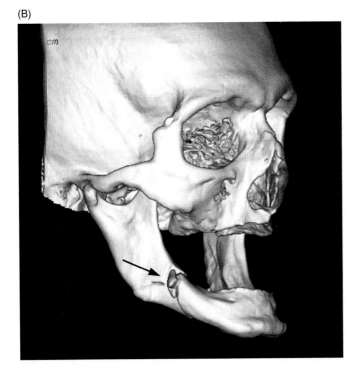

3D surface-rendered CT of the mandible. Oblique 3D CT reconstruction of the edentulous patient shows the fracture (arrow).

Case 15–17

Angle of the mandible fracture

(A)

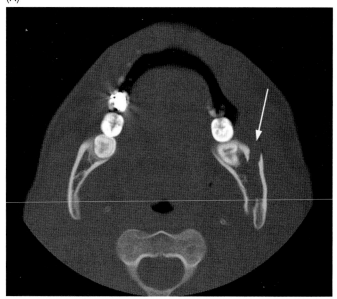

Young man who was beaten in the face. Axial CT of the mandible. Fractures at the angle of the mandible are the second most common, after the body. When two fractures of the mandible are present, they are most often on opposite sides of the symphysis [14]. This patient also had a right parasymphyseal fracture (not shown). Axial CT shows a left mandible angle fracture (arrow).

(B)

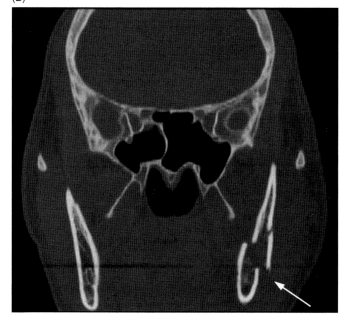

Coronal CT of the mandible. Coronal CT shows the left mandible angle fracture (arrow).

Case 15–18
Coronoid mandible fracture

(A)

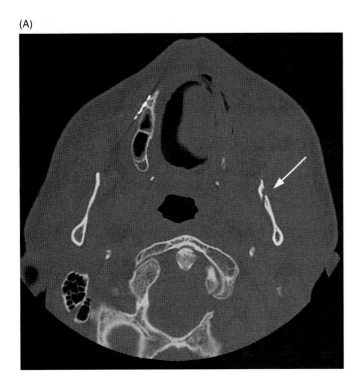

(B)

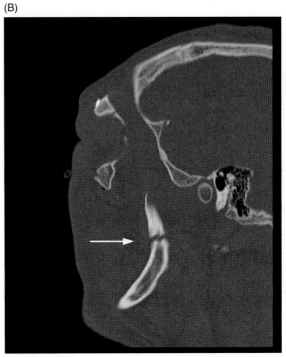

Man who fell on a concrete floor while in custody. Axial (A) and sagittal (B) CT of the mandible. Coronoid process fractures are uncommon, comprising only 1–2% of mandible fractures [12].

Axial and sagittal CTs through the mandible show a fracture at the coronoid process (arrows).

(C)

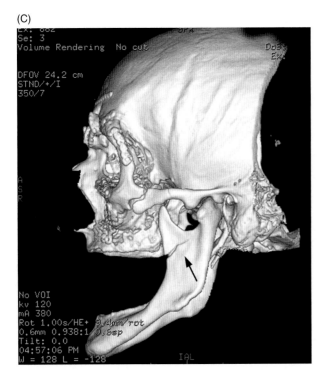

3D surface-rendered CT of the mandible. Sagittal 3D CT reconstruction shows that the fracture line through the coronoid is incomplete (arrow). Multiple other facial fractures with hardware fixation are evident around the orbits.

Case 15–19

Subcondylar mandible fracture

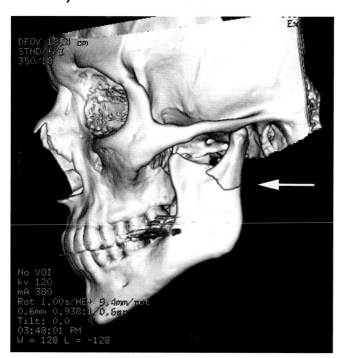

Intoxicated man who fell into a ditch, landing on the left side of his face. 3D surface-rendered CT of the mandible. This sagittal 3D CT reconstruction shows an oblique subcondylar fracture with mild fragment overlap (arrow). Owing to cosmetic deformity and the potential for poor temporomandibular joint function in the long term, these injuries are typically reduced at surgery with either an open or endoscopic-assisted approach [15].

Case 15–20
Condylar fracture of the mandible

(A)

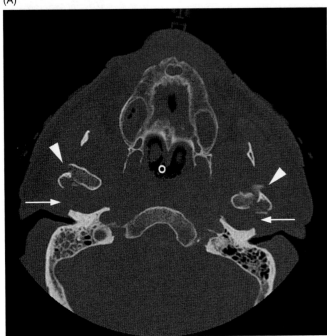

High-speed motor vehicle crash. Axial CT of the mandible. The most common combination of triple mandible fractures is fracture of the symphysis and fractures of both condyles, as seen in this patient. Intracapsular condyle fractures, as in this case, are rare [16]. Axial CT image shows bilateral condylar fractures (arrowheads) with anterior dislocation of each temporomandibular joint (arrows).

(B)

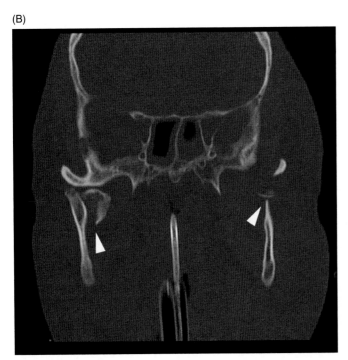

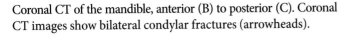

(C)

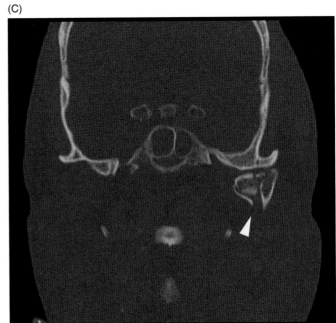

Coronal CT of the mandible, anterior (B) to posterior (C). Coronal CT images show bilateral condylar fractures (arrowheads).

Case 15–21　Flail mandible

(A)

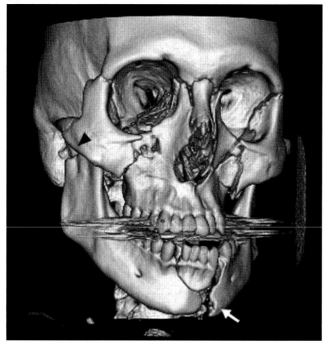

(B)

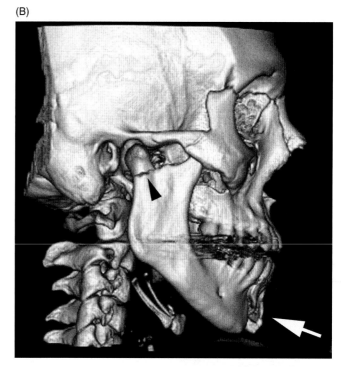

High-speed motor vehicle crash. 3D surface-rendered CT of the mandible, frontal (A) and lateral (B) views. A comminuted fracture of the symphysis (white arrows) is associated with bilateral subcondylar fractures on these 3D CT reconstructions (black arrowhead). These fractures prevent the genioglossus muscles from elevating and protruding the tongue [17]. Loss of support for the tongue can lead to airway obstruction.

References

1. Ellis E III, el-Attar A, Moos KF. An analysis of 2,067 cases of zygomatico-orbital fracture. *J Oral Maxillofac Surg.* 1985 Jun;43(6):417–28. PMID: 3858478.

2. Rhea JT, Novelline RA. How to simplify the CT diagnosis of Le Fort fractures. *AJR Am J Roentgenol.* 2005 May;184(5):1700–5. PMID: 15855142.

3. Sun JK, LeMay DR. Imaging of facial trauma. *Neuroimaging Clin N Am.* 2002 May;12(2):295–309. PMID: 1239163.

4. Kubal WS. Imaging of orbital trauma. *Radiographics.* 2008 Oct;28(6):1729–39. PMID: 18936032.

5. Antonyshyn O, Gruss JS, Kassel EE. Blow-in fractures of the orbit. *Plast Reconstr Surg.* 1989 Jul;84(1):10–20. PMID: 2734385.

6. Rothman MI, Simon EM, Zoarski GH, Zagardo MT. Superior blowout fracture of the orbit: The blowup fracture. *AJNR.* 1998 Sep;19:1448–9. PMID: 9763375.

7. Laine FJ, Conway WF, Laskin DM. Radiology of maxillofacial trauma. *Curr Probl Diagn Radiol.* 1993 Jul–Aug;22(4):145–88. PMID: 8359033.

8. Fraioli RE, Branstetter BF IV, Deleyiannis FW. Facial fractures: Beyond Le Fort. *Otolaryngol Clin North Am.* 2008 Feb;41(1):51–76, vi. PMID: 18261526.

9. Kucik CJ, Clenney T, Phelan J. Management of acute nasal fractures. *Am Fam Physician* 2004;70:1315–20. PMID: 15508543.

10. Bell RB. Management of frontal sinus fractures. *Oral Maxillofac Surg Clin North Am.* 2009 May;21(2):227–42. PMID: 19348989.

11. Hopper RA, Salemy S, Sze RW. Diagnosis of midface fractures with CT: What the surgeon needs to know. *RadioGraphics.* 2006;26(3):783–93. PMID: 16702454.

12. Bormann KH, Wild S, Gellrich NC, Kokemüller H, Stühmer C, Schmelzeisen R, Schön R. Five-year retrospective study of mandibular fractures in Freiburg, Germany: incidence, etiology, treatment, and complications. *J Oral Maxillofac Surg.* 2009 Jun;67(6):1251–5. PMID: 19446212.

13. Alpert B, Tiwana PS, Kushner GM. Management of comminuted fractures of the mandible. *Oral Maxillofac Surg Clin North Am.* 2009 May;21(2):185–92, v. PMID: 19348983.

14. Ellis E III. Management of fractures through the angle of the mandible. *Oral Maxillofac Surg Clin North Am.* 2009 May;21(2):163–74. PMID: 19348981.

15. Lee C, Mueller RV, Lee K, Mathes SJ. Endoscopic subcondylar fracture repair: Functional, aesthetic, and radiographic outcomes. *Plast Reconstr Surg.* 1998 Oct;102(5):1434–43; discussion 1444–5. PMID: 9773997.

16. Laskin DM. Management of condylar process fractures. *Oral Maxillofac Surg Clin North Am.* 2009 May;21(2):193–6, v-vi. PMID: 19348984.

17. Gerlock AJ Jr. The flared mandible sign of the flail mandible. *Radiology.* 1976 119(2):299–300. PMID: 1265259.

Chapter

16

Fractures and dislocations in children

Felix S. Chew, M.D., Catherine Maldjian, M.D., Hyojeong Mulcahy, M.D., and Refky Nicola, D.O.

Case 16–1

Proximal phalanx fracture, salter Type II

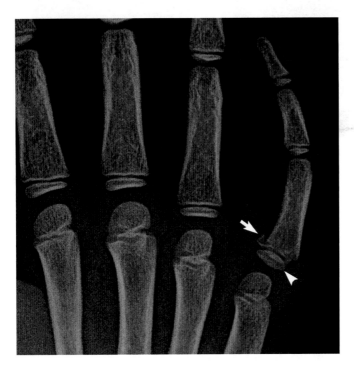

5-year-old girl who fell onto her outstretched hand. PA radiograph of the right hand. There is fracture of the proximal phalanx of the small finger. The fracture passes through the growth plate such that the epiphysis (arrowhead) is slightly offset from the shaft of the proximal phalanx. There is a metaphyseal fragment (arrow) that has displaced with the epiphysis. There are five types of fractures involving the growth plate according to the Salter-Harris classification [1]: Type I fractures pass the growth plate only; Type II fractures pass through the growth plate and the metaphysis; Type III fractures pass through the growth plate and the epiphysis; Type IV fractures pass through the growth plate and both metaphysis and epiphysis; Type V fractures are crush fractures of the growth plate.

Case 16–2
Metacarpal torus fracture

(A)

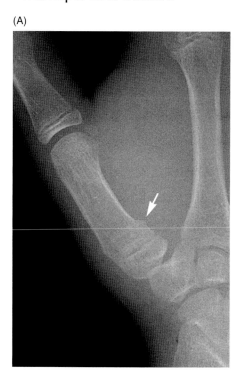

(B)

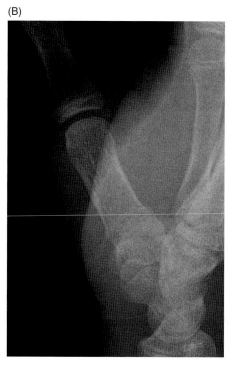

15-year-old male who fell while skiing. Oblique (A) and PA (B) radiographs of the right first metacarpal. There is a torus fracture (arrow) of the proximal shaft of the first metacarpal. The fracture does not involve the nearby physis or joint.

Case 16–3
Scaphoid fracture

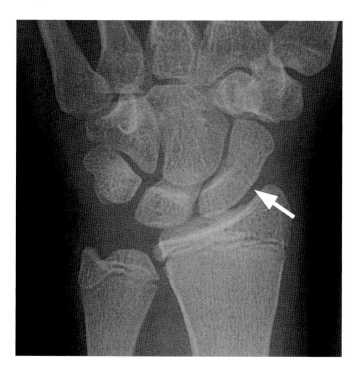

Child who fell on an outstretched hand. PA radiograph of the left wrist. There is a non-displaced waist of scaphoid fracture (arrow) that was seen only on the PA projection. Scaphoid and other carpal bone fractures are infrequent in young children, possibly because the bones are incompletely ossified and are cushioned by cartilage. In the immature skeleton, distal radius fractures are the predominant fractures of the wrist [2].

Case 16–4
Distal radius fracture, salter Type I

(A)

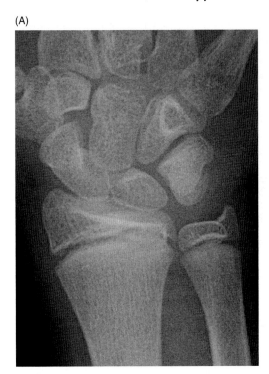

(B)

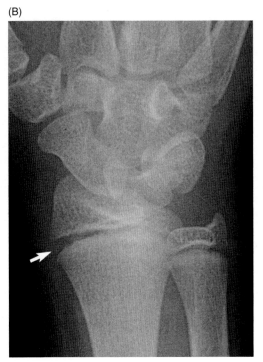

(C)

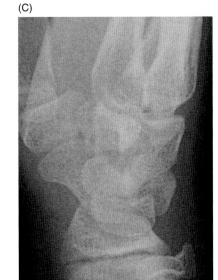

12-year-old girl who fell while attempting a back walkover maneuver on the balance beam, landing on her outstretched wrist. PA (A), oblique (B), and lateral (C) radiographs of the right wrist. There is widening of the distal radial physis laterally (arrow) indicative of a Salter I injury. The bones tend to be stronger in adolescents compared to young children, therefore, while younger ages have radial metaphyseal buckle fractures, adolescents tend to have fractures involving the growth plate rather than the bone, with the majority of wrist fractures in adolescents being Salter I (22%) or Salter II (58%) injuries [3]. A chronic stress injury seen in gymnasts can produce a Salter I injury, which is, however, accompanied by irregularity and sclerosis [4]. Premature physeal closure, radial shortening, and positive ulnar variance may be sequelae of so-called gymnast wrist [5]. (Source: Chew FS. Skeletal Radiology: The Bare Bones. 3rd Edition. Copyright © 2010 by Felix Chew.)

Case 16–5

Distal radius fracture, salter Type II

(A)　　　　　　　　(B)　　　　　　　　(C)　　　　　　　　(D)

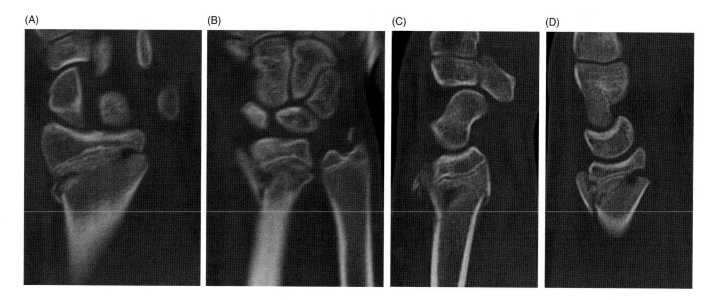

15-year-old male who fell on an outstretched hand. Coronal (A-B) and sagittal (C-D) CT of the right wrist. Coronal CT images show an impacted fracture of the distal radius with comminution of the metaphysis. The fracture extends through the growth plate and there is an accompanying ulnar styloid avulsion fracture. The sagittal CT images show impaction and dorsal angulation of the distal fragment. Ogden [6] extended the Salter-Harris growth plate fracture classification with additional types of periphyseal injuries: Type VI is a peripheral perichondral ring injury (usually open); Type VII is a fracture of the epiphysis only; Type VIII is a metaphyseal fracture; and Type IX is a diaphyseal fracture. The distal radius fracture can be classified as a Salter Type II, and the ulnar styloid fracture can be classified as an Ogden Type VII.

Case 16–6
Buckle fracture of distal radius

(A)

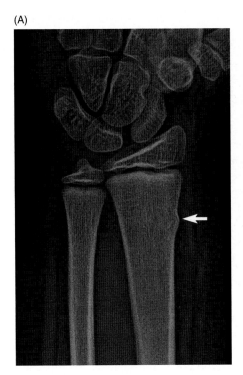

(B)

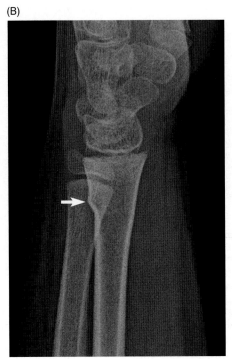

8-year-old girl who fell on her outstretched hand. PA (A) and lateral (B) radiographs of the left wrist. There is buckling of the metaphyseal cortex (arrows), involving primarily the dorsal cortex. If the buckling involved the bone circumferentially, it would have the shape of a torus (similar to a donut). This injury is commonly called a buckle fracture or a torus fracture, with these terms being essentially interchangeable. Children's bones are more pliable, and therefore are more prone to incomplete fractures. Buckle fracture, greenstick fracture, and plastic

bowing deformity represent incomplete fractures unique to children. Greenstick and plastic deformity occur from bending (angulation) forces. Fracture occurring on the tension (convex) side of the bone and not the compression side (concave) gives rise to the greenstick fracture. The tension side would be expected to fail first, as bone is weaker to tension forces compared to compression forces. The mechanism of injury for buckle and torus fractures is compression from axial loading [7].

Case 16–7
Plastic bowing deformity of ulna

(A)

(B)

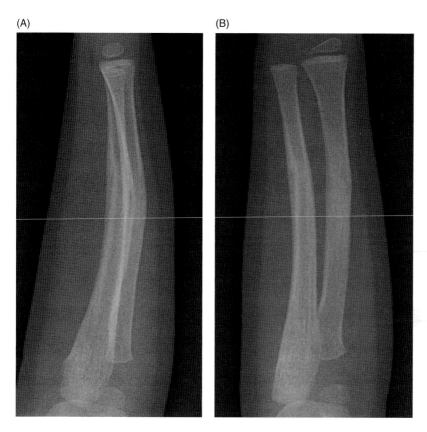

Child who fell on an outstretched hand. Lateral (A) and AP (B) radiographs of the right forearm. Plastic bowing of the ulna and complete fracture of the mid-radius is seen. Bending of the bone with low force is reversible and constitutes elastic deformity. More intense force gives rise to fractures. Forces that exceed those in reversible bending, but fall short of that required to produce a fracture may result in a plastic bowing deformity in children, owing to the increased pliability of their bones. In older children, where much further growth is not anticipated, the deformity will not correct itself and reduction is necessary. Bowing deformity may only be manifest in only one of the two standard radiographic projections, and may therefore be overlooked.

Case 16–8   Greenstick fractures of the forearm

(A)

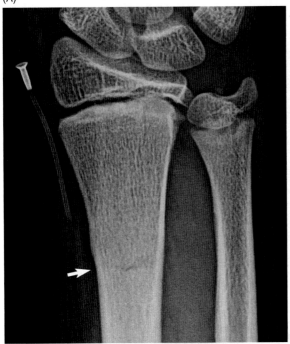

(B)

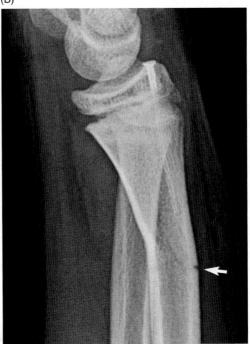

Child who fell on an outstretched hand. PA (A) and lateral (B) radiographs of the right distal forearm. There is an incomplete fracture with cortical break on the tension side and plastic deformity on the compression side in the mid to distal radius and ulna with ulnar angulation, consistent with greenstick fractures. Greenstick and bowing fractures are unique to children, owing to the greater pliability of their bones. When only a single forearm bone is involved, the proximal and distal radioulnar joints are more prone to injury. Isolated ulnar greenstick fracture may represent a Monteggia fracture equivalent where there has been spontaneous radial head reduction.

Case 16–9   Both bones forearm fractures

(A)

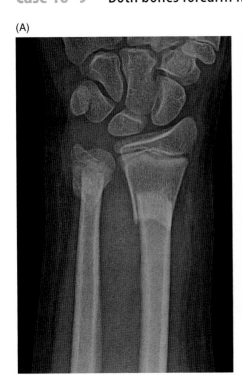

(B)

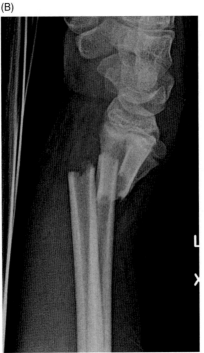

12-year-old boy who fell on an outstretched hand. PA (A) and lateral (B) radiographs of the left distal forearm. On the AP radiograph, there are transverse fractures of the shafts of both the distal radius and distal ulna, neither of which involves the growth plate nor the joint. The lateral radiograph shows that the fractures are dorsally displaced in bayonet apposition, with mild dorsal angulation of the distal fragments. Fractures caused by falls onto an outstretched hand in children are different than those in adults. In children, they are typically growth plate, buckle, or both bones fractures of the distal forearm. In adults, this mechanism is more likely to result in intra-articular fractures of the distal radius or carpal bones.

Case 16–10
Radial head subluxation (nursemaids' elbow)

(A)　(B)

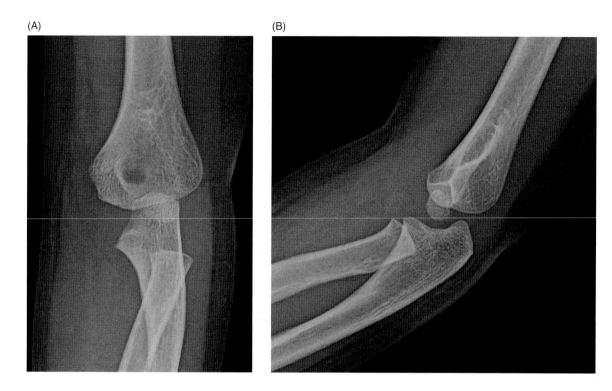

Child who fell while being led by the hand. AP (A) and lateral (B) radiographs of the right elbow. The radius and capitellum should be collinear on all radiographic projections. In this case, the position of the radial head, which is not yet ossified, can be estimated by a line drawn through the axis of the radial neck, which should point directly at the capitellum. Because the line falls posterior to the capitellum, there is posterior subluxation of the radial head. This is known as nursemaids' elbow.

The mechanism is from pulling a toddler's hand by an adult. Before 5 years of age, the annular ligament is relatively lax and the radial head may subluxate when the forearm is pronated and pulled [8]. Supination and flexion may return the radial head to its proper location, and therefore the initial subluxation may be undetected on radiographs when interval supination has occurred.

Case 16–11   Supracondylar humerus fracture

(A)

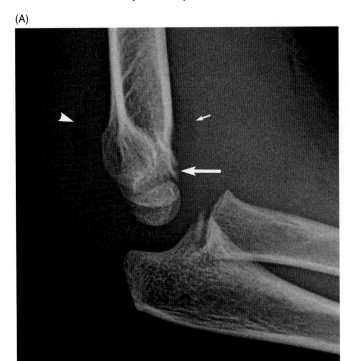

(B)

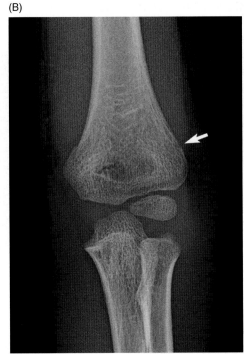

5-year-old boy injured in fall. Lateral (A) and AP (B) radiographs of the left elbow. There is a joint effusion, manifested by posterior fat pad sign (arrowhead) and elevation of the anterior fat pad (small arrow). The fracture (arrows) itself may be difficult to see on radiographs. The fracture traverses the condyles and passes across the olecranon and coronoid fossae. The

mechanism is fall on an outstretched hand. These are among the most common fractures seen in children. A potential complication is radial artery injury with Volkmann's contracture of the forearm and hand. The posterior fat pad sign is highly associated with fracture (70–90%) in children and adolescents [9–11].

(C)

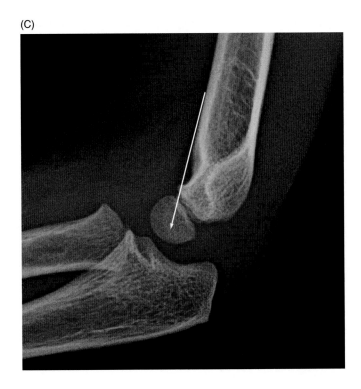

Lateral radiograph of the right elbow. Contralateral elbow obtained for comparison is normal. Supracondylar fractures are posteriorly angulated relative to the normal alignment of the distal humerus, but because the normal distal humerus is itself anteriorly angulated, the abnormal angulation of the distal fragment may not necessarily be angulated relative to the humeral shaft. A line drawn along the anterior cortex of the distal humeral shaft (anterior humeral line) would normally intersect the middle third of the capitellum (long, long arrow). If the anterior humeral line intersects the anterior third of the capitellum or misses it altogether, a posteriorly angulated fracture is presumably present [12].

Case 16–12

Lateral condylar humerus fracture

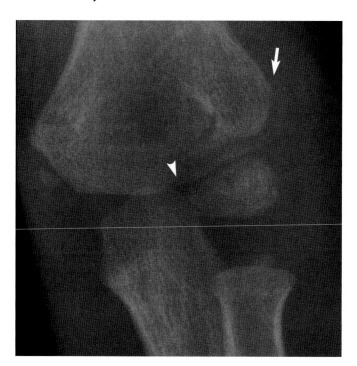

Primary school-aged child who fell. AP radiograph of the left elbow. There is a fracture at the lateral condyle, beginning at the lateral aspect of the metaphysis (arrow) and extending medially to the midportion of the humerus (arrowhead) and then distally into the cartilaginous portion of the epiphysis (Salter Type IV). After supracondylar fractures, lateral condylar fractures are the next most frequent elbow fractures and make up 15–20% of childhood elbow injuries [1, 13]. The fracture fragment includes the lateral metaphysis, capitellum, and lateral trochlea. A fall on an outstretched hand with forearm supination and elbow varus angulation is the mechanism. Pull from the extensor attachment at this site contributes to the fracture and may cause distal and posterior displacement of the fragment. The oblique view is best suited for detecting this fracture. (Source: Chew FS. Skeletal Radiology: The Bare Bones. 3rd Edition. Copyright © 2010 by Felix Chew.)

Case 16–13
Medial epicondyle humerus fracture

(A)

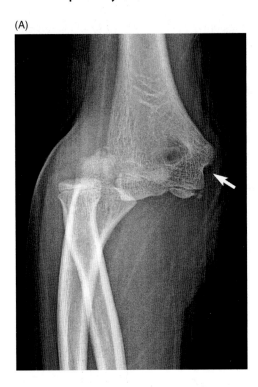

(B)

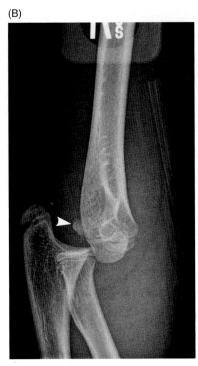

11-year-old boy injured in fall while playing basketball. AP (A) and lateral (B) radiographs of the right elbow. There is posterior dislocation of the elbow. At the medial aspect of the distal humerus, the apophysis of the medial epicondyle is absent (arrow). At this age, all of the apophyseal and epiphyseal centers should be ossified. On the lateral view, the displaced medial epicondyle is partially visible (arrowhead).

(C)

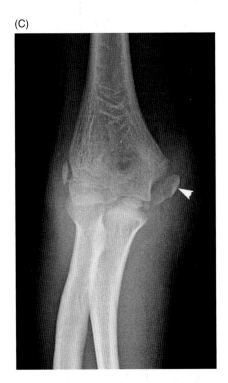

AP radiograph of the right elbow following reduction of the elbow dislocation. The elbow has been reduced. However, the medial epicondyle has only been partially reduced, and multiple fragments are now evident (arrowhead). The common flexor-pronator tendons and medial ulnar collateral ligament originate at the medial epicondyle. As such, it is extra-articular and may be injured without resulting in an elbow effusion [14]. The medial epicondyle is an apophysis, because it does not participate in increasing bone length. Repetitive valgus force with traction from the flexor-pronator tendons may give rise to a chronic avulsion injury, a condition known as little leaguer's elbow, owing to its historical frequency in child baseball pitchers.

Case 16–14

Medial epicondyle humerus fracture

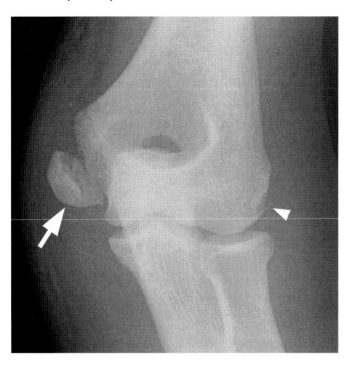

13-year-old girl injured during gymnastics. AP radiograph of the left elbow. An elbow dislocation (not shown) was been previously reduced before this radiograph was obtained. There is a displaced avulsion fracture of the medial epicondyle (arrow), with proximal retraction and marked overlying soft tissue swelling. There is also an avulsion fracture at the proximal attachment of the ulnar collateral ligament (arrowhead). A potential complication is entrapment of the avulsed ossification center in the joint when reduction is attempted. The ulnar nerve, which runs posterior to the medial epicondyle, may also be injured. Note that at this age in an adolescent female, some but not all of the epiphyseal and apophyseal ossification centers have closed.

Case 16–15

Clavicle fracture

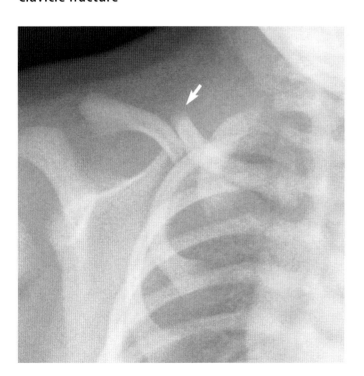

Newborn girl who was not moving her right arm following vaginal delivery. AP radiograph of the right clavicle. There is an acute displaced mid-shaft fracture of the clavicle. The clavicle is the most commonly fractured bone during vaginal birth, with an incidence of about 0.5% [15]. They may be initially undetected [16].

Case 16–16
Atlanto-occipital dissociation

(A) (B) (C)

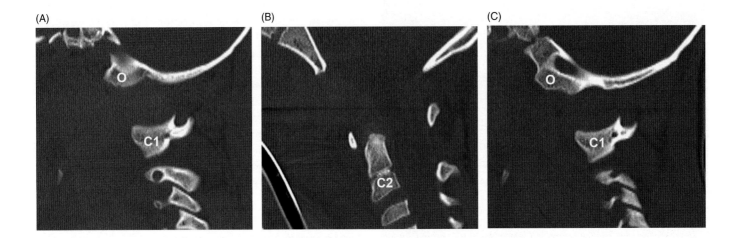

5-year-old child retrieved from severe motor vehicle crash. Sagittal CT of the upper cervical spine, left (A) to right (C). The skull is separated from the cervical spine. There is marked retropharyngeal soft tissue swelling, as demarcated by the endotracheal tube. The left (A) and right (C) occipital condyles are dislocated from the superior articular facets of C1, and separated by approximately 15 mm. The midline image (B) shows marked displacement of the skull base from the top of the cervical spine. The patient did not survive. Atlanto-occipital dissociation is more common in children than adults owing to smaller occipital condyles, larger relative head size, and weaker soft tissue supports.

Case 16–17
Jefferson fracture C1

(A)

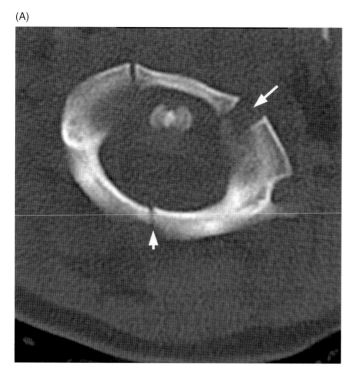

(B)

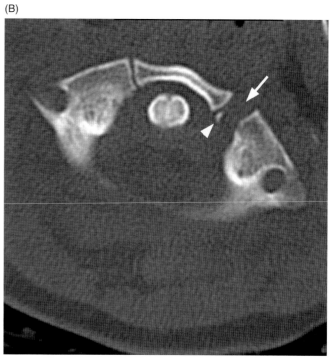

(C)

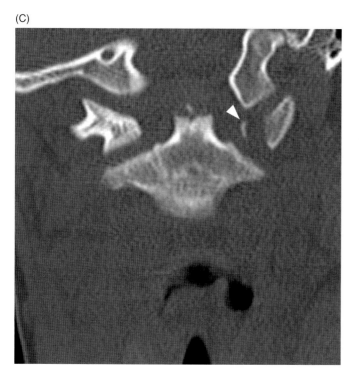

5-year-old child who fell on his head. Axial (A-B) and coronal (C) CT of the upper cervical spine. There is separation of the left anterior C1 synchondrosis (arrow) on the left side. There is a minimally displaced fracture through the posterior arch of C1 (short arrow). Axial CT image shows an avulsion fracture fragment (arrowhead) and separation of the synchondrosis (arrow) on the left side. Coronal CT image shows the avulsion fracture fragment (arrowhead) at C1 on the left.

Case 16–18

Odontoid fracture, Type I

(A)

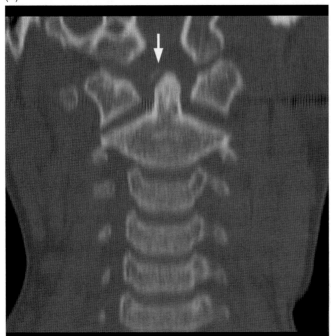

(B)

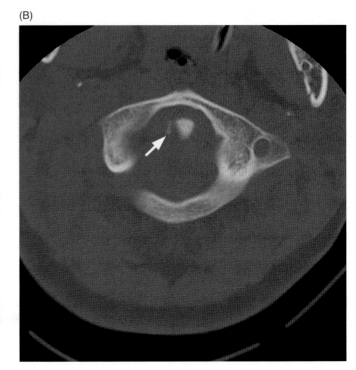

10-year-old child who was struck by a car. Coronal (A) and axial (B) CT of the upper cervical spine. There is a small, laterally displaced, avulsion fracture fragment (arrow) at the tip of the odontoid process. Axial CT image through the ring of C1 shows a small, laterally displaced, avulsion fracture fragment (arrow) at the tip of the odontoid process. Anderson and

D'Alonso Type I fractures of the odontoid process are very rare. The mechanism of injury is thought to be an avulsion of the ligamentous attachments of the odontoid process. A pedestrian child struck by a car from the left is likely to suffer severe left lateral flexion of the upper cervical spine, perhaps explaining this right-sided Type I odontoid fracture.

Case 16–19   Vertebral body fractures C6-C7

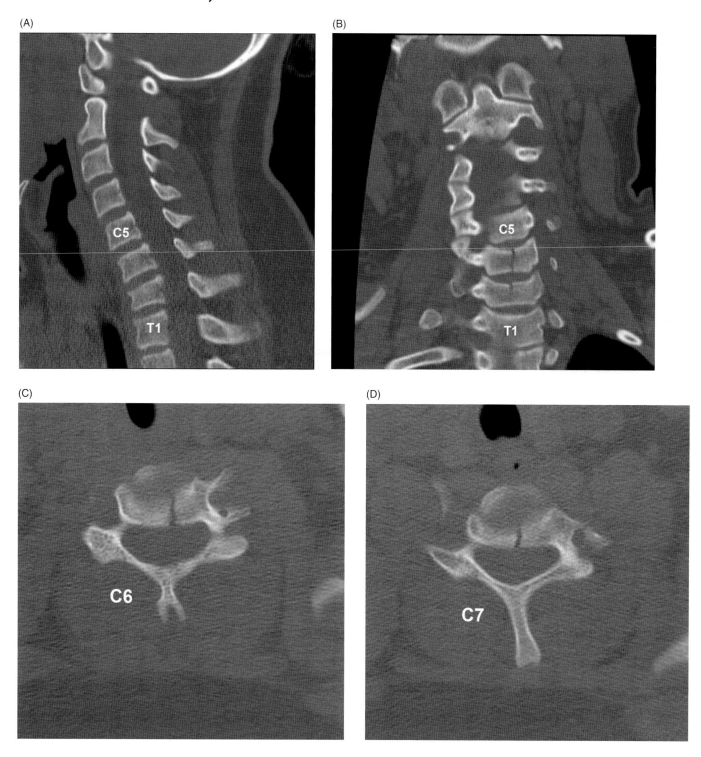

(A)

(B)

(C)

(D)

12-year-old girl who hit a metal pipe with her head while sledding. Sagittal (A), coronal (B), and axial (C-D) CT of the cervical spine. A fracture in the sagittal plane divides the C6 and C7 vertebral bodies in half. Compressive forces in this plane cause acute intervertebral disc herniation, which is responsible for this fracture pattern. This is a subtle fracture that may be occult on lateral radiographs and difficult to identify even on the AP radiographs. CT should be obtained when cervical spine fracture is suspected. 44% of cases of flexion teardrop also demonstrate sagittal fractures. Usually, 2 levels are involved. There is a high association of sagittal vertebral body fractures in the cervical spine with spinal cord injury [17].

Case 16–20   Pelvic ring injury

(A)

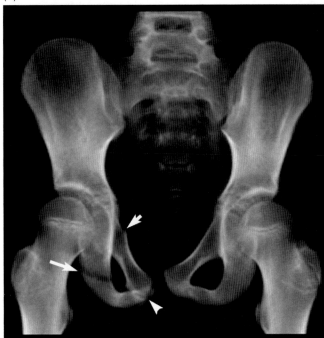

(B)

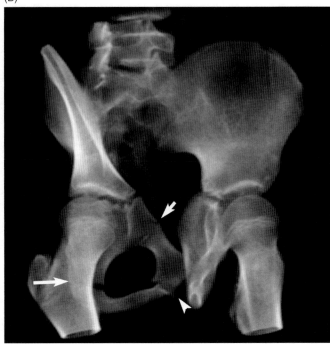

7-year-old girl who was a pedestrian struck by a car. 3D volume-rendered CT of the pelvis, AP (A) and oblique (B) views. There is mild offset of the symphysis pubis. There are fractures of the right obturator ring, including the ischium (long arrow), the superior pubic root (short arrow), and the pubis (arrowhead).

This patient also sustained a right femoral shaft fracture (not shown). Pelvic ring fractures in children are relatively uncommon [18], in part because the skeletally immature pelvis is less rigid and brittle than that of an adult and in part because they do not drive cars and therefore have less exposure to major trauma.

(C)

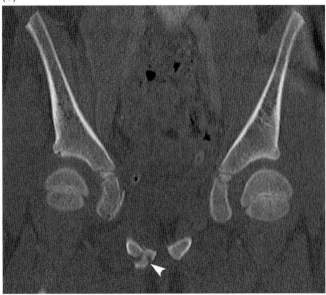

(D)

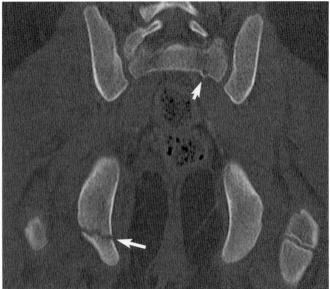

Coronal CT of the pelvis, anterior (C) and posterior (D). There is a buckle fracture of the left sacral wing (short arrow) and a minimally displaced fracture of the right ischium (long arrow).

The more anterior slice shows comminuted fractures of the right pubis (arrowhead).

Case 16–21
Anterior inferior iliac spine avulsion fracture

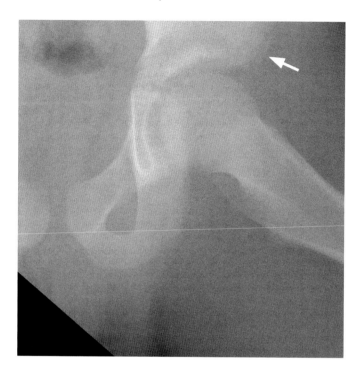

Adolescent male with athletic injury. Frog lateral radiograph of the left hip. There is a subtle avulsion fracture of the left anterior inferior iliac spine (arrow). This injury represents a cortical avulsion fracture of the straight head of the rectus femoris muscle. This injury occurs during forceful extension of the hip.

Case 16–22
Anterior iliac crest avulsion fracture

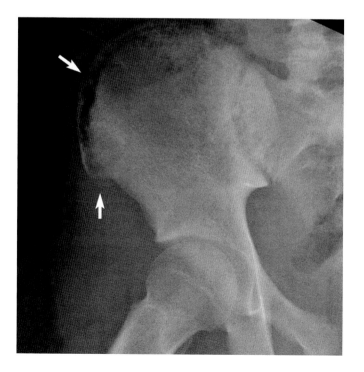

Adolescent male with athletic injury. AP radiograph of the pelvis. There is a mildly displaced avulsion fracture of the anterior superior iliac spine that extends through the anterior portion of the right iliac crest apophysis (arrows). The sartorius muscle and the tensor muscle of the fascia lata originate from the anterior superior iliac spine. The external oblique, internal oblique, and transverse abdominal muscles attach to the iliac crest.

Case 16–23

Anterior superior iliac spine avulsion fracture

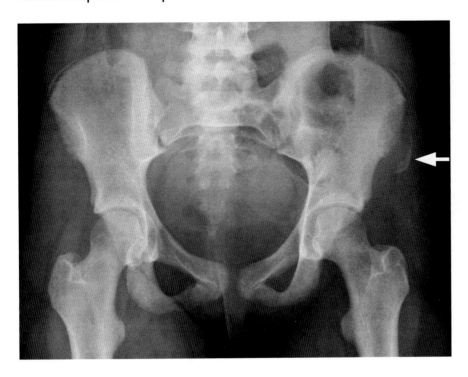

Adolescent female with athletic injury. AP radiograph of the pelvis. There is a displaced avulsion fracture of the anterior superior iliac spine (arrow). These injuries result from forceful extension at the hip, as might occur with sprinting.

Case 16–24

Ischial tuberosity avulsion fracture

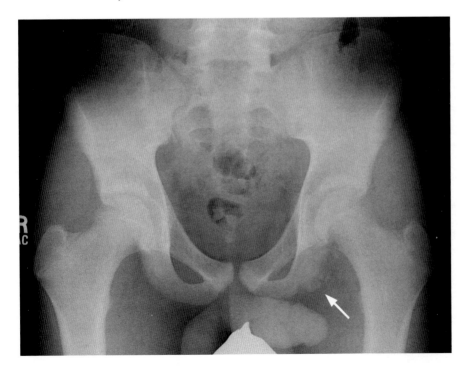

Adolescent male with athletic injury. AP radiograph of the pelvis. There is fragmentation at the left ischial tuberosity (arrow), the result of avulsion of the origin of the hamstring muscles. Avulsion fractures that result from extreme active hamstring muscle contractions may occur in activities such as sprinting [19–20].

Case 16–25
Ischial tuberosity avulsion fracture

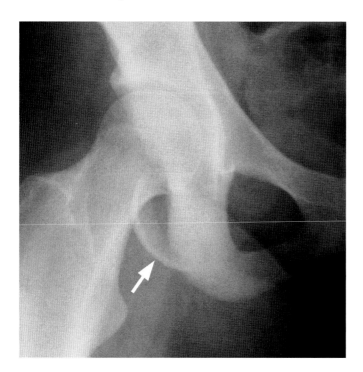

15-year-old female with trampoline injury during side-split maneuver. AP radiograph of the right hip. There is an avulsion fracture of the right ischial tuberosity apophysis (arrow). Sudden, extreme passive tension on the hamstrings may result in ischial tuberosity avulsion fractures; activities such as cheerleading and dancing are associated with this injury [19–20]. (Source: Chew FS. Skeletal Radiology: The Bare Bones. Copyright © 1989 by Felix Chew.)

Case 16–26

Femoral neck fracture, Salter Type I

(A)

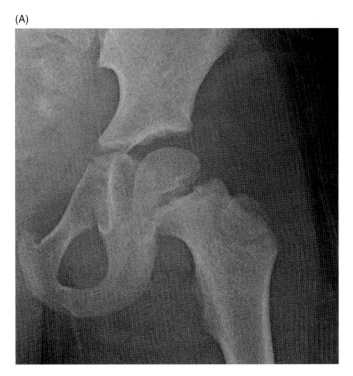

(B)

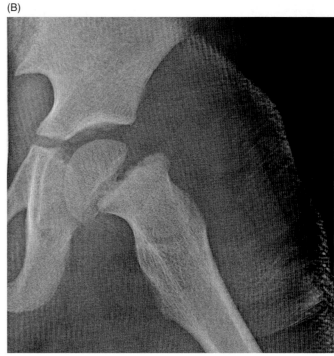

6-year-old boy who was riding his bicycle when he was struck by a car backing up. AP (A) and frog lateral (B) radiographs of the left hip. The AP radiograph shows widening of the proximal femoral physis. The lateral radiograph shows displacement of the femoral neck with the epiphysis remaining in its anatomic location within the acetabulum. There are no fractures involving the ossified portion of the epiphysis or the metaphysis. Pelvic ring injuries were also present in this patient, but are not visible on these views.

(C)

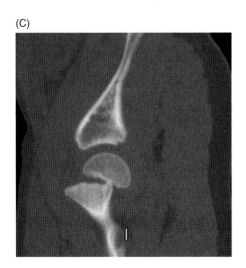

(D)

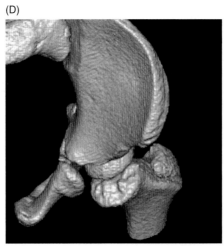

Sagittal CT (C) of the left hip and 3D surface-rendered reconstruction of the left hip (D). There is separation of the epiphysis from the metaphysis at the physis, with anterior displacement of the metaphysis. Because there are no associated epiphyseal or metaphyseal fractures, this injury would be classified as a traumatic Salter Type I fracture. The injury in this case may be distinguished from slipped capital femoral epiphysis on the basis of the traumatic mechanism and the young age of the patient. The 3D reconstruction shows the anterior displacement of the metaphysis from the femoral head. The fracture was reduced and internally fixed. Avascular necrosis and premature osteoarthritis are potential complications of this injury.

Case 16–27

Shaft of femur fracture

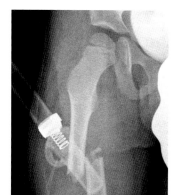

3-year-old pedestrian struck by a truck. AP radiograph of the right femur. There is a transverse mid-shaft femur fracture with a small amount of comminution.

Case 16–28

Newborn femur fracture from birth trauma

(A)

(B)

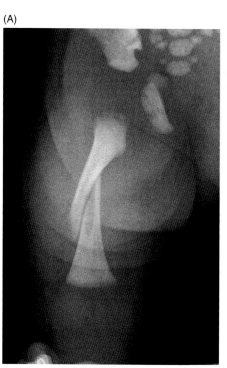
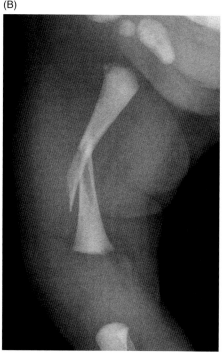

Newborn baby girl who was delivered by cesarean section after breech presentation. Crepitance was noted over the right knee. AP (A) and lateral (B) radiographs of the right femur. There is a long, oblique fracture of the middle third of the femoral shaft. There is no evidence of underlying bone disease and there is no evidence of healing.

Case 16–29   Battered child

(A)

(B)

(C)

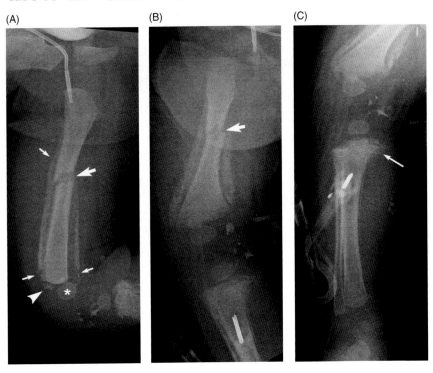

9-week-old baby girl with suspected nonaccidental trauma. Radiographs of the right lower extremity, lateral femur (A), AP femur (B), AP lower leg (C). There is a transverse fracture of the middle third of the femoral shaft (large arrow), with exuberant periosteal fracture healing. There are fractures (small arrows) through the periosteal callus more proximally and more distally, which is indicative of successive episodes of trauma. The distal femoral epiphysis (*) is posteriorly displaced, with small anterior corner fragment (arrowhead). The proximal tibial epiphysis is displaced with bucket handle fractures (long arrow), and periosteal fracture healing is seen in the visualized potions of the tibial and fibular shafts. There is an intraosseous cannula in the tibia for intravenous access.

(D)

(E)

(F)

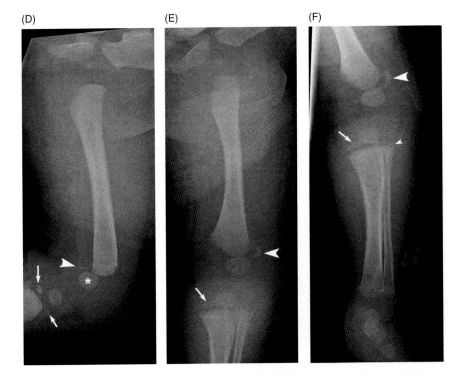

Radiographs of the left lower extremity, lateral femur (D), AP femur (E), AP lower leg (F). There is displacement of the distal femoral (*) and proximal tibial epiphyses, with bucket handle fractures at the distal femur (arrowheads) and proximal tibia (arrows). Early periosteal healing can be seen in the distal femur and proximal tibia. There is a bucket handle fracture of the proximal fibular metaphysis (small arrowhead), even though the epiphysis is not ossified yet. The corner fracture is the classic metaphyseal lesion of child abuse and is called a corner or bucket handle fracture. In this case, it is a corner fracture because the fragment is viewed on end, but with a different radiographic projection, the fragment might appear linear or curvilinear and be called a bucket handle fracture. This lesion is generally considered pathognomonic for nonaccidental trauma and is caused by violent shaking of the infant [21].

Case 16–30
Intercondylar femur fracture

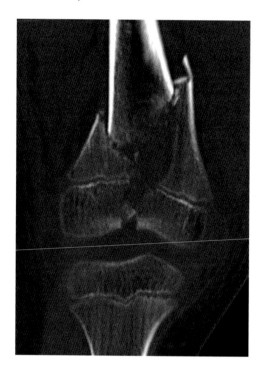

Child in motor vehicle crash. Coronal CT of the right distal femur. There is a Y-shaped fracture extending from the metaphysis across the growth plate and through the intercondylar portion of the epiphysis, separating the medial and lateral condyles into separate fragments. This is a Salter Type IV fracture because the fracture extends through the epiphysis, the physis, and the metaphysis. It requires surgical treatment [22].

Case 16–31   Medial femoral condyle fracture

(A)

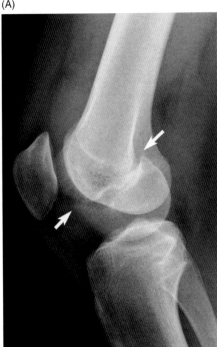

16-year-old male injured while performing gymnastics. Lateral radiograph of the right knee. There is a large joint effusion. There is a mildly displaced fracture extending through the medial femoral condyle in an oblique coronal plane (arrows). The superimposed lateral femoral condyle is intact.

(B)   (C)   (D)

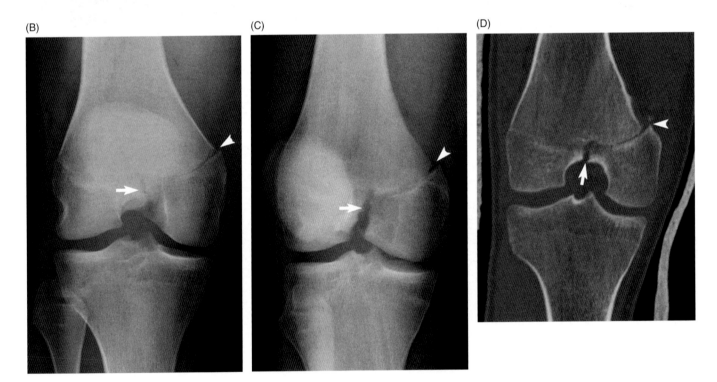

AP (B) and oblique (C) radiographs and coronal (D) CT of the right knee. The fracture of the distal femur traverses the medial portion of the growth plate (arrowhead) and then extends distally through the intercondylar part of the epiphysis (arrow), separating the medial condyle from the remainder of the femur. This is a Salter Type III fracture because the fracture extends through the epiphysis and the growth plate, but not through the metaphysis. The coronal CT shows the intercondylar portion of the fracture (arrow) connecting with the medial growth plate; there is mild medial displacement of the epiphyseal fragment. The lateral portion of the femoral growth plate and the entire tibial growth plate are fused.

Case 16–32
Anterior tibial tubercle fracture

(A)

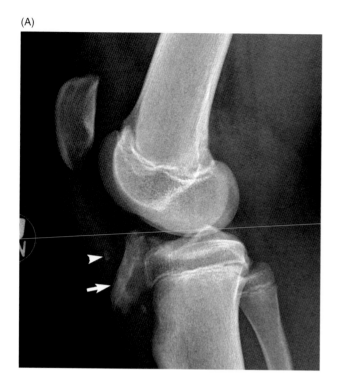

(B)

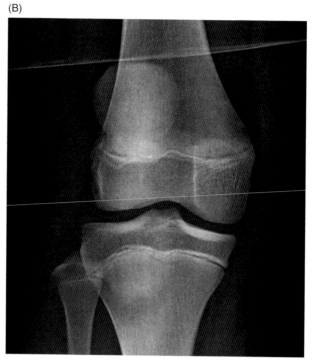

15-year-old female gymnast with knee pain after balance beam maneuver. Lateral (A) and AP (B) radiographs of the right knee. There is an avulsion fracture of the anterior tibial tubercle (arrow) through the open apophyseal plate with proximal retraction by the quadriceps mechanism, resulting in patella alta. The fragment is also rotated because of the inferior location of the infrapatellar tendon on the fragment. The fracture does not extend into the tibial epiphysis. A small ossification within the infrapatellar tendon (arrowhead) is indicative of previous Osgood-Schlatter disease.

Case 16–33   Epiphyseal tibia fracture

(A)

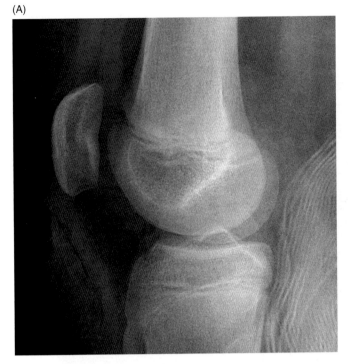

(B)

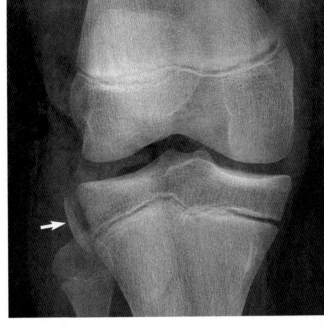

15-year-old adolescent male in a car crash. Lateral (A) and AP (B) radiographs of the right knee. There is a displaced avulsion fracture of the lateral aspect of the tibial epiphysis (arrow).

There is a soft tissue wound over the anterolateral knee and a joint effusion.

(C)

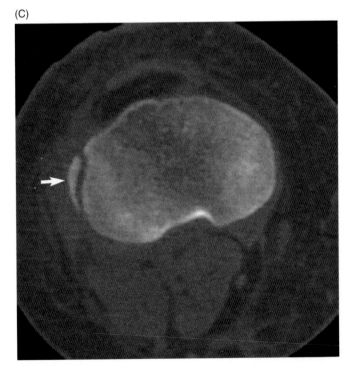

(D)

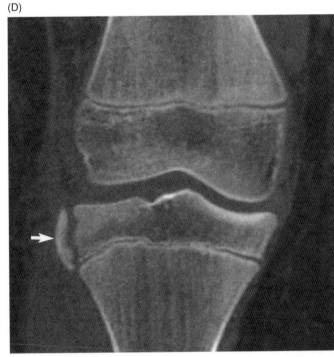

Axial (C) and coronal (D) CT of the right proximal tibia. The lateral tibial epiphyseal fracture (arrow) extends to the growth plate, so that it may be classified as a Salter Type III fracture.

Anatomically, it corresponds to the insertion of the anterolateral ligament of the knee, and is the pediatric analog of the adult Segond fracture [23].

Case 16–34
Plastic bowing deformity of fibula

(A)

(B)

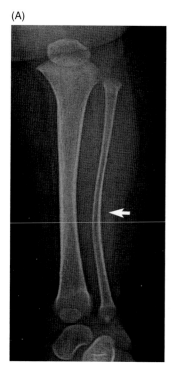
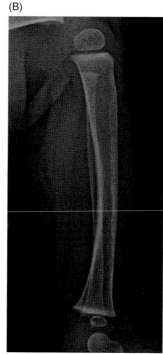

8-month-old infant male who was playing in a baby bouncer; he suddenly began crying and refusing to move the left leg. AP (A) and lateral (B) radiographs of the left lower leg. The fibula is excessively bowed in the coronal plane (arrow). When bone is subjected to excessive loading forces, it deforms before it breaks. With elastic deformation, a process that occurs continuously with physiologic levels of stress, the bone returns to its normal size and shape when it is unloaded. With plastic deformation, the change in size and shape remains when it is unloaded. The plastic bowing deformity is caused by deformation without fracture, and is unique to young children. Their bones have not yet remodeled along lines of stress, so that they function biomechanically more as an aggregate of small units rather than as one larger unit. Adult bones may also undergo plastic deformation but they almost always fracture as well; sometimes the fracture fragments will not fit back together because of the deformation that occurred before the fracture.

Case 16–35
Toddler's fracture

(A)

(B)

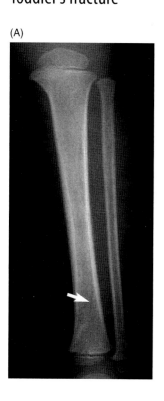
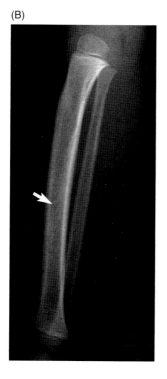

3-year-old child who fell and would not walk. AP (A) and lateral (B) radiographs of the left lower leg. There is a minimally displaced spiral fracture (arrow) of the distal tibial shaft, a so-called toddler's fracture from falling while learning to walk [24]. Toddler's fractures are often difficult to demonstrate by radiographs. It is important to distinguish toddler's fractures from fractures caused by nonaccidental trauma [25].

Case 16–36
Triplane tibia fracture

(A)

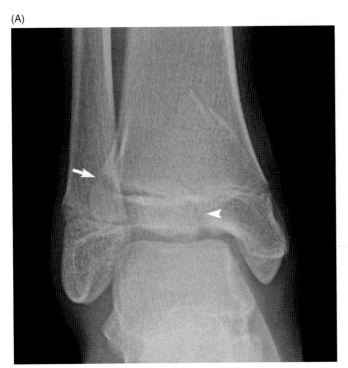

(B)

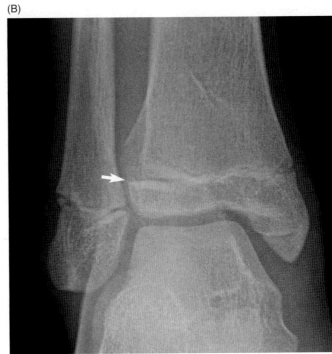

(C)

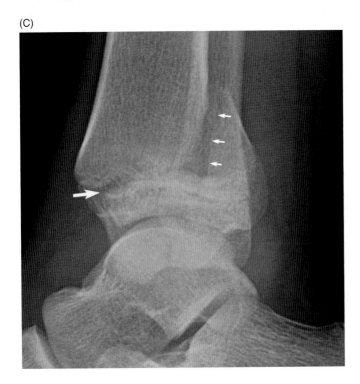

15-year-old adolescent male injured in a fall. AP (A), mortise (B), and lateral (C) radiographs of the right ankle. There is a fracture in the sagittal plane (arrowhead) through the distal tibial epiphysis and widening of the lateral portion of the physis (arrow). Lateral radiograph shows a fracture in the coronal plane (small arrows) extending from the partially closed physis through the posterior aspect of the distal tibial metaphysis. Because the fracture is oriented in the sagittal, axial, and coronal planes, it is called a triplane fracture. Because this fracture can only occur when the physis is partially closed, the age of vulnerability is narrow [26]. This fracture is classified as a Salter Type IV because it involves the epiphysis, the physis, and the metaphysis.

(D)

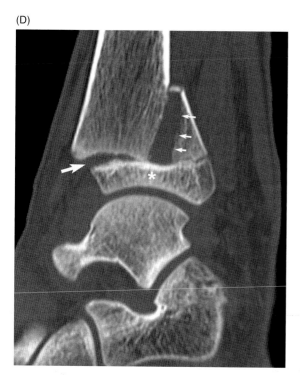

(E)

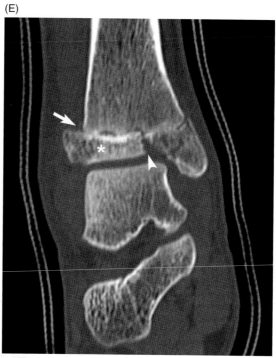

Sagittal (D) and coronal (E) CT of the right ankle. The sagittal CT image shows the displaced fragment (*) with fractures through the physis (arrow) and the posterior metaphysis (small arrows). The coronal CT image shows the laterally displaced fracture through the epiphysis (arrowhead). There are also fractures of the medial malleolus, which are not part of the triplane fracture.

(F)

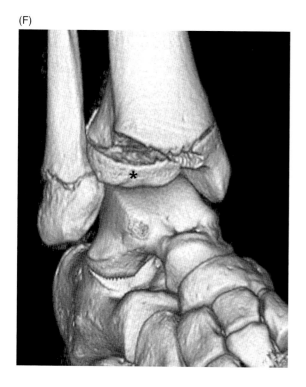

3D surface-rendered CT of the right ankle. The rotatory displacement of the distal triplane fragment (*), still articulating with the talus and lateral malleolus, is easily appreciated.

Case 16–37   Medial malleolar ankle fracture

(A)

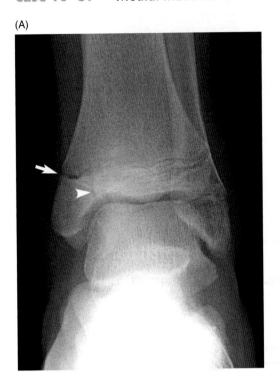

(B)

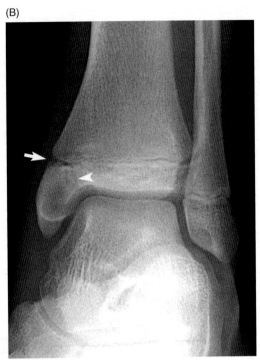

12-year-old boy who turned his ankle. AP (A) and mortise (B) radiographs of the left ankle. There is a fracture of the medial malleolus extending through the partially closed medial physis (arrow) and distally through the epiphysis (arrowhead). This is a Salter Type III fracture.

Case 16–38   Juvenile Tillaux ankle fracture

(A)

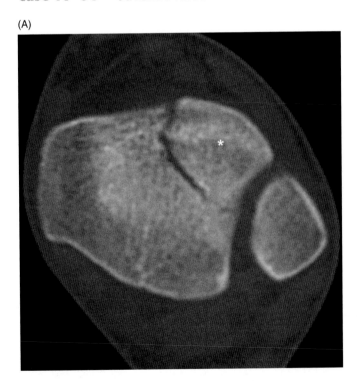

(B)

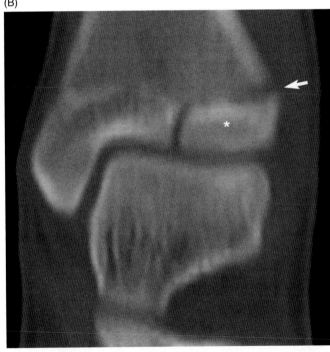

13-year-old girl who fell while participating in cheer squad activities. Axial (A) and coronal (B) CT of the left ankle. There is a mildly displaced fracture of the anterior lateral corner of the distal tibia (*). Coronal CT shows the fracture planes extending in the axial plane through the lateral portion of the physis (arrow) and in the sagittal plane through the epiphysis. The physis is partially closed. This is a Salter Type III fracture that only occurs when the physis is partially closed [27].

Case 16–39
Fifth metatarsal base fracture

(A)

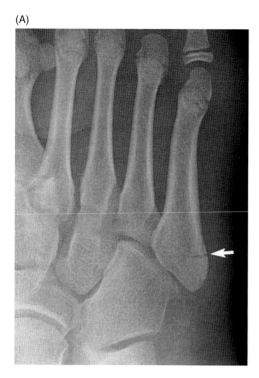

(B)

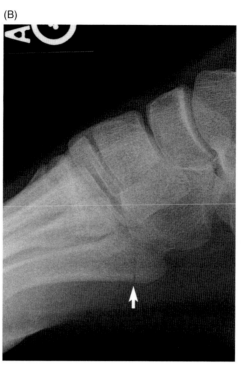

14-year-old adolescent male with right foot injury. The base of his fifth metatarsal was tender to palpation. Oblique (A) and lateral (B) radiographs of the right foot. There is an incomplete fracture (arrow) of the base of the fifth metatarsal extending transversely from the lateral cortex of the styloid process about halfway across the bone. This may be considered a greenstick fracture.

Case 16–40
Fifth metatarsal base fracture

(A)

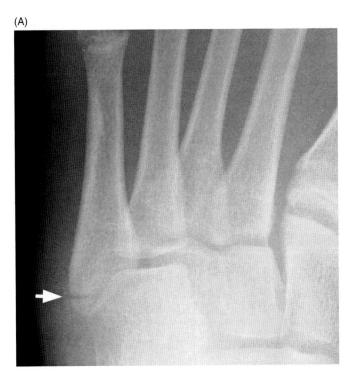

(B)

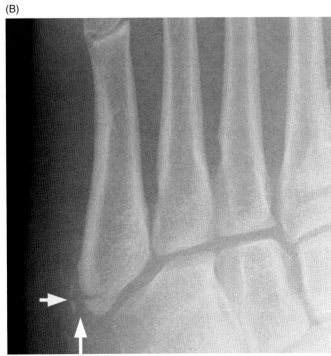

(C)

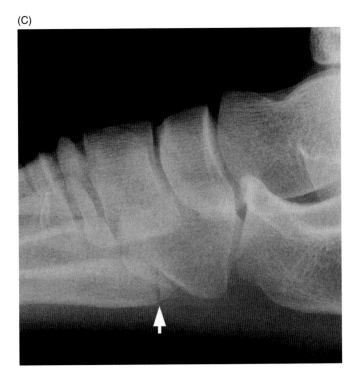

11-year-old boy with an eversion injury of the ankle. AP (A), oblique (B), and lateral (C) radiographs of the left foot. There is a small transverse avulsion fracture (short arrows) at the fifth metatarsal tuberosity, next to the apophysis (long arrow). In children, the longitudinally oriented apophysis found at the lateral margin of the base of the fifth metatarsal may be mistaken for an avulsion fracture. However, apophysis is longitudinally oriented, as opposed to the transverse orientation of a fracture.

Case 16–41

Multiple forefoot fracture-dislocations

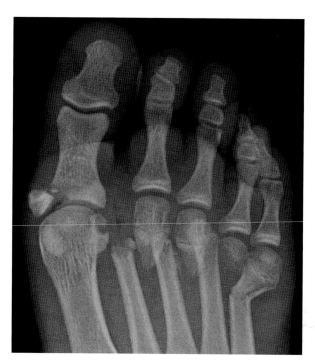

14-year-old boy with foot injury from a crash while competing in motocross. AP radiograph of the right foot. There is an avulsion fracture of the medial margin of the proximal phalanx of the great toe, at the attachment of the medial collateral ligament. The fragment is displaced relative to the remainder of the proximal phalanx, and the articular surface of the proximal phalanx is slightly subluxated in the lateral direction relative to the first metatarsal head. The medial and lateral sesamoids are abnormally separated, suggesting injury of the flexor mechanism of the great toe. The lateral sesamoid appears to be fractured. This combination of features suggests lateral fracture-dislocation of the first MTP joint, with subsequent relocation. There are laterally displaced fractures of the necks of the second through fifth metatarsals, with the MTP joints still intact. The foot is vulnerable in motocross [28], and this injury suggests there was violent abduction of the forefoot as a result of the crash.

References

1. Rogers LF, Poznanski AK. Imaging of epiphyseal injuries. *Radiology.* 1994 May;191(2):297–308. PMID: 8153295.

2. Larson B, Light TR, Ogden JA. Fracture and ischemic necrosis of the immature scaphoid. *J Hand Surg Am.* 1987 Jan;12(1):122–7. PMID: 3805626.

3. Lee BS, Esterhai JL Jr, Das M. Fracture of the distal radial epiphysis. Characteristics and surgical treatment of premature, post-traumatic epiphyseal closure. *Clin Orthop Relat Res.* 1984 May;(185):90–6. PMID: 6705407.

4. Yong-Hing K, Wedge JH, Bowen CV. Chronic injury to the distal ulnar and radial growth plates in an adolescent gymnast. A case report. *J Bone Joint Surg Am.* 1988 Aug;70(7):1087–9. PMID: 3403578.

5. DiFiori JP, Caine DJ, Malina RM. Wrist pain, distal radial physeal injury, and ulnar variance in the young gymnast. Am J Sports Med. 2006 May;34(5):840-9. Epub 2006 Feb 21. PMID: 16493174.

6. Ogden JA. Injury to the growth mechanisms of the immature skeleton. *Skeletal Radiol.* 1981;6(4):237–53. PMID: 7292021.

7. Light TR, Ogden DA, Ogden JA. The anatomy of metaphyseal torus fractures. *Clin Orthop Relat Res.* 1984 Sep;(188):103–11. PMID: 6467706.

8. Salter RB, Zaltz C. Anatomic investigations of the mechanism of injury and pathologic anatomy of "pulled elbow" in young children. *Clin Orthop Relat Res.* 1971;77:134–43. PMID: 5140442.

9. Morewood DJ. Incidence of unsuspected fractures in traumatic effusions of the elbow joint. *Br Med J (Clin Res Ed).* 1987 Jul 11;295(6590):109–10. PMID: 3113624; PMCID: PMC1246979.

10. Norell HG. Roentgenologic visualization of the extracapsular fat; Its importance in the diagnosis of traumatic injuries to the elbow. *Acta Radiol.* 1954 Sep;42(3):205–10. PMID: 13206822.

11. Blumberg SM, Kunkov S, Crain EF, Goldman HS. The predictive value of a normal radiographic anterior fat pad sign following elbow trauma in children. *Pediatr Emerg Care.* 2011 Jul;27(7):596–600. doi: 10.1097/ PEC.0b013e318222553b. PMID: 21712751.

12. Iyer RS, Thapa MM, Khanna PC, Chew FS. Pediatric bone imaging: Imaging elbow trauma in children – A review of acute and chronic injuries. *AJR Am J Roentgenol.* 2012 May;198(5):1053–68. doi: 10.2214/AJR.10.7314. PMID: 22528894.

13. Little KJ. Elbow fractures and dislocations. *Orthop Clin North Am.* 2014 Jul;45(3):327–40. doi: 10.1016/j. ocl.2014.03.004. PMID: 24975761.

14. Silberstein MJ, Brodeur AE, Graviss ER, Luisiri A. Some vagaries of the medial epicondyle. *J Bone Joint Surg Am.* 1981 Apr;63(4):524–8 PMID: 7217118.

15. Beall MH, Ross MG. Clavicle fracture in labor: Risk factors and associated morbidities. *J Perinatol.* 2001 Dec;21(8):513–5. PMID: 11774010.

16. Paul SP, Heaton PA, Patel K. Breaking it to them gently: Fractured clavicle in the newborn. *Pract Midwife.* 2013 Oct;16(9):31–4. PMID: 24358598.

17. Lee C, Kim KS, Rogers LF. Sagittal fracture of the cervical vertebral body. *AJR Am J Roentgenol.* 1982 Jul;139(1):55–60. PMID: 6979865.

18. Holden CP, Holman J, Herman MJ. Pediatric pelvic fractures. *J Am Acad Orthop Surg.* 2007 Mar;15(3):172–7. PMID: 17341674.

19. Stevens MA, El-Khoury GY, Kathol MH, Brandser EA, Chow S. Imaging features of avulsion injuries. *Radiographics.* 1999 May–Jun;19(3):655–72. PMID: 10336196.

20. Waters PM, Millis MB. Hip and pelvic injuries in the young athlete. *Clin Sports Med.* 1988 Jul;7(3):513–26. PMID: 3042159.

21. Nimkin K, Kleinman PK. Imaging of child abuse. *Radiol Clin North Am.* 2001 Jul;39(4):843–64. PMID: 11549174.

22. Tepper KB, Ireland ML. Fracture patterns and treatment in the skeletally immature knee. *Instr Course Lect.* 2003;52:667–76. PMID: 12690891.

23. Porrino J Jr, Maloney E, Richardson M, Mulcahy H, Ha A, Chew FS. The anterolateral ligament of the knee: MRI appearance, association with the segond fracture, and historical perspective. *AJR Am J Roentgenol.* 2015 Feb;204(2):367–73. doi: 10.2214/AJR.14.12693. PMID: 25615760.

24. Dunbar JS, Owen HF, Nogrady MB, McLeese R. Obscure tibial fracture of infants – The toddler's fracture. *J Can Assoc Radiol.* 1964 Sep;15:136–44. PMID: 14212071.

25. Mashru RP, Herman MJ, Pizzutillo PD. Tibial shaft fractures in children and adolescents. *J Am Acad Orthop Surg.* 2005 Sep;13(5):345–52. PMID: 16148360.

26. Patel S, Haddad F. Triplane fractures of the ankle. *Br J Hosp Med (Lond).* 2009 Jan;70(1):34–40. PMID: 19357576.

27. Duchesneau S, Fallat LM. The Tillaux fracture. *J Foot Ankle Surg.* 1996 Mar–Apr;35(2):127–33; discussion 189. PMID: 8722880.

28. Larson AN, Stans AA, Shaughnessy WJ, Dekutoski MB, Quinn MJ, McIntosh AL. Motocross morbidity: Economic cost and injury distribution in children. *J Pediatr Orthop.* 2009 Dec;29(8):847–50. doi: 10.1097/ BPO.0b013e3181c1e2fa. PMID: 19934696.

Fractures and dislocations caused by bullets and blasts (nonmilitary)

Felix S. Chew, M.D.

Case 17–1
Gunshot wound (small finger)

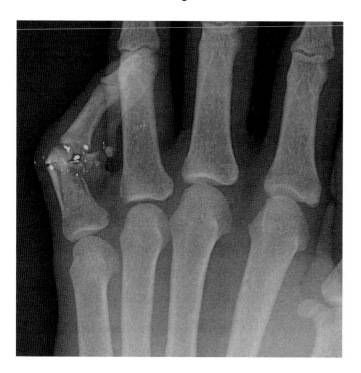

28-year-old man who was shot in the hand. PA radiograph of the left small finger. There is a comminuted fracture of the small finger involving the PIP joint with small bullet fragments.

Case 17–2
Gunshot wound (hand)

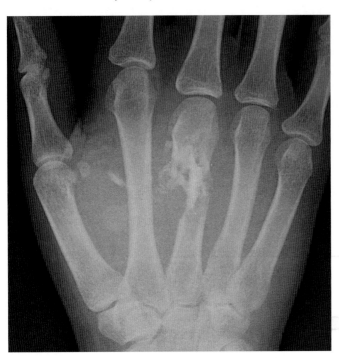

19-year-old man who was shot in the hand. PA radiograph of the right hand. There is a comminuted fracture of the third metacarpal. The bullet passed completely through, leaving only a few small metal fragments.

Case 17–3
Gunshot wound (hand)

(A)

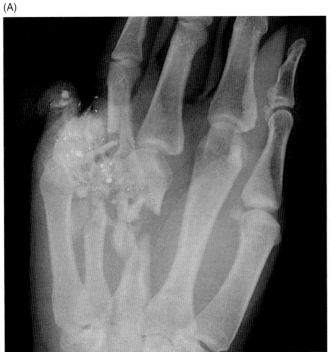

(B)

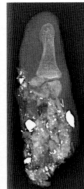

47-year-old man with gunshot wound. PA radiographs of the left hand (A) and left small finger (B). Small bullet and bone fragments are scattered through the hand along the path of the projectile. The bullet entered the hand at the third metacarpal, passed through the fourth MCP joint, and exited through the proximal phalanx of the little finger, amputating it. Low-velocity gunshot wounds have less soft tissue deformity than high-velocity gunshot wounds [1–3]. The mechanism of injury is direct loading along the path of the projectile. Entry and exit wounds may be seen and infection is a potential complication because foreign material is often drawn into the wound. Although the amputated portion of the little finger was recovered at the scene and brought to the hospital with the patient, it was too severely damaged to replant.

Case 17–4   Gunshot wound (carpal bones)

(A)

(B)

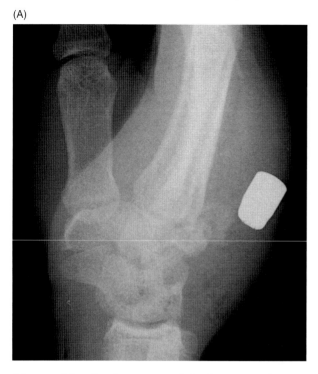
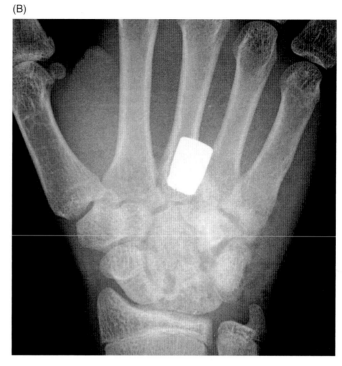

16-year-old male who was struck in the wrist as he attempted to run from gunfire. Lateral (A) and PA (B) radiographs of the right hand. There is a large, intact bullet in the dorsal soft tissues of the left hand. There are comminuted fractures and intercarpal dislocations involving the hamate, capitate, triquetrum, and lunate. There are dislocations of the fourth and fifth

CMC joints. There is marked soft tissue swelling of the dorsum of the hand with pockets of gas. A small amount of gas is also seen in the volar aspect of the wrist, corresponding to the entrance wound. The bullet then passed through the ulnar side of the carpus and came to rest in the subcutaneous tissues of the dorsum of the hand.

(C)   (D)   (E)

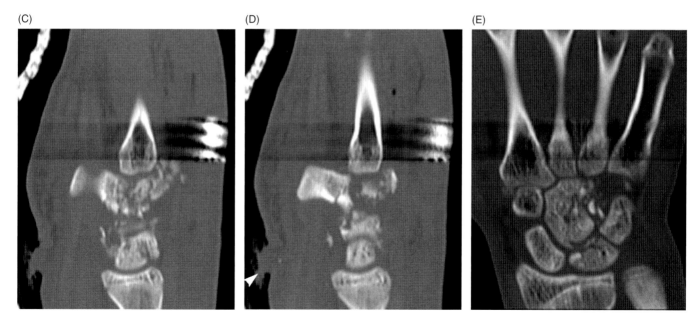

Sagittal (C-D) and coronal (E) CT of the right wrist. There are multiple carpal fractures and a trail of small bone fragments along the trajectory of the bullet. The entry site is at the volar

aspect of the wrist (arrowhead), and the bullet passed through the body of the hamate, fracturing it into small pieces.

Case 17–5

Gunshot wound (hand and wrist)

(A)

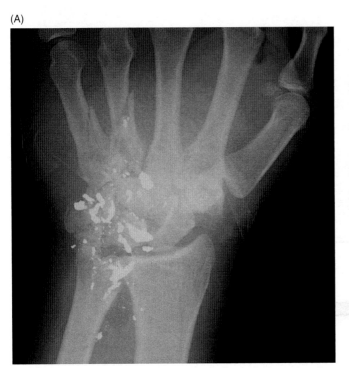

(B)

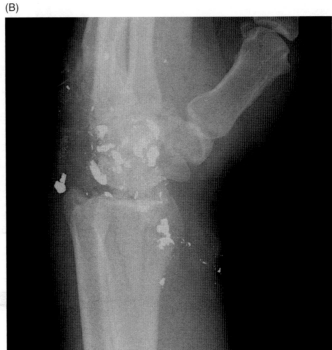

32-year-old man who suffered multiple gunshot wounds. PA (A) and oblique (B) radiographs of the left wrist. Numerous metal fragments obscure the bones and carpal bone fractures are difficult to define, but are undoubtedly present. Fractures of the fourth and fifth metacarpals are evident. The carpal arcs are not clearly delineated and there is some overlap of the proximal and distal carpal row on the PA projection and some ulnar shift of the proximal carpal row as well, which suggests dislocation. Subtle vertical lucencies are seen in the distal radius on the oblique view, indicating additional fractures. Tissue damage sustained by a projectile is governed by several factors, including the kinetic energy of the projectile, propagation of secondary missiles, and cavitation of tissue. The denser the tissue impacted, the greater the transfer of kinetic energy from the projectile, with greater damage to the tissues. Bone, having a relatively high density for biological tissue, sustains greater damage. Fragmentation of the bullet and of the bones, as seen here, releases secondary missiles, which in turn can increase the volume of damage and in some instances cause worse injuries than the primary missile. Low-energy projectiles create cavities only mildly larger than themselves. High-energy projectiles have the capacity to create large cavities and tissue damage and can increase in size even after the projectile has exited. One of the complications with gunshot wounds is infection, a complication seen in about 8% of civilian gunshot wounds to the hand [2].

Case 17–6
Gunshot wound (radius)

(A)

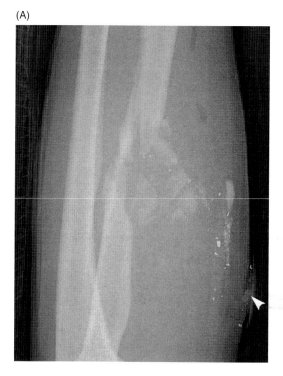

(B)

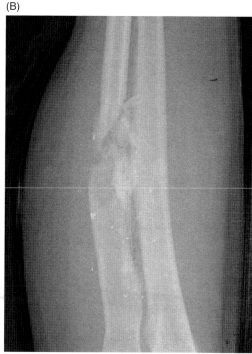

23-year-old woman with gunshot wound. Lateral (A) and AP (B) radiographs of the left forearm. Very comminuted fracture of the mid-shaft of the radius is seen from a gunshot wound. The bullet passed completely through the limb, with a trail of bone and metal fragments leading to the exit wound (arrowhead).

Case 17–7
Gunshot wound (humerus)

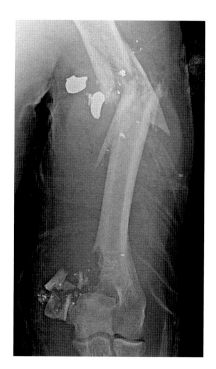

22-year-old man with multiple gunshot wounds. AP radiograph of the left upper arm. There is a comminuted fracture of the humerus at mid-shaft with multiple bullet fragments at the site, two of them large, representing a low-velocity gunshot wound in which the bullet struck the humerus and did not exit. There is a comminuted fracture of the medial condyle of the distal humerus with multiple small bullet fragments, and missing bone fragments, representing a low-velocity gunshot wound in which the bullet passed through and through, taking bone fragments with it. The distal forearm was noted to be poorly perfused, suggesting brachial artery injury at the humeral shaft.

Case 17–8
Gunshot wound (shoulder)

(A)

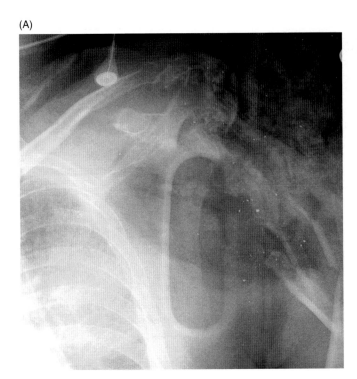

(B)

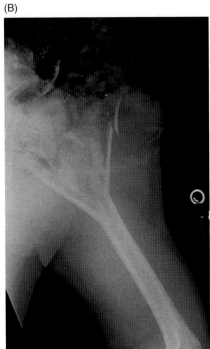

This patient sustained a high-velocity gunshot wound to the shoulder at close range. AP radiographs of the left shoulder (A) and humerus (B). The proximal humerus and surrounding soft tissues have been obliterated, and a temporary dressing packed into the wound at the scene of injury is present. The proximal humeral shaft shows severe splintering with a displacement pattern emanating from the site of entry. The projectile passed completely through the tissues, leaving only a few small fragments of metal.

Case 17–9
Gunshot wound (lumbar spine)

(A)

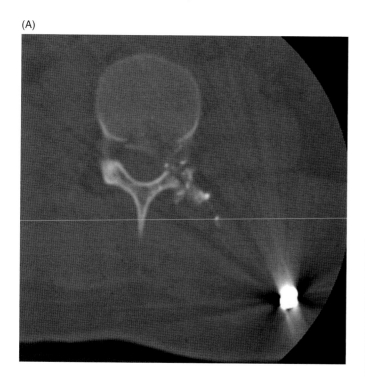

(B)

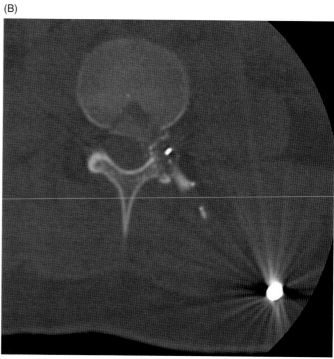

20-year-old man who was shot in the abdomen. Axial CT of the lumbar spine at L3, superior (A) to inferior (B). The entry wound was in the right abdomen, and the bullet passed through L3 vertebral body and left facet joint, coming to rest in the left posterior abdominal wall. A fragment of the vertebral body is displaced into the spinal canal.

Case 17–10

Gunshot wound (pelvis)

(A)

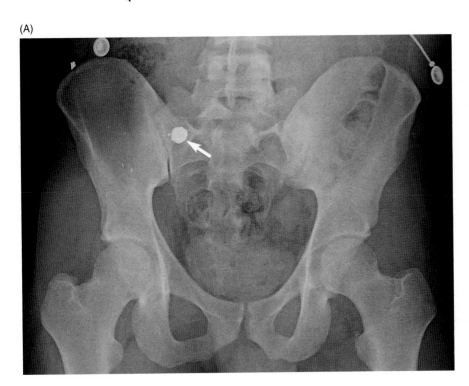

28-year-old man who was shot in the right buttock with a handgun. AP radiograph of the pelvis. The bullet (long arrow) overlies the right sacroiliac joint. The entrance wound has been marked at the skin by the radiologic technologist by a small arrow. There are a few small metal fragments along the path of the bullet.

(B)

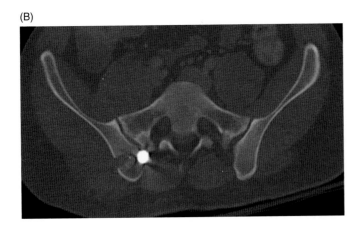

Axial CT of the pelvis. There is an entrance wound in the right buttock. The bullet penetrated through the ilium and came to rest at the sacroiliac joint. There is a small amount of comminution and some small bullet fragments along the path of the bullet.

Case 17–11
Gunshot wound (distal femur)

(A)

(B)

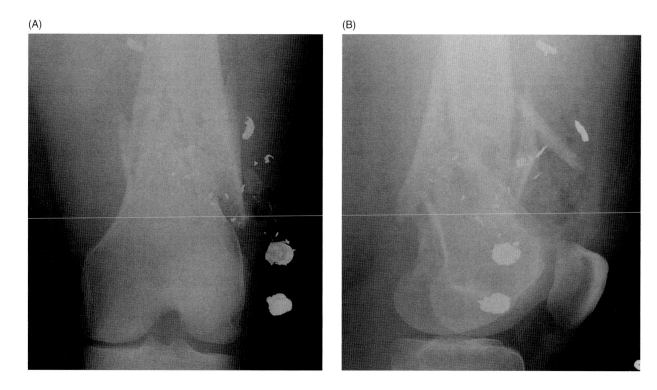

21-year-old man who accidentally shot himself in the thigh with a handgun. AP (A) and lateral (B) radiographs of the left distal femur. There is a comminuted fracture of the distal femoral shaft with bullet fragments. The path of fractures extends from the proximal lateral thigh to the distal medial knee, traversing the bone, consistent with the description of the injury. The morphology of the fractures and the presence of the bullet fragments are indicative of a low-velocity projectile that has expended all of its kinetic energy.

Case 17–12 Gunshot wound (tibia)

(A)

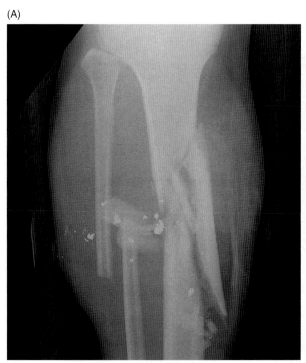

(B)

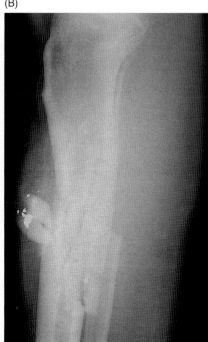

37-year-old man shot in the back of the leg by an assailant with a handgun. AP (A) and lateral (B) radiographs of the right proximal tibia and fibula. There is a gunshot wound involving the tibia and fibula. The pattern of fractures is indicative of a low-velocity projectile, such as from a handgun, with an entry wound from the posterior aspect. The fibula was not struck by the projectile and fractured when the body weight was suddenly transferred from the tibia. Gunshot wounds are open fractures and carry a significant risk of infection. Treatment often includes debridement, external fixation, and antibiotic beads [4].

Case 17–13 Gunshot wound (fibula)

(A)

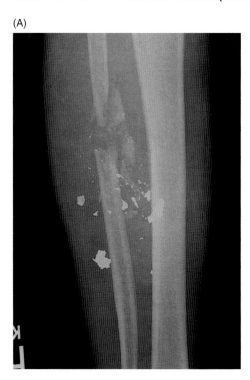

(B)

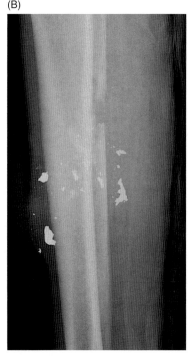

74-year-old man with gunshot wound. AP (A) and lateral (B) radiographs of the right mid-tibia and fibula. There is a gunshot wound involving the shaft of the fibula. The pattern of fractures is indicative of a low-velocity projectile, such as from a handgun, with tissue damage confined to the path of the bullet and the fragments of bone that acted as secondary projectiles.

Case 17–14
Gunshot wound (foot)

(A)

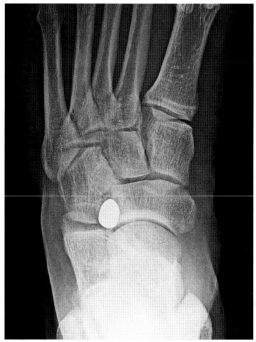

(B)

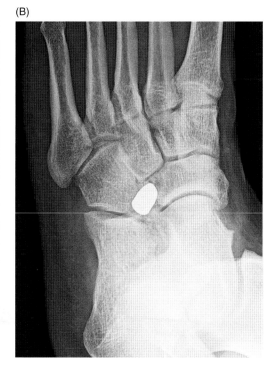

(C)

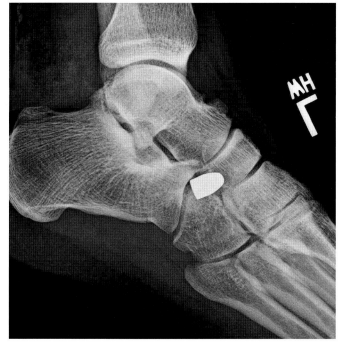

21-year-old man who was standing outside a bar when he heard gunfire and felt sudden ankle pain. AP (A), oblique (B), and lateral (C) radiographs of the left foot. There is a gunshot wound involving the tarsal bones. The bullet is intact and has come to rest in the midfoot.

(D)   (E)

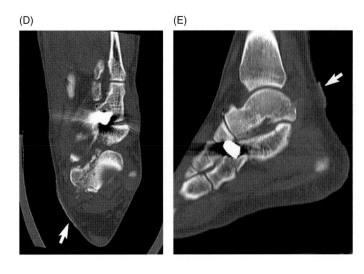

Multiplanar CT of the left foot. The axial CT (D) shows the path of the bullet, with the skin entry site in the posterior ankle, medial to the Achilles tendon (arrow). There are multiple small bone fragments along the track, but the damage appears confined to the path of the bullet. The sagittal CT (E), with the skin entry site marked by an arrow, shows a trail of bone fragments through the talus. Presumably, the weapon was a low-velocity handgun.

Case 17–15
Gunshot wound (foot)

(A)

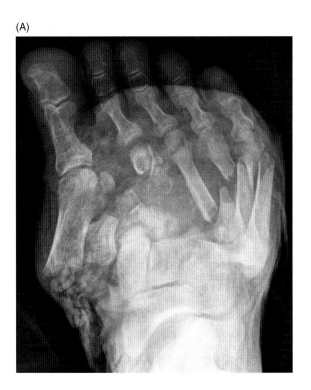

(B)

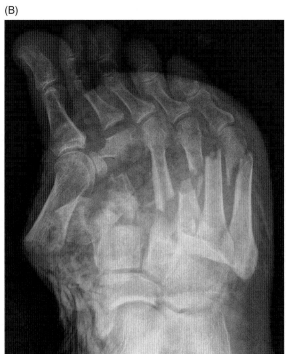

(C)

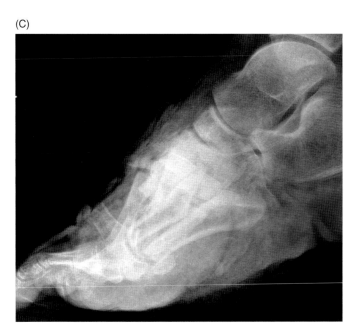

51-year-old man who accidentally shot himself in the foot with an old military rifle. AP (A), oblique (B), and lateral (C) radiographs of the right foot. The projectile has passed through and through the forefoot, without leaving any metal fragments behind. The second metatarsal has been severely fragmented with fragments dispersed in many directions. The third, fourth, and fifth metatarsals are fractured, laterally displaced, and dorsally dislocated at the TMT joints. The first metatarsal is fractured, dorsally displaced, and medially dislocated at the TMT joint. There is gas in the soft tissues.

(D)   (E)   (F)

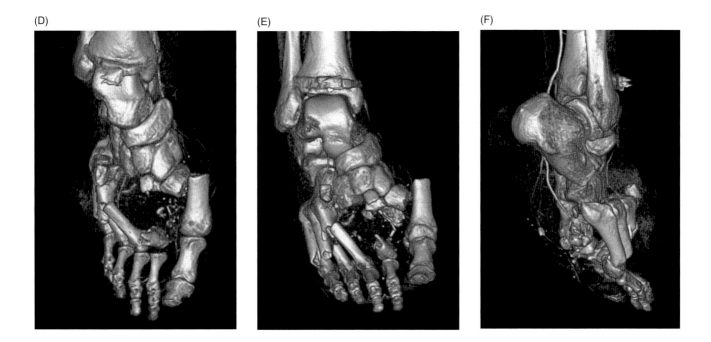

3D surface-rendered CT of the right foot (D-F). The bullet appears to have passed directly through the second metatarsal shaft. The surrounding forefoot structures have been fractured and dispersed away from the entry site by the shockwave and cavitation caused by the high-velocity rifle bullet. The dislocation of the Lisfranc joint is evident. High-velocity weapons include military, hunting, and assault rifles.

Case 17–16   Shotgun wound (shoulder)

(A)

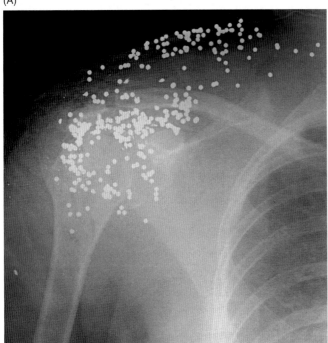

(B)

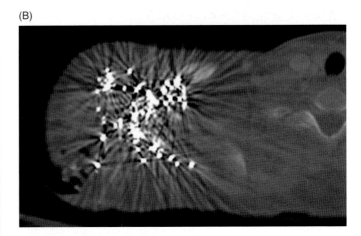

18-year-old hit by gunfire in an urban drive-by incident. AP radiograph (A) and axial CT (B) of the right shoulder. There are multiple shotgun pellets (birdshot) scattered throughout the right shoulder and supraclavicular soft tissues. The shotgun blast arrived from the right side of the patient. CT scan shows that some pellets have penetrated into the humeral head and through the glenoid process.

Case 17–17   Shotgun wound (knee)

(A)

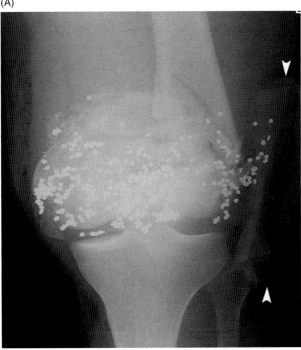

(B)

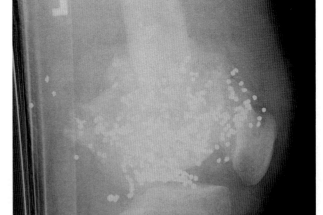

30-year-old man who sustained a shotgun blast to his knee at close range. AP (A) and lateral (B) radiographs of the left knee. There is an open, comminuted fracture of the distal femur with a large number of shotgun pellets. The skin entry site is lateral and covered with a dressing (arrowheads). There is a comminuted distal femoral shaft fracture where the distal femur was translated medially by the force of the shotgun blast.

Case 17–18

Shotgun wound (foot and ankle)

(A)

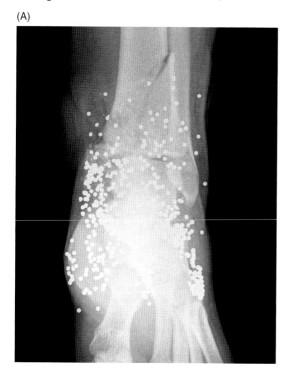

(B)

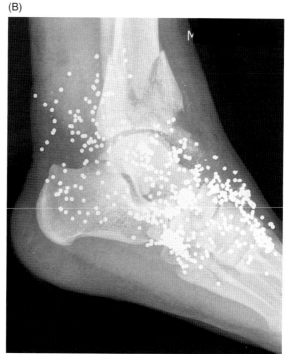

18-year-old man who sustained an accidental shotgun blast to his left foot and ankle. AP (A) and lateral (B) radiographs of the left ankle. There are numerous shotgun pellets (birdshot) throughout the soft tissues of the ankle and foot. There is a comminuted fracture at the distal tibia and fractures of the midfoot are likely to be present but obscured by the projectiles. Shotguns are popular worldwide; in the hands of civilians, more of these weapons exist than the rifled types of long guns. Shotgun wounds differ from those of other missiles because the volume of tissue struck directly by projectiles is large, owing to the fact that the pellets spread apart as they travel away from the barrel. Close-range shotgun wounds can be as destructive as those from a high-velocity rifle, but longer weapon-to-victim distances may produce only minimal injury. The type of shot (size and weight of pellets) used also determines the type of injury, with more serious injuries produced by the larger type of buckshot (greater than 0.14 inches in diameter) [1–3].

Case 17–19   Airgun pellet (knee)

(A)

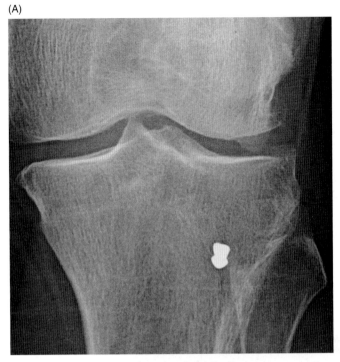

(B)

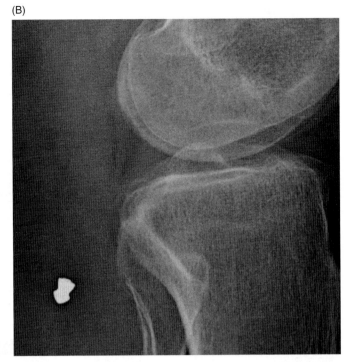

36-year-old man with knee pain. AP (A) and lateral (B) radiographs of the left knee. There is a small metal projectile in the posterior soft tissues of the knee. There are no metal or bone fragments, and the projectile is not deformed. Spring-piston air rifles commonly available in U.S. sporting goods stores typically use .177 cal (4.5 mm) pellets with a muzzle velocity of 1250 ft/s (380 m/s) or less, but other types of projectiles are available, including larger pellets and arrows. Fatalities from airgun wounds have been reported [5].

Case 17–20   Blast injury (hand)

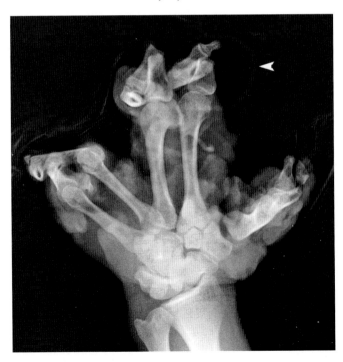

23-year-old man was lighting off fireworks when one of them exploded in his left hand. PA radiograph of the left hand. The hand is severely mangled. The soft tissues are degloved from the bones of the hand. All of the digits have been nearly amputated, but still partially attached by shreds of soft tissue. The soft tissue structure (arrowhead) looped around the index finger is one of the finger tendons. The metacarpals have been violently splayed apart.

Case 17–21
Blast injury (hand and wrist)

(A)

(B)

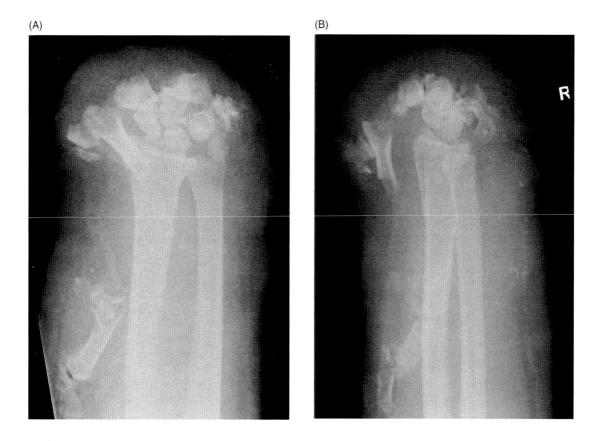

41-year-old man injured in an explosion. AP (A) and lateral (B) radiographs of the right distal forearm. The hand has been mangled, with large and small fragments of the digits and distal carpal bones overlying the proximal wrist and forearm. Most of the digits and metacarpals are absent. The soft tissues are largely obscured by a bulky dressing that was placed in the field. Holding an explosive device in a tightly closed fist might be the expected mechanism for a severe injury like this [6], but the patient could not remember what happened. The absence of metal fragments is characteristic of a nonmilitary device.

Case 17–22
Blast injury (knee)

(A)

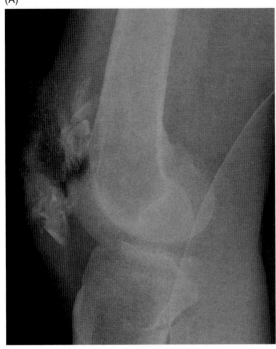

(B)

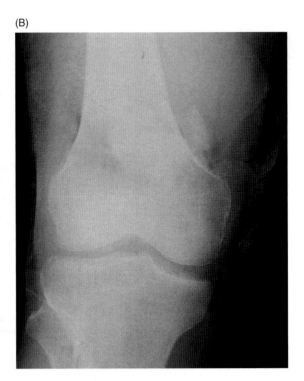

42-year-old man injured in a pyrotechnic explosion. Lateral (A) and AP (B) radiographs of the right knee. There is a highly comminuted open fracture of the patella with dispersed fragments. The injury also involves the anterior aspect of the lateral femoral trochlea.

References

1. Hollerman JJ, Fackler ML, Coldwell DM, Ben-Menachem Y. Gunshot wounds: 2. Radiology. *AJR Am J Roentgenol.* 1990 Oct;155(4):691–702. PMID: 2119096.

2. Ordog GJ, Wasserberger J, Balasubramaniam S. Shotgun wound ballistics. *J Trauma.* 1988 May;28(5):624–31. PMID: 3285016.

3. Kiehn MW, Mitra A, Gutowski KA. Fracture management of civilian gunshot wounds to the hand. *Plast Reconstr Surg.* 2005 Feb;115(2):478–81. PMID: 15692353.

4. Olson SA, Schemitsch EH. Open fractures of the tibial shaft: An update. *Instr Course Lect.* 2003;52:623–31. PMID: 12690887.

5. Milroy CM, Clark JC, Carter N, Rutty G, Rooney N. Air weapon fatalities. *J Clin Pathol.* 1998 Jul;51(7):525–9. PMID: 9797730; PMCID: PMC500806.

6. Adhikari S, Bandyopadhyay T, Sarkar T, Saha JK. Blast injuries to the hand: Pathomechanics, patterns and treatment. *J Emerg Trauma Shock.* 2013 Jan;6(1):29–36. doi: 10.4103/0974-2700.106322. PMID: 23492853; PMCID: PMC3589855.

Index